The Psychiatry of Late Life

The Psychiatry of Late Life

EDITED BY

Raymond Levy

PhD MB ChB FRCP(Ed) FRCPsych
Consultant Psychiatrist

Felix Post

MD FRCP FRCPsych
Emeritus Consultant Psychiatrist

The Bethlem Royal Hospital
and the Maudsley Hospital
London

Blackwell Scientific Publications

OXFORD LONDON EDINBURGH
BOSTON MELBOURNE

© 1982 by
Blackwell Scientific Publications
Editorial offices:
Osney Mead, Oxford OX2 0EL
8 John Street, London WC1N 2ES
9 Forrest Road, Edinburgh EH1 2QH
52 Beacon Street, Boston,
   Massachusetts 02108, USA
99 Barry Street, Carlton
   Victoria 3053, Australia

First published 1982

Set by Southline Press Ltd., W. Sussex

Printed in Great Britain at the
University Press, Cambridge

DISTRIBUTORS

USA
   Blackwell Mosby Book Distributors
   11830 Westline Industrial Drive
   St Louis, Missouri 63141

Canada
   Blackwell Mosby Book Distributors
   120 Melford Drive, Scarborough
   Ontario M1B 2XA

Australia
   Blackwell Scientific Book
   Distributors
   214 Berkeley Street, Carlton
   Victoria 3053

British Library
Cataloguing in Publication Data

The Psychiatry of late life
   1. Geriatric psychiatry
   I. Levy, Raymond   II. Post, Felix
   618.97′689   RC451.4.A5
ISBN 0–632–00962–4

Contents

Contributors

Tom Arie FRCPsych FFCM MRCP
Professor of Health Care of the Elderly, Nottingham University

David Jolley BSc FRCPsych DPM (Manchester)
Consultant Psychiatrist, Honorary Lecturer, Manchester University

John Grimley Evans FRCP MFCM
Professor of Medicine (Geriatrics), University of Newcastle upon Tyne

Loïc Hemsi MRCP FRCPsych DPM
Consultant Psychiatrist, St George's and Springfield Hospitals and Senior Lecturer in Psychogeriatrics, St George's Hospital Medical School, London

Malcolm Lader DSc PhD MD FRCPsych DPM
Department of Pharmacology, Institute of Psychiatry, London

Raymond Levy PhD FRCP(Ed) FRCPsych
Consultant Psychiatrist, The Bethlem Royal and the Maudsley Hospitals, London

Elaine Perry BSc PhD
Research Associate, Pathology Department, Newcastle General Hospital

Robert Perry MB ChB MRCP MRCPath
Clinical Scientist, Honorary Neuropathologist, MRC Neuroendocrinology Unit, Newcastle General Hospital; and Honorary Lecturer, University of Newcastle, Newcastle upon Tyne

Felix Post MD FRCP FRCPsych
Emeritus Consultant Psychiatrist, The Bethlem Royal and the Maudsley Hospitals, London

Robert Woods MA MSc ABPsS
Lecturer in Clinical Psychology, Institute of Psychiatry, London

Preface

The recent growth of interest in the psychiatry of old age has been reflected in the increasing number of publications in the field. There have appeared several valuable small books addressed to medical students, general medical practitioners, and other health workers in contact with the elderly. There have also been monographs dealing with specific aspects of the subject, as well as multi-author texts reporting or summarising the results of research. Finally, there is a recent large American handbook of mental health and ageing with exhaustive international multidisciplinary contributions.

There has, however, not been available for some years a textbook for psychiatrists-in-training and for practising psychiatrists wishing to inform themselves on the subspeciality which psychogeriatrics, in spite of its ugly name, has become. The present volume attempts to fill this gap, and we are grateful to Mr Per Saugman, as Chairman and Managing Director of Blackwell Scientific Publications, for inviting us to make this attempt, and also to the firm's Mr Jony Russell for guiding and assisting us during the editing process.

Reviewers often complain of the lack of uniformity of multi-author works, but here we have deliberately avoided such uniformity. In particular, more space has been allocated, and a more detailed presentation has been asked for, in the case of neuropathology, of psychology, and of the practical aspects of psychogeriatrics because these would seem to be areas in which most of our intended readers may have relatively little knowledge. On the other hand, the authors of the more descriptive clinical chapters have assumed much basic knowledge of general psychiatry. All our authors were encouraged to forego exhaustive lists of references documenting every single statement. Instead, an attempt has been made to select publications which would prove to be points of departure for more detailed study, and these include review articles and chapters of books.

We would like to express the hope that this book may also prove helpful to non-medical readers working with the elderly, and useful to psychiatrists beyond the confines of the United Kingdom. Our authors obviously reflect experience in Britain but have attempted, where possible, to relate this to an international context.

Finally, we would like to express our gratitude to Mrs I.V. Clarke for her help with the typing and Miss Anne Dobson for patiently going through successive drafts, collating editorial suggestions and keeping us in touch with all the other contributors.

Raymond Levy   *The Bethlem Royal and*
Felix Post   *the Maudsley Hospitals 1981*

CHAPTER 1

The Ageing Brain and its Pathology

Robert & Elaine Perry

The brain is in some respects as old as the organism itself since its key constituents — nerve cells — do not divide after the neonatal period. This often-stated dogma seems at first sight to offer a rather gloomy prospect for the ageing individual, although in fact age-associated changes following maturation are probably no more prevalent in the brain than they are in most other tissues of the body. The majority of the human race is not destined to develop serious psychiatric problems in old age and, in the elderly, obvious malfunction of the brain generally occurs, as it does with other organs, in conjunction with distinct disease processes.

In the absence of routine biopsy, conventional neuropathological studies of the brain are of little value to the psychiatrist in providing a diagnosis or assisting in the management of particular diseases. There is however no doubt that neuropathological investigations of postmortem brain tissue have, in conjunction with previous clinical assessments, provided invaluable information on the incidence of various diseases in the population and on the likely association between particular clinical symptoms and specific neuropathological abnormalities. One such example is in the classification and incidence of dementia. Further, in the field of neurology, combined neuropathological and neurochemical investigations of the postmortem brain in Parkinson's disease have been even more fruitful. In this now classical instance, deficits due to the loss of dopaminergic neurons in the substantia nigra can, to a certain extent, be countered by appropriate chemical intervention. No such example as yet exists in any psychiatric disease although specific neuropathological and, to a lesser extent, neurochemical abnormalities have been characterised. Useful treatments of psychiatric diseases in young or old patients are in general either available through serendipitous observation (as in the so-called functional psychoses) or are not yet available at all (as in the organic type of brain disease). In psychiatric disease, the ultimate goal of neuropathological investigation of the brain, if it is to emerge from the realm of the academic, must be the description of morpho-

9

logical or neurochemical changes which may provide a rational basis for
therapy.

Traditional neuropathological assessment of the brain involves several
routine procedures. Intitally, at autopsy the brain is weighed, examined for
surface abnormalities, and suspended in 10% formalin. After a period of
fixation for at least 4–6 weeks, the brain is sectioned and macroscopic
lesions documented. Samples of tissue are then taken from abnormal areas,
or areas of interest, for subsequent processing and histological examination.
Finally, after microscopic observations, the various findings are combined
into an overall neuropathological assessment of the normality or specific
diseased state of the brain. Further quantitative neuropathological techniques, applied to the fixed brain, have provided a means of distinguishing
between those age-associated changes which occur in many normal old
people and those which are related to specific psychiatric diseases.

The contents of this chapter are perhaps best viewed as a description of
the principal morphological changes found in old age, and in various
psychiatric diseases, and should provide the clinician with a clearer understanding of the problems which arise in classifying mental diseases in the
elderly. The material has been divided into three main sections. First those
morphological changes which occur in the brains of elderly people who are
not generally considered to be psychiatrically abnormal are described. Then
morphological abnormalities which have been associated with well defined
psychiatric diseases, known as organic brain syndromes, are discussed.
Where they do exist, many of the neuropathological features of organic
psychiatric diseases are evident, to a lesser extent, in old age and the
distinction between structural changes in the first and second sections is
somewhat arbitrary being principally based on quantitative as opposed to
qualitative differences. A certain amount of overlap between these two
sections is unavoidable as, for example, in the descriptions of histological
features which distinguish multi-infarct dementia and senile dementia of
Alzheimer type from changes found in normal old age. The last main section
includes briefly those diseases in which structural abnormalities have not as
yet been consistently described — diseases generally regarded as of the
functional or non-organic type.

MORPHOLOGICAL CHANGES IN THE AGEING BRAIN

Cerebral atrophy

It is now well established that, following maturation, a reduction in brain size
occurs with increasing age. It has, however, proved much more difficult to
quantify the extent of this atrophy in individual cases and to assess the
precise relation between brain atrophy and intellectual function in elderly

people. The weight of the brain provides the simplest measure of brain substance and most, if not all, investigations in which brain weight has been measured have demonstrated a significant decline with age, amounting on average to between 5 and 10% from maturity to the ninth decade (Blinkov & Glezer 1968; Dekaban & Sadowsky 1978). In the female brain however this decline is slightly less pronounced (Hoch-Ligeti 1963). There are in fact drawbacks to using brain weight alone as an index of atrophy and a number of factors limit its value in assessing atrophy in individual cases. These include: a marked variation in individual brain weights; the inclusion of trapped or retained CSF in cerebral ventricles, fissures and sulci; the absence of information on brain size prior to atrophy; and the lack of specificity regarding the extent of atrophy in particular brain regions. A further complicating factor which arises in the elderly is the inadvertent inclusion of clinically or pathologically abnormal individuals within the 'normal' control group. If such cases are strictly excluded on the basis of careful clinical and neuropathological assessments, the decline in brain weight with age may not actually be as extensive as has generally been reported (Tomlinson *et al* 1968).

The recent study of Davis & Wright (1977), in which atrophy was assessed by comparing cranial cavity volume with brain volume, has partially overcome some of these limitations and is probably the most reliable estimate of brain atrophy in the elderly to-date. This study demonstrated that atrophy of brain tissue did not reach significant proportions until the middle of the sixth decade and that, beyond this age, the rate of decline appeared to be exponential. A similar age-related decline was, infact, reported in the volume of the fixed cerebral hemispheres by Miller *et al* (1980) in investigations using image analysing techniques. In the latter investigation, if allowance was made for a proposed secular increase in brain size throughout this century, atrophy of the cerebral hemispheres commencing after the age of 50 was found to proceed at a steady rate of 2% per decade. In contrast to the findings of Davis and Wright, the decline was linear rather than exponential and, interestingly, in the elderly, it apparently occurred predominantly in cerebral white matter. Hubbard & Anderson (1981) have reported a 5% total loss of brain tissue in advanced old age in a study which utilised the techniques of Davis and Wright to compare brain volume with cranial capacity. Few reports have commented on possible regional variations in the degree of cortical atrophy in the aged although Tomlinson *et al* (1968) noted that gyral atrophy was more extensive in parasaggital frontal and parasaggital parietal regions in 11 out of 28 non-demented people.

In the clinical situation, observations using X-ray computed tomography (CT) provide a potential basis for assessing brain size without the complications of terminal physical illness or postmortem pathological artefact such as brain swelling (Messert *et al* 1972). Current reports (Gonzales *et al* 1978, Jacoby *et al* 1980) on age-related changes in brain size in the elderly using such tomographic techniques, are generally in broad agreement with previous and recent pathological findings. These measurements are, however, handicapped by the limited ability of presently available CT apparatus to delineate accurately grey and white matter and to compare quantitatively cortical atrophy and ventricular size. In the recent report of Jacoby *et al* (1980) in which particular care was taken to scan a mentally normal population, cerebral atrophy significantly increased over the age range 60–89 years and a small, but significant, reciprocal relationship was found between the degree of cortical atrophy and performance before death in a memory and information test. It is probably important not to overinterpret the significance of atrophy in the individual case since a moderate or even marked degree of atrophy may occur in psychiatrically assessed normal elderly individuals.

Cell populations

Two types of cell, the neuron and astrocyte, have received most attention with respect to changes in the ageing brain. Neurons, by virtue of their unique role in transmitting impulses and conveying information, have been most intensively studied. Since neuron numbers do not increase after the neonatal period, the object of many studies has been to determine whether the numbers of nerve cell bodies decrease substantially with increasing age. Fewer studies have attempted to answer equally important questions regarding the integrity of the two types of neuronal processes— axons and dendrites. Alterations in the number or arborisation of these processes, occurring in the absence of marked perikaryal changes, could obviously influence neuronal function and interaction. Amongst non-neuronal cell types, astrocytes have featured most extensively in ageing studies since they frequently respond to neuronal loss or degeneration either by an increase in absolute numbers or by hypertrophy of the astrocytic cell body and its processes.

Nerve cell bodies

Most investigators have assessed neuronal populations by direct manual counts of cell perikarya in standard histological sections prepared by formalin fixation, paraffin embedding and subsequent cresyl fast violet (Nissl) staining. Recently such studies have been extended by the introduction of automated image analysing techniques. It is worth noting that both manual and automated counts provide an estimate of cell body numbers per unit area in a brain section. They thus represent a measure of neuronal 'packing' density which may require adjustment for brain atrophy or volume changes which occur after fixation.

The occurrence and extent of neuronal loss in the aged human brain has been a controversial topic for many years although various reports in the last 20 years have at least partially defined the natural history of certain neuronal populations. In many parts of the brain, especially the cerebral cortex, neurons do decrease substantially in numbers with age. This decrease however is often non-linear, with minimal changes between the third and sixth decades and maximum losses occurring between the seventh and tenth decades. In contrast, certain neuronal populations or nuclei, principally situated in the brain stem, apparently remain stable throughout life.

Interest in the neuronal population of the cerebral cortex stems partly from the enormous development of the neocortex in the human and its assumed major role in cognitive function and behavioural patterns. Brody, who pioneered detailed neuronal counts in the human cortex throughout life, examined 20 cases (Brody 1955) with ages ranging from birth to 95 years and 18 cases (Brody 1970) with ages ranging from maturity to old age (41–87 years). In the first investigation areas investigated included pre- and post-central gyri, temporal lobe and occipital lobe and, in the later study, the frontal lobe. The general conclusion which was drawn from these original studies was that a progressive neuronal loss of between 40 and 50% occurs in certain regions of the cerebral cortex with increasing age. Similar cell losses were later reported by Colon (1972), although the decline was slightly less, and also by Shefer (1973). The more recent investigations of Henderson *et al* (1980) and Terry *et al* (1977), using automated image analysis techniques, have generally confirmed and extended these various observations. In the study of Henderson *et al*, 64 normal cases (age range 16–95 years) were investigated and, as with Brody's original investigation, the regions of cortex sampled were restricted (8 out of 11 areas being derived from the specialised motor and sensory cortex, the remainder from the temporal lobe and the gyrus rectus). Neuron loss occurred in all these areas but its degree varied. The loss was pronounced in motor and sensory cortex and least obvious in the inferior temporal gyrus and gyrus rectus. Loss of large pyramidal neurons was reported to be greater than small neurons; it ranged from 44 to 53% and followed the pattern for neurons as a whole — being pronounced (around 50%) in the pre- and post-central gyri and least in the temporal cortex. Beyond the age of 65 years the rate of decline of large neurons decreased, possibly reflecting a stabilisation in neuronal density. The density of small neurons was found to be more stable throughout life. Indeed in this particular study the decline in the latter was not statistically significant in either the gyrus rectus (12%) or inferior temporal gyrus (20%), although it reached significance (41%) in the post-central gyrus. According to Brody (1978), however, numbers of small neurons in the internal and external granule cell layers in the cortex do tend to decline quite extensively with advancing age.

These studies in the neocortex, whilst clearly supporting the general concept of a decline in neuronal numbers throughout life, have demonstrated variations in the vulnerability of different types of neurons in different cortical areas. It is interesting to note that neuron loss is apparently extensive in the highly specialised motor and sensory cortex. Whether a similar decline occurs in the large 'association' areas of frontal, temporal, parietal and occipital lobes, and whether variations in neuronal populations in these areas can be related to clinical measures of intellectual function or behavioural patterns remains to be determined.

Neurons in the neuromelanin pigmented locus coeruleus, which lies as a bilateral column of cells lateral to the brain stem aqueduct, show a similar age-dependent loss to that seen in pyramidal neurons in the cerebral cortex, amounting to between 30 and 40% (Vijayashankar & Brody 1973, Brody 1978) by the eighth decade. A slightly less extensive age-related decline has recently been reported by Tomlinson *et al* (1981) who also noted the presence of extra neuronal pigment in the elderly group and identified occasional neurofibrillary tangles in the large pigmented locus coeruleus cell bodies. Since it is now established that this brain stem nucleus provides the source of most, if not all, of the noradrenergic nerve fibres found within the different layers of the cerebral cortex, it will be of interest to determine to what extent the age-related loss of neuronal cell bodies correlates with the levels of cortical noradrenergic biochemical markers and whether a relationship exists between the decline in locus coeruleus cell bodies and the disturbances in memory or cognition, both of which are common in old age.

In the cerebellar cortex, as in the cerebral cortex, there is evidence of an age-dependent loss of Purkinje cells of about 30% (Ellis 1920) which is most obvious beyond the age of 60 years (Hall *et al* 1975). Similar conclusions have also been reached with regard to anterior horn cells in the spinal cord (Tomlinson & Irving 1977). The effect of ageing on neuronal populations in the basal ganglia and thalamus are not as well characterised as in cortical areas. In the brain stem a number of investigators have quantified the effects of ageing on neuronal populations and nuclei which are of more relevance to motor or sensory function and co-ordination than to cognitive processes. Discrete nuclei in the brain stem which are stable into old age include the abducens (Vijayashankar & Brody 1971) and trochlear nuclei (Vijayashankar & Brody 1973) and the ventral cochlear nucleus (Konigsmark 1969), whilst the facial nucleus shows a small age-related decline (Maleci 1934) and evidence regarding the inferior olive is controversial. Monagle & Brody (1974) reported no change with age, in contrast to Sandoz & Meier-Ruge (1977) who found 20% loss between 20 and 50 years. Obviously many more brain stem nuclei and other regions remain to be investigated in the ageing human brain as a function of increasing age. With advancing immunocytochemical techniques, future studies may be directed towards establishing the numerical status of particular transmitter and neuropeptide associated neurons which will hopefully provide a much clearer picture of the effects of age on specific neuron types.

Dendritic processes

Studies on dendritic process in the ageing brain, which may reflect the ability of the brain to adapt and respond to stimulation, are sparse. This relative paucity of information is largely due to methodological difficulties. Conventional neuropathological stains do not delineate dendritic processes in either a qualitative or quantitative fashion. The Golgi–Cox impregnation technique selectively demonstrates dendritic arbors, although only in a small percentage of the total neuron population of a given brain area. Despite difficulties in applying this technique to postmortem human brain, observations (Scheibel *et al* 1975, Scheibel 1978) in 20 patients (age range 4–102 years) have demonstrated apparently sequential dendritic abnormalities in pyramidal and granule cell neurons in the frontal and temporal cortex, and hippocampal regions. The earliest visible change is a loss of dendritic spines, and therefore presumably also of synapses especially in the horizontal dendritic process. The dendrites subsequently develop swelling and varicosites with loss of horizontal dendritic components. In addition the cell body swells, distortion in the apical dendritic shaft becomes visible and eventually the cell body disappears altogether. These changes are generally most pronounced in the third (pyramidal) neuron layer but are also common to the Betz cells in the fifth layer of the motor cortex.

Astroglia

Compared with our present knowledge on neuronal populations in the aged, far less information is available on alterations occurring in the supportive but no doubt equally important astrocytic populations. Hypertrophy of astrocytes and their processes, which has been observed in the cerebral hemisphere in old age, is most obvious in subpial and subependymal regions and within the cortex itself (Corsellis 1976a, Terry *et al* 1981) where it may represent a secondary reaction to the cortical neuron loss which occurs in the elderly. There is evidence to suggest that the absolute numbers of glial cell bodies do not alter substantially from maturity to old age and only a 15% decrease in glial cells has been recently reported in one of the few studies of this subject (Henderson *et al* 1980). In this investigation, which utilised an automated image analyser, all cells below 12 μm in size were regarded as astrocytes. It should be noted that the numbers of glial calls do not appear to increase in conjunction with neuronal loss occurring with age, despite their probable hypertrophy. This contrasts with the situation in some but not all diseases (see pp. 39 and 47) where neuronal loss is accompanied by an increase in astrocytic numbers.

Pigmentations and depositions

Various organic pigments and minerals accumulate in the human brain throughout life. In many sites these depositions appear to be relatively innocuous and have not yet been associated with specific age-related brain syndromes or with psychiatric diseases. Examples of such depositions include the ferrocalcareous material, which is present in the media and adventitia of striatal blood vessels, and the formation of corpora amylacea in sites such as the periventricular regions. In contrast, the deposition of lipofuscin in neurons throughout life has attracted considerable attention and, at one time, its effect was considered to be so deleterious that various theraputic regimens were suggested to minimise or reduce its accumulation. At the light microscopic level, lipofuscin is usually seen as yellow or brown granules in the cell body region, which may occupy a considerable volume (up to 75%) of cytoplasm. Ultrastructurally it is recognised as membrane bound, granular, lamellar, and particulate bodies.

The formation of lipofuscin has been associated with lysosomal function, partly because lipofuscin and lysosomes are anatomically contiguous at the ultrastructural level. It seems likely that the pigment is a byproduct of general protein, lipid or lipoprotein metabolism. Chemically the constituents of lipofuscin are ill defined, although they include lipids and proteinaceous material (Pearse 1972). In the central nervous system, certain neurons or nuclei appear particularly prone to accumulate lipofuscin and in the neurons of for example the inferior olive, dendate nucleus, globus pallidus and anterior horn cells of the spinal cord large amounts are often seen. The extent to which lipofuscin interferes with physiological processes is not known with certainty, although it probably does not decrease protein synthesis. It has been pointed out that the relative stability of neuronal numbers in the inferior olive, despite the accumulation of large quantities of lipofuscin with advancing age, suggests that lipofuscin does not have a direct toxic effect on metabolic processes in neurons (Monagle & Brody 1974, Tomlinson 1979) although physiological normality of neuronal function has not been established.

The pigment neuromelanin has, unlike lipofuscin, a restricted distribution in the brain. It accumulates to the greatest extent in the perikarya of neurons in the substantia nigra whilst axons and dendrites in this region appear largely free of this pigment. Neuromelanin formation is almost certainly related to catecholamine transmitter function, particularly that of dopamine neurons in the substantia nigra.

Senile plaques

Senile plaques are recognised microscopically as minute areas of abnormal tissue or neuropil which develop within the cortical grey matter and occasionally in other brain regions. They are generally considered to be a degenerative change. In some people plaques may be present at a relatively early age and have been seen from the fourth decade onwards (Tomlinson 1979), when they are most frequently found in medial temporal lobe structures such as the amygdaloid and hippocampus (Dyan 1970a). In neocortical brain regions including all four cortical lobes, senile plaques are found in increasing numbers with advancing age and are present to a greater or lesser extent in approximately 80% of normal elderly people beyond the eighth decade. Quantitative studies, in which the number of plaques has been estimated in low power fields (each 1.3 mm across) from many cortical areas have shown that they may be unevenly distributed throughout the neocortex. In a series of 28 psychometrically assessed elderly people (Tomlinson 1968), the mean neocortical plaque count was found to be between 3 and 4 per low power field. Approximately two-thirds of these cases (20 out of 28) showed very few or no neocortical plaques whilst, in the remaining third, the mean plaque density ranged between 6 and 13. At this density plaques were generally found between the third and fifth neuronal layers in the cortex. Despite this relatively low mean plaque density, a considerable variation was found in plaque numbers both between the various neocortical lobes and within a particular neocortical region. The latter was such that occasional low power microscopic fields showed over 50 plaques — an appearance which can suggest to the unwary observer a diagnosis of Alzheimer's

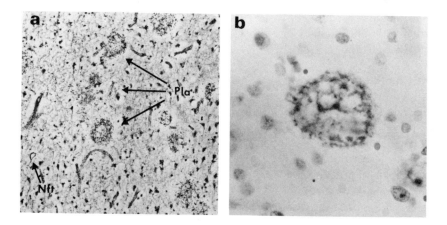

Fig. 1.1 (a) Senile plaques (Pla) in the temporal cortex of an 82-year-old female with senile dementia of Alzheimer type. This photomicrograph is taken from cortical layers 3–5 and includes a neurofibrillary tangle (Nft). (von Braunmühl ×160).
(b) Acetylcholinesterase demonstrated histochemically in a senile plaque. The histochemical techniques for acetylcholinesterase demonstration are given in Perry *et al* (1980).

disease. Such an error is much more likely to arise if only one or two cortical areas are examined.

Senile plaques are not readily identified histologically with conventional paraffin embedded material and, for their consistent demonstration, frozen sections and silver staining techniques are required. Using silver stains, such as von Braunmühl, the size of typical senile plaques ranges from 20 μm to 200 μm. In transverse section they appear circular (Fig. 1.1a) often with a more densely staining amyloid-containing centre or core. At the periphery the plaque edge is well defined yet not sharply demarcated from adjacent neuropil. Small senile plaques consist of abnormal neuronal processes, referred to as neuritic processes or neurites, intermingled with astrocytes or microglia. In larger plaques, the neuritic processes are concentrated at the periphery and the central region contains many amyloid fibres. Senile plaques do not appear to have a significant relationship to either neuronal cell bodies or blood vessels.

Support for the neuronal origin of the majority of processes observed in senile plaques derives mainly from electron microscopic observations (Kidd 1964, Terry *et al* 1964) which have identified many of the neuritic processes as presynaptic, unmyelinated axonal terminal or boutons. Many of these axonal terminals contain abnormal mitochondria, lamellar lysosomes, and paired helical filaments. In addition to glial processes postsynaptic (dendritic) neuronal processes have been observed electron microscopically although, in contrast to axonal processes, they appear morphologically to be relatively normal (Gonatas *et al* 1967). Despite numerous light and electron microscopic observations, the pathophysiological significance of senile plaques remains obscure. The histochemical demonstration of several enzyme activities within plaques (Josephy 1949, Friede 1965, Perry *et al* 1980) suggests that they are not wholly degenerative in nature and may infact partially represent an abortive attempt at regeneration. In the hippocampal formation the localisation (Fig. 1.1b) of acetylcholinesterase to senile plaque neuritic processes suggests that some of these may be proliferating terminal cholinergic processes derived from the septum (Perry *et al* 1980) and in the neocortex similar cholinergic processes may have an origin in the basal nucleus of Meynert. Although there is a paucity of information on the status of neuronal processes in the ageing brain, both the abnormal neuritic processes which are present in senile plaques and the volume of neuropil occupied by senile plaques is likely to be associated with deranged synaptic function in that area of brain.

Neurofibrillary tangles

Neurofibrillary tangles are abnormal intracellular structures which can be identified at the light microscopic level using conventional silver stains (e.g. Bielschowsky or Glees & Marsland) as aggregated bundles of filaments within the perikaryon of pyramidal neurons (Fig. 1.2a). Although these structures were first associated with presenile dementia by Alois Alzheimer (1907) they have since been identified in other pathological conditions (reviewed by Wiśniewski *et al* 1979) and their development in the normal ageing brain has been the subject of many investigations. Regional distribution studies (see for example Tomlinson 1972) have identified medial temporal lobe structures as areas which are particularly prone to develop tangles. In approximately 5% of apparently normal individuals neurofibrillary tangles are evident by the fifth decade of life. The numbers of neurofibrillary tangles then increase in a linear fashion and their presence in these regions is almost universal by the ninth or tenth decades (Dayan 1970a, Ball 1976, Tomlinson 1979). Although hippocampal neurofibrillary tangles are present in the vast majority of elderly people, their density is substantially lower than in cases with senile dementia of Alzheimer type (see p. 32). In contrast to the hippocampus, neocortical neurofibrillary tangles are infrequently found in the normal elderly populations (Tomlinson *et al* 1968, Dyan 1970a) and, if they are readily identifiable in the neocortex either in biopsies or at post-mortem, they are almost always associated with clinical dementia of Alzheimer type. Neurofibrillary tangles in the neocortex do not therefore increase in density with age as they do in the hippocampus, and in this respect their age-related distribution differs.

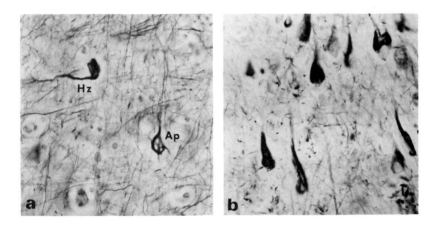

Fig. 1.2 (a) Neocortical neurofibrillary tangles *(left)* generally have a curved or curvilinear form and may extend into apical (Ap) or horizontal (Hz) dendrites. Neurofibrillary tangles in pyramidal cells of the hippocampus *(right)* are straighter and generally extend into the apical dendrite. (Glees & Marsland ×400.)
(b) In the hippocampal formation, the structures shown in Fig. 1.2a react histochemically for acetylcholinesterase. (Acetylcholinesterase ×640.) Both sets of photomicrographs are taken from elderly patients with senile dementia of Alzheimer type.

At the ultrastructural level, early observations on neurofibrillary tangles in 1963 revealed twisted fibrils or tubules with a maximum diameter of approximately 22 nm (Kidd 1963, Terry 1963) as the main structural feature. The nature of these twisted fibrils has been a matter of controversy but present evidence suggests that each twisted fibril is composed of a pair of filaments wound round each other helically and each measuring between 10 and 13 nm across. There is also evidence that some tangles contain straight, non-twisted, tubular elements (Yagishita *et al* 1980). Chemical isolation and physical analyses indicate that neurofibrillary tangles are composed primarily of protein (Iqbal *et al* 1974, 1975) probably consisting of aggregated subunits arranged in a β-pleated conformation. The origin and significance of neuro-fibrillary tangles are still unknown and, although they are generally regarded as primarily degenerative structures, the histochemical demonstration of enzyme activity such as nucleoside phosphatase and acetylcholinesterase (Fig. 1.2b) in association with neurofibrillary tangles suggests that they may not, at least initially, be as inert as was formerly believed. Several groups have examined the obvious possiblilty that neurofibrillary tangles are derived from neuronal neurofibrils or neurotubules (Iqbal *et al* 1978, Gambetti *et al* 1980, Grunde–Iqbal *et al* 1979). This is, however, still an unresolved issue since attempts to localise neurofilament or neurotubulin antigens on neuro-fibrillary tangles have produced conflicting reports. Other investigators have suggested that neurofibrillary tangles accumulate as a result of deranged protein synthesis (De Boni & Crapper 1978).

Granulovacuolar degeneration and Hirano bodies

In the brains of many elderly and, to a lesser extent, younger people distinctive vacuoles, each with a haemotoxophilic staining central granule, are present in pyramidal cells of the hippocampus (Fig. 1.3). These intra-cytoplasmic vacuoles — appropriately termed granulovacuolar change — were first identified by Simchowicz in 1910. Despite the many intervening years of light and electron microscopic observations (Hirano *et al* 1968) on these structures, their precise nature and significance remains obscure. Their presence in the elderly and increase in density in senile demetia of Alzheimer type suggest that they represent a form of degenerative change and, in many neurons, the vacuoles are present in sufficient numbers to occupy most of the neuronal perikaryon.

Hirano bodies are eosinophilic, generally ovoid structures which, like granulovacuolar degeneration, are more common in the hippocampal reg-ion of the elderly brain than elsewhere (Fig. 1.4). Although first described by Hirano in the brains of cases with the parkinsonian–dementia complex of Guam (Hirano 1965), they are infact more widely distributed than granulo-vacuolar degeneration. Their presence in normal brains from the third

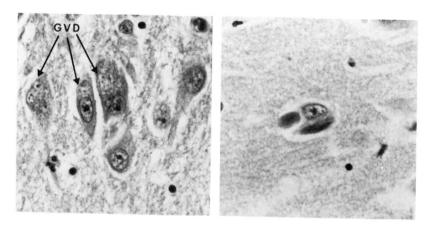

Fig. 1.3 *(Left)* Granulovacuolar degeneration (GVD) in pyramidal neurons of the hippocampal formation in a man of 79 years with senile dementia of Alzheimer type. Arrows indicate affected cells. (H. & E. ×640.)

Fig. 1.4 *(Right)* Hirano bodies situated in the hippocampal pyramidal layer in a man of 79 years with senile dementia of Alzheimer type. (H. & E. ×640.)

decade onwards and their increase in numbers in the elderly in senile dementia of Alzheimer type and in other disease processes is now well established (Ogata *et al* 1972). Electron microscopic observations have demonstrated that Hirano bodies are ordered, paracrystalline structures which may lie both within neuronal cytoplasm and in other cell processes.

Amyloid

Amyloid is an apparently insoluble, extracellular, fibrillary material which accumulates, often with deleterious effect, in visceral organs, blood vessels and the brain. It is associated both with specific diseases and with increasing age. A recent comprehensive review on the distribution and nature of amyloid was provided by Glenner (1980a and 1980b). There appears to be no single disease process which gives rise to amyloid deposition and its classification is somewhat arbitrary. All types of amyloid appear microscopically as an eosinophilic extracellular material reacting with specific stains such as Congo red and thioflavin-T. The green bi-refringence which is seen when amyloid, stained with Congo red, is viewed with polarised light indicates a regular β-pleated sheet type of intermolecular bonding. Under the electron microscope, amyloid consists of bundles of fibres, the individual components of which can be resolved to linear, non-branching fibrils between 7 and 10 nm in width.

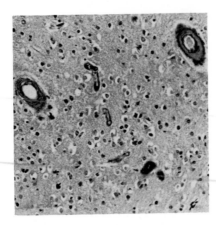

Fig. 1.5 Small and medium sized cortical blood vessels showing prominent vessel walls due to vascular and perivascular amyloid deposition. (H. & E. ×160.)

In the elderly human brain, the majority of amyloid deposition occurs in association with senile plaques and cerebral vessels. In both cases the incidence of amyloid increases with age (Wright *et al* 1969) although plaque amyloid appears to be quantitatively greater than vessel amyloid (Tomlinson 1979). There are, however, individual cases in which amyloid is almost exclusively located in vessels and perivascular regions (Fig. 1.5) and to these the term 'congophilic angiopathy' (Pantelakis 1954) has been applied. Within senile plaques amyloid is located predominantly in the central or core region of the plaque although, in some cases, amyloid may not be visible at the light microscopic level. Electron microscopic observations have suggested that, in the early development of senile plaques, abnormal neurites are present before amyloid fibrils can be identified (Terry & Wiśniewski 1970).

More is known about the distribution and physicochemical characteristics of amyloid deposits in the brain than about its origin or pathophysiological significance. However one consequence of the elucidation of the intermolecular configuration — the β-pleated sheet — is that proteins or peptides which are suggested as candidates for the formation of amyloid must obviously be capable of associating in a β-pleated sheet configuration. In this connection it is of interest that several neuropeptides, including substance P and cholecystokinin octapeptide, have been shown to be capable of self-association into fibrillary forms (Fig. 1.6) which have a similar dimension to amyloid fibrils and a probable β-sheet configuration (Candy *et al* 1981a, Perry *et al* 1981a). It is not yet known if such neuropeptides, or their pro-forms, or breakdown products are related to brain amyloid or amyloid formation at other sites. More general currently held views as to the origin of plaque amyloid in the brain include a derivation from immunoglobulin, hormones, viruses, or peptides and proteins secreted by APUD-type cells and glial cells. (APUD is an acronym given to cell types common to various visceral organs which have, amongst other charateristics, an ability to secrete peptide hormones (reviewed by Gould 1978).)

Support for the hypothesis that plaque amyloid is associated with immunoglobulin molecules or their fragments derives from several sources. In the first instance a direct analogy exists with certain systemic amyloid diseases, in which it has been reported that the chemical composition of amyloid appears to be similar to light chain fragments of immunoglobulin (Glenner *et al* 1971, 1972). Secondly there is the more specious analogy with cerebral amyloid deposits in transmittable diseases (such as scrapie in sheep)

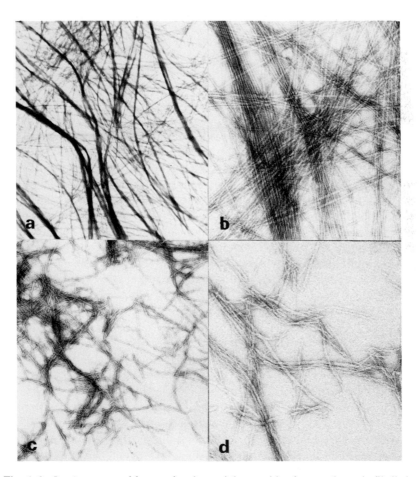

Fig. 1.6 *In vitro,* several low-molecular-weight peptides form polymeric fibrils in saline solutions. Fibrillary forms of the neuropeptide substance P (composed of 11 amino acids) are laterally aggregated in **a** and can be resolved into individual fibrils **(b).** Similar fibrils are formed by cholecystokinin derived peptides such as cholecystokinin-8. The non-sulphated fibrillary form of this peptide is illustrated at low **(c)** and high magnification **(d). a** × 8000, **b** × 100 000, **c** × 66 000, **d** × 185 000.

in which it is postulated that amyloid represents forms of immunoglobulin produced against the putative transmittable agent or even represents the agent itself. Thirdly, immunocytochemical reaction of plaque amyloid with antisera raised against immunoglobulins such as IgG has been demonstrated (Ishii & Haga 1976). In spite of such indirect evidence suggesting a link between amyloid and immunoglobulins, direct evidence is lacking. The possibility that the formation of some amyloid fibrils follows disturbances in non-immunoglobulin protein synthesis or protein metabolic processes has been suggested (Glenner 1978), although evidence to support this possibility is not available. The formation of amyloid fibrils could, for instance, follow the excessive production of a specific protein, hormone or peptide, or alternatively it could follow a disturbance of proteolysis whereby protein or peptide, fragments, produced as a result of proteolysis, self-associate into insoluble β-sheets. A further possibility is that peptide fragments which inhibit or facilitate β-sheet formation in other proteins or peptides are, respectively, decreased or increased in the plaque region. Although vessel amyloid has similarly not been characterised, there is theoretically a stronger case for considering such amyloid fibrils as being derived from serum proteins or from proteins or peptides which are specifically associated with vessels. The chemical nature of both plaque and vessel amyloid will probably not be finally elucidated until pure preparations of each type are isolated and analysed.

The demonstration of an association between the clinical degree of dementia and the mean density of senile plaques provides circumstantial evidence that amyloid, particularly plaque amyloid, may be deleterious to cerebral function. Direct evidence for such a concept is, however, still lacking and such pathophysiological disturbances as may result from amyloid deposition are likely to remain speculative until the origin and nature of amyloid fibrils are known.

Cerebrovascular degeneration

The term cerebrovascular degeneration or disease, interpreted literally, refers to arteriosclerotic degeneration and related diseases which primarily affect cerebral arteries. Generally, however, the term is more widely applied in the context of brain damage (either infarction or ischaemia) associated with impairment or cessation of cerebral blood flow. Although local thrombus formation in cerebral vessels undoubtedly causes cerebral infarction (Moosy 1971), many authorities maintain that a substantial proportion of cerebral infarcts are not caused by locally developing thrombi in cerebral arteries but result either from arterial constriction or from emboli or thromboembolic aggregates which originate from proximal sites and impact in distal arterial branches, usually the small terminal branches but occasionally in larger vessels (Fisher 1951, Hutchinson & Yates 1957, Schwartz & Mitchell 1961,

Blackwood *et al* 1969, Jörgensen & Torvik 1969, Lhermitte *et al* 1970). These emboli may arise from ulcerated atheromatous plaques sited in extra-cranial vessels such as the carotid bifurcation or, less frequently, may be derived from the heart. Other cardiac disorders such as dysrhythmias, hypo- or hypertension may also impair cerebral blood flow and the numerous, rarer, causes of cerebral infarction are described in standard neurological texts.

Cerebral vessels

Several different techniques are available for the postmortem assessment of the degree of arterioslcerosis in cerebral vessels (Moosy 1971) and no single method is entirely satisfactory. Ideally, clinical observations should be used to supplement pathological data. Arteriosclerosis is usually investigated at postmortem by making a qualitative or semi-quantitative assessment of the state of the vessels (atheromatous degeneration, arterial wall thickening, and lumen size) at the base of the brain and also, by the more diligent pathologist, in the cervical, extracranial course of cerebral arteries, such as the carotid bifurcation. These assessments may be supplemented by the histological examination of vessels or by the use of more sophisticated techniques such as the postmortem injection of arteries with radio-opaque contrast medium. However, none of these methods succeeds in pinpointing those crucial factors, such as the extent of collateral circulation and the effects of temporary diminution in cerebral blood flow, which may deter-mine whether or not blood flow is sufficiently impaired in life to produce irreversible cerebral ischaemia.

Cerebral infarcts

The majority of cerebral infarcts are caused, directly or indirectly, by cerebrovascular degeneration. Measuring the extent and distribution of cerebral softenings therefore provides a useful practical measure of the effects of cerebrovascular disease in the elderly brain. Large cerebral infarcts are easily recognised on the surface of the unfixed brain where they may be related to a particular branch of the cerebral arteries. Quantitatively, how-ever, cerebral infarcts are best assessed in the fixed, sectioned brain. In the method employed by Tomlinson *et al* (1968), which is probably the most satisfactory so far devised, visible infacts are charted onto idealised drawings of standard coronal brain sections. Such a chart can provide information on the site of an infarct, its approximate original size (in ml), and its arterial distribution.

Incidence

Regardless of the mechanism of production of a cerebral infarct, the incidence of cerebrovascular disease is clearly increased in the elderly compared to younger age groups. At the pathological level, Tomlinson *et al* (1968) investigated the incidence of cerebral infarcts or softenings in a group of 28 hospital patients (mean age 75 years, range 65–92 years) who died with various illnesses. All except one of these cases were considered, on the basis of a psychometric assessment, to be intellectually normal (the exception may have had early dementia). Visible cerebral softenings, other than minute lesions, were noted in 13 (47%) of this group. Of the remainder, 15 (28%) had no ischaemic lesions and only 7 (25%) had occasional softenings below 1 mm in size. In the 13 cases with readily identified visible softenings, the volume of brain involved ranged from 2 to 91 ml (mean 13.2 ml). The mean volumes of visible cortical infarcts in patients dying with physical illness, terminal confusion, and depression were 20.3 ml, 7.0 ml and 14 ml respectively. In nearly two-thirds of these 13 cases with visible lesions, the basal ganglia contained small softenings. The majority of the larger infarcts were situated in the cerebral cortex, frequently on one side of the brain only and had occurred predominantly in the distribution of the middle and posterior cerebral arteries. Frontal lobe lesions were rare and extensive white matter lesions not encountered. The frequency of cerebral infarcts in the elderly may have been over-represented in this series since, to some extent, stroke patients were deliberately included. In spite of any such limitation several conclusions may be drawn from this and the related studies. In the first instance cerebral softenings of small or moderate size are not infrequent in intellectually preserved people. Secondly a relatively large amount of cortical tissue (up to at least 50 ml) can apparently be destroyed without resulting in obvious intellectual impairment. Thirdly the site of an ischaemic lesion may, in general, be less important with regard to the production of intellectual impairment than its size.

Miscellaneous

Tumours

Of the various benign CNS tumours which may occur in the elderly, in the absence of clinical signs and symptoms, the commonest is the meningioma. This usually arises above the tentorium and it is worth noting that, in elderly people who develop meningiomas, age-associated brain atrophy may actually be beneficial. The larger cranial capacity : brain volume ratio allows meningiomas to reach a larger size in the elderly, compared with younger patients, before focal brain compression and raised intracranial pressure develop.

Subdural haematoma

Both unilateral and bilateral subdural haematomata occur more commonly in the elderly compared with younger age groups. The majority of such haematomata follow episodes of mild or relatively trivial cerebral trauma and it is likely that the lax subdural space, which accompanies cerebral atrophy, contributes towards the increased incidence in the elderly (p.48).

Other morphological aspects

Amongst those morphological aspects of the ageing brain which have not been described, Lewy bodies, neuro-axonal spheroids, and Marinesco bodies are discussed elsewhere (Tomlinson 1979). Information at the subcellular level on, for example, axonal processes, synapses (receptor size, number of vesicles), nuclei, nucleoli, and mitochondria would be of great value in understanding the life history of the neuron but such studies are, to-date, sparse or absent.

Chemical aspects

Neurochemical estimation of the levels of putative chemical markers have been used by some investigators to provide quantitative indices of cell numbers (Bowen & Davison 1980) in old age. The validity of this technique is open to question since the levels of chemicals can change extensively and reversibly in the absence of actual changes in cell numbers. Even assessments of nuclear DNA — which is a relatively constant cell constituent — are not necessarily useful since reductions in this nucleic acid due to neuronal loss may occur in conjunction with increased levels due to glial proliferation.

Investigation of the chemical changes associated with ageing after maturation has largely depended on advancing knowledge and techniques available for estimating the different chemical systems of the brain. Thus earlier studies tended to concentrate mainly on general chemicals such as lipids, carbohydrates, proteins (including many enzymes), and nucleic acids. More recent studies have included classical neurotransmitter systems (such as noradrenaline, dopamine, 5-hydroxytryptamine, acetylcholine and γ-aminobutyric acid) and also the various neuropeptides which have now been shown to exist in many brain areas. Activities associated with these numerous different chemical systems have generally been investigated in postmortem human brain and it is probably true to say that most appear to decline, to a greater or less extents, across the sixth to tenth decades of life. Exceptions to this trend do exist and include an increase in, for example, the activity of monoamine oxidase (an enzyme which degrades both noradrenaline and 5-hydroxytryptamine). In this respect the proposition (Robinson *et al* 1972) that a concomitant decline in these monoamines may lead to an increased incidence of depression in the elderly is interesting although still controversial. As far as they have been investigated, neuropeptide concentrations in the human brain have not yet been shown to decline with age although this is still a largely unexplored area.

Clinically it is difficult to ascribe alterations in particular brain functions (which no doubt depend on the integrity of various different neuronal systems) to specific age-related chemical changes. The precise function of, for instance, the different cerebral transmitter systems in the brain is not yet understood. Nevertheless several groups of workers have demonstrated anatomical differences in the stability of certain transmitter systems in the ageing brain which may shed some light on age-associated changes in brain function. For example age-related decreases in the enzyme synthesizing γ-aminobutyric acid (glutamate decarboxylase) are apparently particularly pronounced in the thalamus which may account for decreasing ability to process sensory information (McGeer & McGeer 1976). Decreasing choline acetyltransferase — the cholinergic transmitter synthesizing enzyme — is most pronounced in the hippocampus and certain areas of cerebral cortex (Perry *et al* 1977, Davies 1978) which may, in turn, be related to impairments of short-term memory function and other cognitive aspects common in old age.

A key change associated with ageing is likely to be specific alterations in protein synthesis occurring as a result of alterations in the rates of transcription (the production of RNA from DNA). Whilst reductions in RNA with age have been widely observed in the ageing brain, interpretation of changes in overall levels of RNA is difficult without further information on the state of the different forms of messenger, transfer, and ribosomal RNA. Specific messenger RNA molecules are, for example, responsible for the production of each of the numerous proteins (enzymes, receptors, structural proteins, and proteins involved in transport, uptake and release mechanisms) which govern neuronal and glial cell function. No doubt it will ultimately be possible to identify and quantify the transcriptionally active RNAs coding for those different molecules and so assess the influence of age on the brain at the molecular level.

MORPHOLOGICAL ABNORMALITIES ASSOCIATED WITH PSYCHIATRIC DISEASE

Dementia of Alzheimer type

Comparison of presenile and senile dementia of Alzheimer type

Presenile Alzheimer's disease, occurring before the age of 60 or 65 years, presents no difficulties in pathological diagnosis. The brain is atrophied with wide sulci, narrow convolutions, decreased white matter and lateral ventricular enlargement. Characteristic senile plaques and neurofibrillary tangles are invariably present in large numbers in the cortex and are particularly obvious in medial temporal, limbic brain areas such as amygdaloid and hippocampus. In the latter region the additional histological abnormalities of granulovacuolar degeneration and Hirano body formation are found. Severely affected cortical areas may also show a degree of vacuolation of the neuropil, astrocytic reaction and, in silver stained sections, apparent fragmentation and distortion of neuronal processes. Cortical neuronal loss almost certainly accompanies presenile Alzheimer's disease.

In contrast to presenile Alzheimer's disease, the pathological diagnosis of senile dementia of Alzheimer type (SDAT — occurring over the age of 65 years) is often more difficult. Thus whilst more obvious and quantitatively greater changes are present in the younger age groups, in the senium the distinction between normality and SDAT may be obscured by the presence, in non-demented individuals, of age-associated changes such as brain atrophy and the formation of senile plaques and neurofibrillary tangles. Additional factors which complicate the diagnosis of SDAT are the increased incidence of cerebrovascular disease in the elderly (Corsellis 1962) and the possibility that in the very elderly the amount of 'senile degeneration' which is necessary to produce dementia is less than in younger age groups (Constantinidis 1978, Tomlinson 1980). For many years difficulties encountered in assessing elderly brains obscured the relationship between clinical aspects of senile dementia and pathological changes. The use of semi quantitative or quantitative techniques in assessing pathological features has, however, provided a much more scientific basis for investigating this relationship (Neumann & Cohn 1953, Corsellis 1962, Tomlinson *et al* 1970, Dyan 1970b, Ball 1976).

Incidence

In the elderly the incidence of dementia increases from the seventh decade onwards and above the age of 80 years approximately 25% of the population is affected. Many pathological studies have established that SDAT is the largest single cause of dementia in the elderly being responsible for between 50 and 80% of the dementias in old age (Tomlinson *et al* 1970). In a recent series of 73 elderly cases of dementia (mean age 77 years; Tomlinson 1980) 38 (53%) were considered, pathologically, to have either SDAT or probable SDAT and a further 12 cases (16%) showed Alzheimer-type changes in association with ischaemic cerebral lesions. In approximately 80% of demented individuals in this series, therefore, significant Alzheimer type pathological changes were present and in 50% they constituted the main neuropathological abnormality.

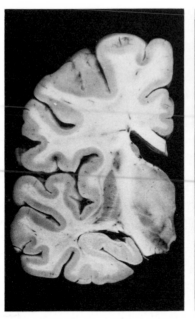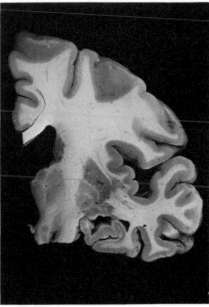

Fig. 1.7 Fixed coronal sections derived from the left hemisphere *(left)* of an elderly normal individual and right hemisphere *(right)* of an aged matched case of senile dementia of Alzheimer type. These photographs illustrate the lack of diagnostic features when cases of Alzheimer-type dementia and non-demented individuals are compared macroscopically. (Two-thirds actual size.)

Macroscopic features

Whilst cortical atrophy has been justifiably considered to be a characteristic feature of presenile Alzheimer's dementia, it has not generally been appreciated that a straightforward association between atrophy and dementia does not extend into the elderly, senile period (Fig. 1.7). In several investigations, assessments of cerebral atrophy made simply from measurements of brain weight have not reliably differentiated between elderly demented and non-demented individuals (Jacob 1952, Tomlinson *et al* 1970, Bondareff 1981), and rather surprisingly if males alone were compared (Tomlinson *et al* 1970), the mean brain weight was actually found to be slightly, though not significantly, higher (by nearly 40 g) in the demented group. It is likely that these findings partly reflect the limitations of using brain weight alone as an index of cerebral atrophy since recent, more refined, quantitative investigations on the extent of cerebral atrophy in senile dementia have demonstrated that, despite a degree of overlap, there are significant differences between SDAT and controls. In one of these investigations, Hubbard & Anderson (1981) quantitatively compared cerebral atrophy in age matched, neuropathologically assessed normals and dements by assessing the degree of atrophy (using a point counting morphometric technique in various brain regions) and relating this to the cranial capacity as a measure of the original size of the brain (see p. 11). Cerebral cortical atrophy in demented individuals between the ages of 67 and 79 years ranged in this study from 13% in the frontoparietal region to 18% in the temporal lobe; the mean cortical atrophy was 14.4%. An analysis of white matter in this series revealed a similar mean (11.8%) but greater range of atrophy extending from 8.5% in the occipital lobe to 26% in the temporal lobe. Total cerebral tissue (both grey and white matter) was significantly reduced by 12.7% in the demented group and the ventricular size was increased by 53%. The latter is similar to the increase in ventricular size previously recorded in demented individuals by Tomlinson *et al* (1970). Beyond the age of 80 years (and up to 92 years) Hubbard & Anderson (1981) found that only the temporal cortex was significantly atrophied in demented individuals. The ventricles in this more elderly group were increased by 9.3% in size compared to controls, although this trend did not reach significance. Temporal lobe atrophy of both grey and white matter is also pronounced before the age of 80 years and atrophy of this particular area appears to be a frequent and characteristic feature of SDAT as has been pointed out by Tomlinson *et al* (1970). Miller *et al* (1980), using an automated visual analysis technique to assess atrophy in the fixed brain, noted a reduction in average hemisphere volume (both grey and white matter) of 18% in demented individuals compared to an age-matched control group.

Clinical reports of brain size in senile dementia, based on computed tomography, have upheld the overall concept of atrophy in SDAT but have also emphasised the extent of individual variation (Jacoby & Levy 1980a). It has additionally been claimed that the CT 'density' of the brain is reduced in presenile and senile dementia (Naeser *et al* 1980) although, in this particular study, only one aged-matched control case was examined. In general, however, both clinical and pathological investigations support the thesis that cerebral atrophy is not so pronounced in senile dementia as it is in presenile dementia and that assessments of atrophy must be used cautiously if they are intended as a means of diagnosing SDAT either clinically or pathologically. Although in individual cases it is not possible to make a diagnosis of SDAT by assessing the extent of brain atrophy at postmortem, a careful macroscopic examination of the fixed, sectioned brain is still an essential step in the pathological assessment of brains from suspected demented individuals since it reveals the presence of cerebral infarcts (see p. 25) and other lesions which may have contributed to or caused clinical dementia.

Microscopic features

All the histological features of SDAT are found to a lesser extent in some normal elderly people and are described in detail on pp. 16–24. In the present section, the microscopic abnormalities of the brain in SDAT are mainly described from the viewpoint of neuropathological diagnosis.

Biopsy

Little justification exists for performing cerebral biopsies to diagnose or classify dementia in the elderly since the treatable causes that occur in this age group can usually be identified by other means. The pathologist who is presented with a cortical cerebral biopsy may, however, make a reasonably confident diagnosis of SDAT on the basis of either a high density both of neurofibrillary tangles and senile plaques or of a high density of neuro-fibrillary tangles and a moderate or low number of plaques. Given the presence of these histological abnormalities in a biopsy specimen, the only proviso which should be added is the possibility of the case being one of mixed or combined dementia (see p. 39) since it is obviously not possible, on the basis of a single biopsy, to exclude the existence of ischaemic lesions elsewhere in the brain. If, in a biopsy specimen, senile plaques are present in the absence of neurofibrillary tangles or if both are present in small num-bers, diagnostic difficulties arise. The differential diagnosis then includes the presence of age-associated senile degenerative changes (without sufficient histological abnormalities to warrant a diagnosis of SDAT) or of SDAT in which less severe histological abnormalities are present in the particular area of brain biopsied.

Postmorten

Compared with cerebral biopsy, the pathological diagnosis of senile demen-tia of Alzheimer type can be made with much more certainty after death, following brain fixation and histological examination. In most laboratories the diagnosis is based on the distribution and density of senile plaques and neurofibrillary tangles in archi- and neocortical brain regions. In the neocor-tex, qualitative histological assessments of samples from the four cortical lobes (ideally taken bilaterally) provide a sufficient basis for the accurate diagnosis of the majority of severe or moderately severe cases of SDAT. Neurofibrillary tangles and senile plaques in such cases are present in large numbers and the identification of areas of plaque fusion (which often occurs if plaques exceed 25 per low power field), or of senile plaques throughout all cortical layers (which frequently occurs if plaques exceed 30 per low power field), and fragmented or disrupted neuropil, serve as confirmatory features. In medial temporal lobe structures the presence of numerous neurofibrillary tangles in the posterior (as opposed to the anterior) segment of the hippocampus is said to be a distinctive feature of SDAT (Ball 1976). Those brains showing less extensive cortical changes require the employment of quantitative or semiquantitative techniques if senile dementia of Alzheimer type is to be reliably distinguished from non-demented elderly people. The criteria used for such quantitative assessments depend on individual laboratories. In the investigations of Tomlinson *et al* (1970) equal, if not greater, importance has been attached to the presence of neocortical neurofibrillary tangles than to the actual plaque density, although the latter exceeded a mean of 14 per lower power field in the neocortex of SDAT cases. Similar quantitative techniques have also been applied to archicortical regions (such as the hippocampal formation) to diagnose and grade the severity of senile dementia of Alzheimer type (Dyan 1970b, Ball 1976); in these areas a quantitatively greater density of granulovacuolar degeneration (Woodard 1962, Tomlinson *et al* 1970) and Hirano body formation (Gibson & Tomlinson 1977) are also found. Quantitation of senile degenerative change further enables the pathological severity of the Alzheimer disease process to be assessed and allows a correlation to be made with clinical measures of dementia and also, more recently, with indices of different neurochemical systems in the brain (Perry *et al* 1978, 1982).

Whatever the number and distribution of senile plaques and neurofibrillary tangles, the diagnosis of SDAT can only be maintained if ischaemic lesions (see pp. 25–6) do not exceed approximately 50 ml in volume and if any ischaemic lesions which are present are not situated in critical brain areas such as the hippocampal formation or the corpus callosum. If such ischaemic lesions are found, then the possibilty of a mixed (multi-infarct and Alzheimer type) dementia arises. Similarly macroscopic and microscopic examination of other areas should be undertaken to exclude other disease or lesions which may contribute to the dementing syndrome such as old traumatic injury or Wernicke's encephalopathy. Even with the benefit of quantitative and qualitative pathological assessments it is not always possible to state unequivocally whether or not SDAT is present. This results from a degree of overlap which exists pathologically between mild cases of SDAT and a small percentage of non-demented individuals. The uncertaintity of diagnosis in these cases was recognised in the classification adapted by Tomlinson *et al* (1980), in which a distinction was drawn between, on the one hand, those cases with an unequivocal diagnosis of SDAT in whom the histological changes exceeded those encountered in a clinically assessed normal group and, on the other hand, cases with a probable diagnosis of SDAT. In the latter category were placed cases where histological changes exceeded those found in the majority of normals but which were similar to those encountered in the occasional normal or non-demented individual. In individuals who fall, pathologically, into the category of probable SDAT, it is possible that other factors have contributed to the precipitation of the dementing features observed during life.

Involvement of non-cortical or non-limbic regions in SDAT

The deep grey matter of the cerebral hemispheres such as basal ganglia and thalamus, do not show extensive abnormalities in SDAT and the substantia nigra also appears to be spared. In the brain stem, however, neuronal loss in the neuromelanin pigmented locus coeruleus undoubtedly occurs in some cases of SDAT (Forno 1966, 1978, Mann *et al* 1980, Tomlinson *et al* 1981, Bondareff *et al* 1981). This particular nucleus is considered to be the site of origin of many of the noradrenergic fibres of the brain (see p. 14) and cell loss in this nucleus in SDAT is consistent with several reports that chemical abnormalities of noradrenaline or related neurochemical activities are present in the neocortex (p. 35). It is of some interest that locus coeruleus neuronal loss may not occur to the same extent in all cases of SDAT and it has been recently suggested that two subgroups of the disease may exist (Bondareff *et al* 1981). In one group of patients, cell counts are apparently in the normal or near-normal range, whereas in the other, neuron loss is extensive. The extent of the locus coeruleus neuron loss appears to correlate with the degree of the dementia as assessed pathologically by a senile plaque count (Tomlinson *et al* 1981) or clinically from a dementia score (Bondareff *et al* 1981).

In several brain areas not obviously affected neuropathologically in Alzheimer's disease, the volume of neuronal nucleoli and levels of cytoplasmic RNA have been reported to be decreased (Mann & Sinclair 1978). These reports, if confirmed, raise the possibility of abnormalities in protein synthesis occurring in areas of the brain not obviously involved in the process of Alzheimer's disease.

Cortical cell populations in SDAT

Loss of neurons in SDAT is accepted almost without question by many people, although the actual evidence supporting such a concept is surprisingly sparse. Neuronal loss is certainly not as extensive in SDAT as it is, for instance, in Pick's disease or Jakob–Creutzfeld disease and it is probable that neuronal loss, per se, is not a direct cause of the dementing process. In 1973, Shefer compared neuronal numbers in six cases of SDAT (mean age 79 years) with those in ten control or normal patients and six patients with a vascular dementing process. Neuronal counts in the third cortical layer (obtained from six cortical areas) and in the hippocampal subiculum were consistently lower in SDAT, especially in the latter area. The actual loss in SDAT was between 20 and 50% and, in this investigation, only the subiculum showed a marked decrease in cortical grey matter thickness. This neuronal loss is unlikely to be due to lipofuscin accumulation since the latter is not increased in SDAT (Mann & Sinclair 1978). In 1977, Terry *et al* maintained, in an automated image analysis investigation of three cortical regions, that no significant neuronal loss occurred in SDAT. However a more recent report (Terry *et al* 1981) from this group refers to a significant loss of large cortical pyramidal neurons amounting to between 40 and 46% and accompanied by astrocytic hyperplasia in SDAT. In the former study, the thickness of the grey matter was apparently not significantly reduced in SDAT and this observation accords with those of Shefer (1973). It is unlikely that such cortical neuronal loss as occurs in SDAT is directly related to the cholinergic derangement — indicated recently by neurochemical analysis (see below) — since intrinsic cholinergic neurons are either sparse or absent in the cortex and the majority of cholinergic nerve processes in this brain region are terminal axonal processes thought to be derived, on the basis of animal studies, from cell bodies situated in the nucleus of Meynert. The latter is a poorly circumscribed group of large, polymorphic neurons which extend throughout most of the substantia innominata region. Histochemical observations and microchemical analysis of the latter region in the human brain (Candy *et al* 1981b) are compatible with this nucleus having a major cholinergic function. Whether or not the nucleus of Meynert is involved pathologically in SDAT is not yet known with certainty although assessments of this nucleus reveal a moderate cell loss in some, but not all, cases of SDAT (Perry, unpublished observations). If a consistent cortical neuronal loss can be established in SDAT it will obviously be of great interest to determine whether particular neuronal (transmitter or peptide) types are selectively affected.

Chemical aspects

Clear and consistent evidence of a cholinergic abnormality in SDAT, which appears to be related to the severity of the disease has recently stimulated interest in the biochemistry of this disorder. The enzymes choline acetyltransferase and acetylcholinesterase (but not the muscarinic cholinergic receptor) are substantially reduced in many brain areas, particularly in the cortex and hippocampus (Perry & Perry 1980). Whether this is a primary change relating directly to the disease process and whether it is amenable to appropriate pharmacological intervention (in at least early cases) are, at present, unanswered questions. The involvement of at least one other major neurotransmitter system — the noradrenergic system — is indicated by both the pathological evidence discussed above (p. 34) and biochemical estimations of noradrenergic-related activities in cortex (Adolffson *et al* 1978, Cross *et al* 1981). However these may be relatively non-specific changes since they are seen in other disorders, e.g. Parkinson's disease. Neuropeptide abnormalities (including reductions in the concentration of somatostatin) have also been recorded recently (Davies *et al* 1980, Rossor *et al* 1980) although, on the basis of present evidence, these alterations appear to occur at later stages in the disease process (Perry *et al* 1982). Future investigations should establish whether Alzheimer's disease, like Huntington's chorea, is associated with widespread chemical changes which are not readily amenable to treatment or whether, like Parkinson's disease, it may be possible to pinpoint a particular neurochemical deficit which may be countered pharmacologically.

Multi-infarct dementia

Incidence

The relationship between cerebrovascular degeneration and psychiatric abnormalities is not as well characterised as that between cerebrovascular degeneration and neurological syndromes (the latter is discussed in detail in standard neurological texts). A small proportion of individuals with ischaemic cerebral lesions will undoubtedly develop dementia although the incidence of the syndrome in the general population is not as great as was

infarcts are found in the elderly (pp. 25–6), multi-infarct dementia unaccompanied by senile degenerative change only accounts for between 15 and 20% of dementing illnesses in the elderly (Tomlinson *et al* 1970). A further 10–15% of cases show a significant degree of cerebral infarction co-existing with senile degenerative change (p. 39). This latter group is classified as combined or mixed dementia. The precise neuropathological features which determine the onset of multi-infarct dementia are not clearly established but major factors associated with its aetiology are likely to include the involvement of particular brain areas and the destruction of a critical quantity of tissue. The clinical symptomatology of multi-infarct dementia differs sufficiently from that of senile dementia of Alzheimer type to allow distinctions between the two to be made, in some cases, before death (Roth & Morrissey 1952, Rosen *et al* 1979, Blessed 1980). There is also evidence that multi-infarct dementia develops, on average, in a slightly younger age group, that the male population is more vulnerable, and that it often occurs in the presence of hypertension (Corsellis 1962).

Quantitative aspects

In both clinical and pathological studies, caution should be exercised in attributing a dementing syndrome to multi-infarct dementia on the basis of the demonstration of small infarcts in the brain. Single or multiple cerebral infarcts, below 50 ml in total volume, are unlikely to give rise to dementia unless co-existing Alzheimer type changes or other destructive or degenerative lesions are present. Similarly, whilst the demonstration of single or multiple infarcts with a volume greater than 50 ml is sufficient to diagnose multi-infarct dementia in the majority of cases, unless co-existing senile dementia of Alzheimer type can be excluded the possibility of a mixed dementia has to be considered.

It has been known for many years that destruction of cerebral tissue resulting from cerebral ischaemia and infarction may be associated with a dementing syndrome; however, the concept that infarction of a critical quantity of tissue may be required before dementia supervenes, has only emerged from the more recent studies of Tomlinson *et al* (1968, 1970). In nine demented patients in whom cerebral infarction was felt to be the major neuropathological lesion responsible for dementia, the average volume of cerebral tissue destroyed amounted to 150 ml (range 60–412 ml) (data recalculated from Tomlinson *et al* (1970)). This mean of 150 ml volume represents approximately 15% of the total volume of the cerebral hemi-spheres and contrasts with a much smaller volume of infarcted tissue (mean 9.6 ml) measured in the brains of 27 psychometrically assessed normal cases. Analysis of individual cases examined in these particular studies suggested that cerebral infarcts of between 50 and 100 ml are likely to be associated with some degree of intellectual decline and dementia, whereas infarcts totalling 100 ml or more are almost always seen, in the elderly, in conjunc-tion with an established dementing syndrome.

Regional aspects

Multi-infarct dementia offers a unique opportunity to investigate the role of different cerebral areas in some of the intellectual and other functions in the human brain. Observations on the regional distribution of cerebral infarcts in elderly cases of multi-infarct dementia have demonstrated an almost invariable involvement of the cerebral cortex; however there is little neuro-pathological support for the assertion (Hachinski *et al* 1974) that the com-monest cause of vascular dementia in the elderly is the development of widespread multiple small infarcts (producing the morphological picture of état lacunaire or état criblé). The majority of cases of multi-infarct dementia in the elderly prove to have several cerebral infarcts of a moderate or large size rather than multiple separate lesions, and in most cases both hemi-spheres are affected — although not necessarily equally or symmetrically. More rarely, vascular lesions confined to one hemisphere produce dementia and occasionally a single large infarct will be found to constitute the main lesion in terms of the volume of tissue involved (Fig. 1.8). Analysis of the distribution of infarcts in the various cortical lobes suggests that lesions in the frontal lobes, especially the rostral or anterior areas, are less frequently associated with dementia than infarcts in parietal, occipital, or temporal lobes. The degree to which infarcts in non-cortical areas, such as the basal ganglia or diencephalon, contribute to multi-infarct in the senium is not well

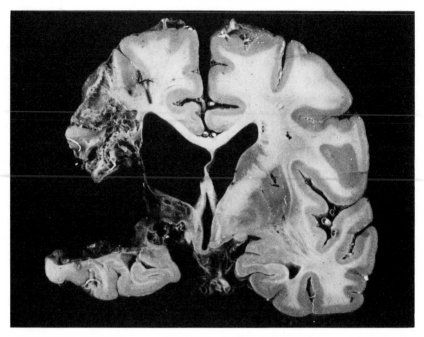

Fig. 1.8 In this unusual case the large infarct, in the territory of the middle cerebral artery, constituted the main ischaemic lesion in a 75-year-old male with multi-infarct dementia. Several smaller softenings were present in the opposite hemisphere. The cerebral arteries in this case were injected with radio-opaque material. (Two-thirds actual size.)

established. Multiple small basal ganglia infarcts may be present in cases of multi-infarct dementia but, since they occur quite frequently in non-demented old people, their presence cannot be directly related to the development of a dementing syndrome. In occasional presenile cases, bilateral thalamic infarcts are associated with cognitive impairment, although pathological studies in the senile age group indicate that such cases are rare. Ischaemic lesions which affect the hippocampus bilaterally may, by virtue of a disturbance of memory function, produce a dementing-type syndrome and involvement of the corpus callosum (the main commissural tract in the brain) has been noted in some of the cases originally investigated by Tomlinson *et al* (1970). These findings support the common observation that certain brain regions are closely involved in normal intellectual and memory function and that damage to these areas is more likely to be associated with dementia than cerebral destruction sustained elsewhere. The relative involvement of grey and white matter has not been assessed in multi-infarct dementia and both cortical and white matter destruction contribute to the localised cerebral shrinkage and dilated ventricles which are usually found in this disease.

In the presenile period and occasionally over the age of 60 years, cerebral softenings may predominate in, or exclusively involve, the white matter alone. This is seen in the rare 'Binswanger's encephalopathy' — a dementing illness in which bilateral white matter lesions are associated with hypertension and thickened cerebral arterioles. Clinically this condition pursues a more protracted course than the more common dementias and has characteristic features on computed tomography (Rosenberg *et al* 1979). The use of computed tomography and other tomographic techniques should, in the future, enable the natural history and the importance of the size and sites of ischaemic lesions to be more thoroughly assessed. However, CT scanning is not yet as sensitive in identifying cerebral hemisphere infarcts as neuropathological examination since the incidence of ischaemic lesions in the general elderly population seems to be higher when assessed neuro-pathologically than when assessed by current tomographic techniques. More accurate delineation of the brain itself, and lesions within it, may follow the introduction of scanning techniques based on positron emission tomography or nuclear magnetic resonance.

Combined Alzheimer-type and multi-infarct dementia

The simultaneous presence of several pathological processes is a well recog-nised feature of general geriatric practice and, in pathological studies, the co-existence of vascular and senile degenerative brain disease (Corsellis 1962, Tomlinson *et al* 1970) is not unexpected. In the series of 73 elderly dements (mean age 77 years) reported by Tomlinson (1980), significant senile degenerative change (senile plaques and neurofibrillary tangles) was present in two-thirds and significant cerebrovascular disease in one-third. In 16% of cases these two groups overlapped; dementia could therefore be attributed to the combined effects of two pathological processes. In approx-imately half of such combined cases the severity of either pathological process, if present alone, would be sufficient to cause a dementing process. In the remainder the extent of pathological changes, assessed quantitively, was generally between that of the normal group and that clearly associated with dementia. Clinically it has proved difficult to diagnose patients with mixed or combined senile dementia (Blessed 1980) although the pattern of their clinical decline should, at least theoretically, contain identifying features.

Pick's disease

This form of dementia is comparatively rare in the elderly, partly because its peak incidence occurs in the sixth and seventh decades but also because it is less common than other forms of dementia such as Alzheimer's disease or multi-infarct dementia. As with other dementias, progressive intellectual decline and behavioural abnormalities constitute the major clinical features of Pick's disease. In this disorder, however, frontal lobe symptomatology, repetitive behaviour, and a facetious mood are often prominent in the clinical presentation and enable the diagnosis to be suspected in life. The disease pursues a more protracted clinical course than Alzheimer's disease and a family history of Pick's disease may be present.

The neuropathology of the disease has been reviewed in detail by Corsellis (1976a). The macroscopic appearance is frequently diagnostic and led both to the initial recognition of the disorder and to its early description as 'progressive circumscribed cerebral atrophy'. Brain atrophy is often extensive but may be confined to particular regions of the cerebral cortex where cortical gyri may be markedly shrunken (Fig. 1.9). Such circumscribed atrophy may be present in temporal, frontal, parietal or, very occasionally, occipital lobes but it is most characteristic in the anterior (rostral) part of the

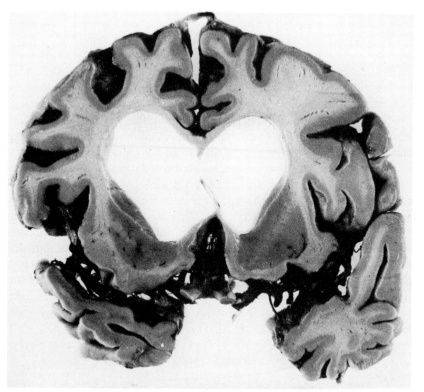

Fig. 1.9 Coronal section through the fixed cerebral hemispheres of a case of Pick's disease showing ventricular dilatation and considerable cortical atrophy. Bilateral atrophy is also present in the caudate nucleus. (Actual size).

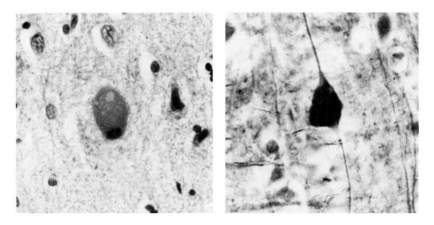

Fig. 1.10 Pick bodies. These distinctive neuronal abnormalities can be demonstrated *(left)* with conventional (H. & E.) or *(right)* silver (Glees & Marsland) stains. Both photomicrographs are from neocortical neurons. The silver stained neuronal process suggests that the neuron involved is bipolar in type. (× 640.)

superior temporal gyrus. Occasional central nuclei, such as the caudate or putamen, are also atrophic and in some cases white matter is severely affected.

Microscopically the most consistent findings are of cortical neuron loss and gliosis in affected areas of cortex; however a more striking histological abnormality — and one which is restricted to Pick's disease — is the presence of Pick bodies or Pick cells. These are abnormally expanded neurons showing an accumulation of material in the immediate perikaryal region of the cell (Fig. 1.10). They are found in the neocortex in small granule-type neurons and in deeper brain structures such as the basal ganglia. Electron microscopic observations on these abnormal neurons have revealed vesiculated cytoplasm with accumulations of neurofilament and neurotubules (Schochet *et al* 1968). Whilst the morphological abnormalities in typical cases of Pick's disease are readily recognised and present no difficulties in diagnosis, in other instances one or more of the characteristic features may be absent. Such atypical cases are frequently classified as Pick's disease even though the pathological justification for making this diagnosis is open to question. Neurochemical observations in Pick's disease are sparse. Several groups have reported reductions in muscarinic receptor binding in the absence of decreased choline acetyltransferase (White *et al* 1977, Yates *et al* 1980) suggesting the involvement of non-cholinergic neurons in the disease process. Further neurochemical and histochemical studies are required to shed light on the specific involvement of particular neuron types.

Huntington's disease

Although most cases of Huntington's disease develop in the fourth and fifth decades of life, occasional cases present later. Clinically, disorders of movement are characteristic of the syndrome with psychiatric symptoms (e.g. hallucinations, irritability, paranoia, and depression) frequently occurring in the initial stages. At some stage or other dementia is usually a major feature of the illness.

Morphological abnormalities of the brain are invariably present in established cases and are macroscopically visible in the striatum as areas of atrophy, especially in the head of the caudate nucleus. Less severe atrophy may also be seen in the putamen and a variable degree of neocortical atrophy is often found in the frontal and temporal lobes. The presence of atrophic neocortical areas neuronal loss is most prominent in layers II and in the disease, although the relationship between the extent of neocortical atrophy and the degree of dementia has not yet been established. In these neocortical atrophic areas neuronal loss is most prominent in layers II and IV often in association with reactive gliosis. Microscopic abnormalities in the caudate nucleus and putamen are particularly striking. The numerous small neurons in these nuclei, which are probably mainly interneurons, are considerably decreased in number and, in severe cases, it is often only the large neuronal perikarya and astrocytes which survive. The prominence of astrocytes in the caudate and putamen was originally considered to be a reactive gliosis but recent quantitative estimates of astrocytic numbers in the caudate show that the increased density of astrocytes is due to tissue shrinkage and atrophy rather than astrocytic proliferation (Thörner *et al* 1977).

Earlier neurochemical studies in Huntington's disease demonstrated a loss of GABA-related activities in several brain areas including the caudate and putamen (Perry *et al* 1973, Bird & Iversen 1974). However, hopes that this might be a primary and treatable abnormality have faded in the face of the lack of clinical response to GABA agonists and of newer findings that a number a different transmitter and neuropeptide systems are apparently affected by the disease. Since neuropathological changes are anatomically widespread, chemical changes which are distributed in all affected areas (including, for example, the cortex) may be particularly important. It is therefore of interest that a significant, though moderate, loss of the glial enzyme, glutamine synthetase, has recently been demonstrated in all brain areas investigated, including frontal and temporal cortex (Carter *et al* 1981). This enzyme is involved in the metabolism of the amino acid transmitter candidate glutamic acid. Glutamic acid itself may be involved in the disease process since experimental kainic acid lesions (the action of which includes destruction of neuronal cell bodies with glutamate receptors) mimic some of the pathological changes in Huntington's chorea.

Alcoholism

Clinically the deleterious effects of excessive alcohol consumption can be seen at all ages, although the diagnosis of alcoholism in the elderly may be obscured by the presence of personality change and intellectual decline. Neuropathologically there are several alcohol-associated brain conditions of relevance to psychiatry which may be subdivided as follows:

1   cerebral changes which are directly related to alcohol consumption, the best known of which is Wernicke's encephalopthy;

2   changes which arise as a consequence of the effects of alcohol consumption on other organs, such as hepatic encephalopthy;

3   consequences of cerebral trauma;

4   less well established states such as the association between alcohol intake and a 'dementing syndrome' or 'alcoholic defect state'.

Many other specific alcohol-associated syndromes, such as cerebellar degeneration, amblyopia and peripheral neuropathy, present primarily as neurological syndromes rather than psychiatric diseases and will not be discussed.

Specific alcohol-associated syndromes

Wernicke's encephalopathy, described originally in 1881, is a well established pathological complication of alcoholism. The characteristic clinical symptomatology of short-term memory loss accompanied by confabulation in an alert consciousness (Korsakoff's psychosis) and the pathological involvement of restricted areas of brain have interested psychiatrists, psychologists, and neuropathologists for many years. The brain is involved in a pathologically distinct and virtually diagnostic pattern. In cases dying in the acute or chronic phases of the disease, symmetrical paraventricular or periaqueductal lesions are found in the thalamus, hypothalamus, midbrain, and mammillary bodies. It is probable that the distinctive regional distribution of this disease is due to a susceptibility of different brain regions to a metabolic derangement induced by nutritional deficiency factors related to thiamine metabolism. In the acute phase, the affected areas are macroscopically haemorrhagic with microscopic areas of necrosis and dilated, congested small vessels. Those cases surviving the acute phase develop atrophy and gliosis in the affected areas. The bilateral involvement if mammillary bodies in the Korsakoff–Wernicke syndrome is generally held to be responsible for the memory disorder associated with this condition, although other authorities (citing the involvement of the medial dorsal nucleus of the thalamus and apparent normality of the mammillary bodies in cases with an amnestic syndrome) have cast doubt on the primary role of these in memory dysfunction (Victor *et al* 1971).

Two distinctive, but rare, demyelinating or degenerative conditions affecting white matter — central pontine myelinolysis and Mar-chiafava–Bignami disease — have also been associated with, but are not exclusively confined to, excessive alcohol consumption. Clinical symptoms of the former, in which demyelination occurs in central pontine regions, include a flaccid tetraplegia, bulbar paralysis and coma. In Mar-chiafava–Bignami disease a combination of neurological and psychiatric symptoms may occur: dementia, emotional disorders, and frontal lobe symptoms have been variously observed (Victor & Banker 1978). Patho-logically, degeneration of the central portion of the corpus callosum with sparing of the ventral and dorsal surfaces was originally described by Mar-chiafava & Bignami (1903). These same authors later described similar lesions in the anterior commissure, middle cerebellar peduncles and subcor-tical white matter. Microscopically, demyelination and a variable degree of axonal loss and blood vessel proliferation are the most salient features. As with Wernicke's encephalopathy, nutritional deficiencies have been impli-cated in the pathogenesis of this syndrome but the precise cause remains obscure.

Hepatic encephalopathy

The various neuropsychiatric symptoms and signs which characterise this disorder are generally held to reflect the toxic effect which certain chemicals (principally ammonia) exert on the brain in the absence of adequate liver function. The condition is not confined to alcohol-induced liver disease and may occur as a complication of liver failure from whatever cause. Patho-logically, morphological changes are usually identifiable within the brain although they are not extensive and may not immediately be appreciated. Protoplasmic astrocytic hypertrophy can be demonstrated in the cerebral cortex, diencephalon, midbrain, and the brain stem. A variable degree of neuronal degeneration in the cerebral cortex has been reported by some investigators.

Cerebral trauma in alcoholism

Compared to his sober counterpart the inebriated alcoholic has an increased risk of head injury and is more susceptible to the complications of cerebral trauma. Episodes of head trauma in alcoholics tend to be poorly documented and, initially at least, may be disguised or unrecognised because of alcohol intoxication. Some of the direct and late consequences of cerebral trauma are discussed on pp. 48–50 and apply equally to the alcoholic and the non-alcoholic. In the elderly alcoholic, however, traumatic cerebral damage may contribute towards an already compromised brain (in terms of age-dependent changes and alcohol-associated syndromes) and be a con-tributing factor in the development of the 'alcohol defect state'. An additional infrequent but important complication which is seen more often in alcoholics is the development of uni- or bilateral subdural haematomata following relatively mild or trivial injury. In the presence of a dilapidated personality and intellect, the symptoms of subdural haematoma may be initially unrecongnised.

Alcoholic defect state

The so-called 'alcoholic defect state' is not easily defined clinically nor have consistent features been identified at the neuropathological level. Chronic inebriation or repeated episodes of acute inebriation can, but not always do, produce an apparent disintegration of personality, habits, and intellect. In a clinical survey, at least 10% of alcoholics showed such features (Horvath 1975). The lack of inevitable progression and the improvement generally seen following complete abstinence distingusih 'alcoholic dementia' from other forms of progressive degeneration and dementia such as Alzheimer's disease and multi-infarct dementia. Pathologically, it has not been resolved whether this state is either a distinct entity (related perhaps to directly toxic effects of alcohol on the neuron) or a combination of other alcohol-associated syndromes (such as Wernicke's encephalopathy, anoxic encephalopathy (following seizures), mild hepatic encephalopathy, cerebral trauma, or nutritional deficiencies).

In addition to this clinical syndrome there is evidence of more widespread morphological changes associated with alcoholism in various clinical radiological reports (B. M. J. 1981, Brewer & Perrett 1971, Haug 1968, Fox *et al* 1976, Epstine *et al* 1977, Cala *et al* 1978, Ron *et al* 1980, Carlen *et al* 1981) and pathological studies (Courville 1966, Victor *et al* 1971). These have suggested that brain atrophy may be present in a larger proportion — approximately 50% of alcoholics — occurring as non-specific ventricular dilatation or localised to specific brain regions such as the frontal lobes and the cerebellar vermis. Whilst these investigations have mainly been conducted on young or middle aged alcoholics, there is no reason to believe that the elderly are not equally affected. The histological counterpart of this atrophy has not been precisely defined although some authorities (Victor & Banker 1978) consider it to be a reflection of established alcohol-associated syndromes such as Wernicke's encephalopathy. In the elderly alcoholic, the occurrence of age-associated brain disease are factors which complicate both the clinical and pathological assessments of such cases since their presence may be either coincidental or a contributing factor in the development of an 'alcohol defect state'. There is, however, no evidence to suggest that alcohol initiates or contributes to the formation of senile plaques or neurofibrillary tangles. Neurochemical investigations in alcoholism are few although cholinergic and noradrenergic abnormalities have been reported (Antuono *et al* 1980, Nordberg *et al* 1980). It should be noted that the central problem in alcoholism — dependency on alcohol — has no known morphological or chemical substrate.

Parkinson's disease

The peak incidence of this disorder occurs in the sixth and seventh decades, although it is not infrequent beyond the age of 70. Neurological aspects of this disorder are dealt with in standard texts and psychiatric symptoms may also arise. Despite the difficulties which may be encountered in accurately assessing the mental status of patients with Parkinson's disease, there is some clinical evidence to suggest that, as the duration of the disease increases a proportion of patients become demented (Celesia & Wanamaker 1972, Pearse 1974, Marttila & Rinne 1976).

The development of dementia may be related, directly or indirectly, to the loss of dopaminergic neurons in the substantia nigra with consequent neurotransmitter abnormalities in the basal ganglia or neocortex. Other factors must be involved, however, since dementia is not seen in all cases of idiopathic Parkinson's disease, although dopaminergic neuronal loss is a constant finding. It is of interest that a similar dopaminergic neuronal loss has been reported in dementia pugilistica following repeated mild head injury (pp. 49–50).

Pathological evidence has been presented to suggest that Alzheimer-type dementia develops more frequently in Parkinson's disease and contributes to or causes the dementia reported in the latter disorder. In a recent retrospective clinico-pathological survey of 36 cases of Parkinson's disease, it was concluded that 16 (55%) had clinical features compatible with the presence of moderate or severe dementia (Boller *et al* 1979). Neuropathologically, in the nine patients assessed as being severely demented, senile plaques and neurofibrillary tangles were readily identified. Similar neuropathological features were present in several of those cases with moderate clinical dementia. These authors concluded that approximately two-thirds of patients with idiopathic Parkinson's disease were likely to have clinical and neuropathological features of Alzheimer-type dementia at the time of death. It remains to be determined to what extent such changes are an extension of the parkinsonian disease process itself; whether Parkinson's disease predisposes to the development of an Alzheimer-type dementia; and whether the loss of locus coeruleus cells (which occurs in both idiopathic Parkinson's disease and a proportion of cases of SDAT) is associated with a common degenerative process.

Neurochemically the now classical demonstration in postmortem brain tissue of a transmitter defect in Parkinson's disease, which can be countered clinically by replacement therapy, has set a precedent for the chemistry of cerebral disease which has unfortunately not yet been achieved in any other disorder. The loss of dopaminergic neurons, particularly in the substantia nigra, may be the primary lesion in Parkinson's disease but it is certainly not the only chemical change since alterations in, for example, γ-aminobutyric acid, noradrenergic, and cholinergic activities in various brain areas have also been demonstrated. The dopamine deficit, however, is regarded as the most important known aspect of deranged neurochemistry in Parkinson's disease on the basis of the therapeutic success in administering L-dopa. Nevertheless while often relieving symptoms for a considerable length of time, L-dopa does not retard the progress of the disease and future studies need to investigate the factor or factors which determine the degeneration of dopaminergic neurons.

Jakob-Creutzfeld disease

This is an infrequent and unusual disease which generally affects middle aged people although occasional cases occur in the seventh decade. The initial presenting symptoms, though often non-specific, usually include episodes of confusion, memory loss, delirium, and hallucinations. In the later stages of the disease, dementia is invariably present and is usually acompanied by evidence of pyramidal tract involvement, myoclinic epilepsy, and a characteristic EEG. Death occurs, in most cases, between 12 and 18 months after clinical presentation. At postmortem examination, cerebral atrophy, usually of a mild degree, is present — although it may occasionally be quite severe. No diagnostic macroscopic features are present and it is essential to confirm the diagnosis histologically. Even microscopically the diagnosis may not be made easily because the changes are often subtle and not readily appreciated. Three microscopic features are considered to be characteristic of the condition: neuronal loss and degeneration, astrocytic proliferation, and hypertrophy (Fig. 1.11a), and a variable degree of fine or coarse vacuolation (spongiosis) in the neuropil (Fig. 1.11b). These histological features predominate in the cerebral cortex although there may be a considerable variation in the extent of involvement between different neocortical lobes and in various brain regions. For this reason a variety of subgroups have been described.

The morphological basis for dementia in Jakob-Creutzfeld disease is almost certainly related to the extensive neuronal loss and degeneration in the cerebral cortex. Interest in the disease has been stimulated by the demonstration that it can be transferred to animals by inoculation with brain material from affected individuals (Gajdusek & Gibbs 1971). This links Jakob-Creutzfeld diseases to diseases such as scrapie and kuru in which transmittable agents have also been demonstrated, but the precise relationship of Jakob-Creutzfeld disease to these other diseases and, possibly, to familial cases of Alzheimer's disease is not yet established.

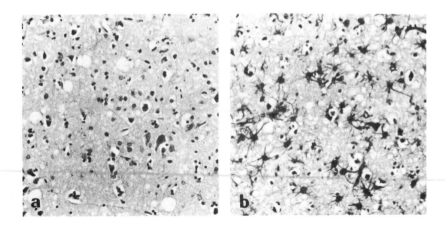

Fig. 1.11 **(a)** Spongiosis in the frontal lobe of a patient with Jacob-Creutzfeld disease. In this case vacuoles were most prominent in the (illustrated) cortical layers 4–5. (H. & E. ×160.) **(b)** This section illustrates hypertrophied and reactive astrocytes in the same area of cortex as **a** (Holzer ×160.)

Trauma

The aged brain, by virtue of its reduced capacity to compensate for the effects of traumatic destructive lesions, is more susceptible to the immediate consequences of cerebral trauma and in certain respects to later developing complications. Chronic subdural haematomata occur more frequently in elderly compared to younger age groups, possibly because of the lax subdural space which accompanies cortical atrophy and the susceptibility of delicate dural or meningeal vessels to tearing by mild traumatic episodes. The clinical presentation of a subdural haematoma may, initially at least, be non-specific and includes psychiatric symptoms such as intermittent episodes of confusion, disorientation, and drowsiness. Neurosurgical intervention in elderly patients with subdural haematoma often produces less recovery than is seen in younger age groups.

In the brain itself, the vulnerability of particular regions to trauma are described below to illustrate the many brain areas which may be involved and their possible relevance to the development of post-traumatic psychiatric symptoms. Although, by their very nature, head injuries occur in unpredictable and variable circumstances, the brain lesions which follow cerebral trauma can usually be found in characteristic and predictable brain areas. Surface cortical contusions in the hemispheres may result from direct or indirect (the so-called contre-coup) impact damage or from the various rotational, torsional, acceleration and deceleration forces which act at the moment of injury. The latter kinetic forces, acting against the irregular bony surface of the floor of the anterior and middle cranial fossae, are largely responsible for the cortical traumatic lesions which so characteristically occur on the inferior and lateral surfaces of the frontal and temporal lobes. Both impact and kinetic forces may disrupt white matter tracts and vessels in the callosal and parasagittal hemisphere regions; at midbrain level similar mechanisms are responsible for severing axonal pathways in laterally situated tracts traversing the upper brain stem. The latter disruption may critically affect cortical or diencephalic brain stem interactions. Additional, but more variable, consequences of cerebral trauma include the development of localised or regional ischaemic lesions and brain stem haemorrhages secondary to tentorial herniation. Whether or not these additional lesions develop depends, amongst other things, on the degree of oedema, haemorrhage, and vessel disruption which has occurred in the cerebral hemispheres.

In view of the diverse brain regions which are susceptible to traumatic damage, it is not surprising that the survivors of the acute phase of mild, moderate, or severe brain injuries often show specific or non-specific psychiatric symptoms in addition to neurological deficits. Non-specific psychiatric symptoms, such as lack of concentration and mild memory disturbances, may reflect the presence of cortical surface contusion or hemisphere white matter lesions even in the absence of a skull fracture or other stigmata of severe head injuries. On the other hand, moderate or severe injuries which result in extensive brain lesions, can be followed by personality changes and intellectual deficits or 'dementia'. Such intellectual deficits may be clinically evident in the immediate post-traumatic period or they may develop much later. The elderly individual with a past history of a moderate or severe brain injury has, theoretically at least, an increased likelihood of developing dementia since, by virtue of a lowered cerebral reserve, he may be more susceptible to senile degeneration in the brain and other age-associated changes.

Falling within a different neuropathological category — and perhaps reflecting different aetiological mechanisms— is the intellectual impairment or partial dementia which develops following repeated mild or moderate head injury. This condition is rare, usually presenting in middle aged boxers (dementia pugilistica) but occasionally in other people with an occupational exposure to head trauma such as jockeys. Amongst several neuropathological abnormalities found in this condition (reviewed pathologically by Corsellis 1978) those which are of academic interest to the study of dementia in old age are the destruction of the septum or adjacent forniceal regions; the development of numerous neocortical neurofibrillary tangles in the absence of senile plaques; and, in most cases, degeneration or loss of dopaminergic cells in the substantia nigra. The fornix contains most of the efferent axons which emerge from the hippocampus to innervate the mammillary bodies and septum. A smaller number of fibres (including cholinergic, noradrenergic, serotonin and substance P fibres) travel in the reverse direction from the septal area to the hippocampus. These fibre tracts are a critical component of the so-called 'limbic region' and their disruption in this form of head injury, with subsequent intellectual or memory impairment, links the syndrome to the amenestic state which develops following bilateral hippocampal or medial temporal lesions (Scoville & Milner 1957, see also Horel 1978). It is not yet known which, if any, of the traumatic morphological derangements contributes to the development of neurofibrillary tangles. Amongst several possibilites their formation may follow disruption of synaptic connections or even interruption and subsequent degeneration of particular neurotransmitter tracts. Although it has been suggested (Roth 1978) that the dementia in boxers supervenes when degenerative ageing processes impose further damage on an already compromised brain, the relatively short time course between brain injuries and the development of clinical symptoms render this explanation unlikely.

Other causes of dementia

In a minority of elderly demented individuals (usually between 5 and 15%) there is no evidence of SDAT or of multi-infarct dementia on neuropathological examination. These cases can be subdivided into two broad categories: one group with well recognised, but rare, diseases or syndromes known to give rise to dementia, and a smaller group in which there are no satisfactory clinical or pathological features to explain the dementing illness. In the group with specific abnormalities, a wide range of disorders may be present including some of those outlined above and others referred to elsewhere (see for example Marsden & Harrison 1972, Tomlinson 1980). Such dementing syndromes may be associated with diseases of an infectious (bacterial) nature, such as the development of GPI in cerebral syphillis; diseases of viral origin, of which the best known is herpes simplex encephalitis; cerebral infarction arising as a consequence of subarachnoid haemorrhage or meningitis; and various manifestations of neoplasia ranging from benign or malignant cerebral tumours to cerebral metastasis or para-neoplastic complications of malignant growths such as limbic encephalopathy.

Other disorders to which dementia has been attributed include syndromes with a less well defined or no morphological pathological basis. In the former category the syndrome of normal pressure hydrocephalus (Adams *et al* 1965) has been diagnosed with increased frequency in the last decade although neuropathological reports on such cases are few. Clinically this syndrome is characterised by a triad of 1 mental symptoms (especially dementia), 2 gait disturbances, and 3 incontinence. In the classical case, which usually presents in the immediate presenile period, enlargement of the lateral ventricle is associated with a normal CSF pressure (at least at the time of diagnosis) and little or no evidence of cortical gyral atrophy. Various radiological techniques exist for diagnosing the condition and CT scanning now plays a major role. Pathologically, a distinction may be made between hydrocephalus arising in the absence of other CNS disorders, the so-called idiopathic variety of normal pressure hydrocephalus, and the obstructive or communicating forms of hydrocephalus which occasionally result from such diverse diseases as subarachnoid haemorrhage, cerebral trauma, or meningitis. The pathological basis for the idiopathic variety of normal pressure hydrocephalus is ill defined and appears to be a consequence of deranged CSF flow over the cerebral hemispheres or impaired absorption of CSF into arachnoid villi. Neurosurgical intervention in cases diagnosed as normal pressure hydrocephalus has not been uniformly sucessful. Only about 25% of cases so diagnosed improve significantly following the insertion of ventriculo-atrial or ventriculo-peritoneal shunts although, in a further 25%, the procedure is felt partly to alleviate the symptoms (Salmon 1969, Gustafson & Hagberg 1978, Black 1980). The inability to reliably predict which patients will respond to ventricular drainage procedures, and the relatively high incidence of complications such as subdural haemorrhage, seizures, cerebral infarction, and infection which follow operative intervention, have limited its application.

Those dementing conditions for which no satisfactory morphological basis has been demonstrated include various 'metabolic' derangements which occur in association with physical disease and deficiency syndromes or endocrinological disturbances such as B_{12} deficiency and myxoedema. Finally, in the smaller group in which no definitive diagnosis can be made, senile degenerative change of Alzheimer type or cerebral infarcts may be present in some cases but to a degree which quantitatively does not exceed those encountered in normal, non-demented individuals. Whether such patients are unduly susceptible to minor degrees of degenerative change or whether other factors contribute to the dementing condition is not known.

PSYCHIATRIC DISEASES WITHOUT ESTABLISHED NEUROPATHOLOGY

Schizophrenia and paraphrenia

Clinical observations suggest there may be several subgroups within the adult schizophrenia syndrome and, in the elderly, the predominance of paranoid symptoms provides a basis for further division. The cause of the disorder or disorders is, as yet, unknown and both genetic and social factors have been variously implicated. In addition many investigators have searched for pathological abnormalities, both within the brain and, for example, in visceral organs such as the heart, kidneys and gastrointestinal tract.

Morphological observations

Almost all areas of the central nervous system have been pathologically investigated in schizophrenia. Based on the assumption that deranged cognition and thought disorders are most likely to originate in neocortical regions, many studies conducted between 1920 and 1950 concentrated on the cerebral cortex. A number of other reports have described abnormalities in a surprisingly large range of central nervous system regions such as the basal ganglia, diencephalon, hypothalamus, mammilliary bodies, cingulum, corpus callosum, choroid plexus, pons, cerebellum, spinal cord and, in the peripheral nervous system, the parasympathetic system. Neuropathological observations have mainly concentrated on the state of neuronal perikarya and relatively non-specific degenerative features have been described including neuronal shrinkage, atrophy, cytoplasmic 'ballooning' or swelling, decreases in cytoplasmic RNA, and lipid accumulation. More specific abnormalities which have been reported in the cortex include the existence of acellular regions (suggesting deranged neuronal development or neuronal loss), areas of infarction, and abnormalities in the various neuronal types of the different cortical layers. Other investigators, arguing that neuronal derangements may be accompanied by an astrocytic reaction, have described alterations in fibrillary and protoplasmic astrocytes and microgliial cells. In addition, reported abnormalities of the white matter include the presence of foci of demyelination, 'grape-like' degeneration and axonal loss. Even the leptomeninges have not escaped the scrutiny of neurosurgeons or neuropathologists who have commented on leptomeningeal thickening in cerebral biopsies from schizophrenics. In a smaller number of investigations, cytoplasmic inclusion bodies have been identified. Summaries and reviews of these various observations have been provided, amongst others, by Dastur (1959), Neito & Escobar (1972), and Corsellis (1976b).

Despite the obvious extent of these many pathological investigations there is, as yet, no firm neuropathological basis for relating morphological abnormalities to the schizophrenic or paraphrenic syndromes. Many people have questioned the validity of the various pathological findings in schizophrenia on the basis that adequate control groups have not been included and that most of the observations are probably more subjective than scientific. More recent reports, based on CT scanning, of cerebral atrophy in a subgroup of schizophrenic patients, have regenerated considerable interest in the question of gross structural brain changes in schizophrenia. As assessed by CT scans or pneumoencephalopathy, lateral ventricular size has been found by some groups to be significantly increased in a proportion of schizophrenic cases (Huber 1958, 1961, Haugh 1962, Asano 1967, Johnstone *et al* 1978, Golden *et al* 1980, Tanaka *et al* 1981), although others (Storey 1966) have found no difference between schizophrenics and controls. The question of whether atrophy occurs in schizophrenia below the tentorium, in the cerebellum, is still a controversial issue and various inconsistent clinical reports have appeared (see, for example, Nasrallah *et al* 1981). Since both ventricular dilatation and cerebellar atrophy have been reported to occur in other neurological and psychiatric diseases — such as cerebellar atrophy in both alocholism (Allen *et al* 1979) and mania (Nasrallah *et al* 1981) — the question of the specificity of these findings arises. The underlying pathological abnormalities need to be determined if such gross structural lesions are to shed light on the nature of the schizophrenic disease process. It is also worth noting that, before the advent of CT scanning, neuropathological assessments provided little or no evidence of substantial cerebral atrophy in schizophrenics. Two investigations which utilized brain weight as an index of brain size (Broser 1949, Rosenthal & Bigelow 1972) did not demonstrate differences between schizophrenics and controls; while a postmortem analysis of elderly patients with schizophrenic and paranoid disorders by Corsellis (1962) noted slight cerebral atrophy in 50–66% of cases and no instances of severe atrophy. In respect to this atrophy, the schizophrenic and paranoid groups did not apparently differ from a group with affective psychoses.

Whether or not specific brain regions are specifically involved in the genesis of the schizophrenic syndrome is an unresolved question. The development of schizophrenia-like symptoms in patients with temporal lobe lesions or epilepsy (Hillbom 1951, Slater *et al* 1963, Taylor 1975), although possibly reflecting a predisposition to the disease in certain patients, suggests that the temporal lobe and adjacent limbic regions may be more closely involved in schizophrenia than other areas. An analysis of this and related topics has been provided by Davison & Bagley (1969).

Chemical aspects

The literature on the biochemistry of schizophrenia is vast and often confusing. Numerous hypotheses abound but consistent observations are generally rare. A particularly attractive notion has been that of a defective indole-N-methylating system leading to the production of hallucinogenic-type amine derivatives. However, there is not yet any clear-cut evidence of such a defect in postmortem schizophrenic brain. The dopamine hypothesis (which proposes an overactivity of dopaminergic transmitter systems, particularly in limbic forebrain systems) has enjoyed much popularity recently. It is consistent with the efficacy of drugs which block dopamine receptors and with recent findings of increased dopamine receptor binding in postmortem brain tissue from affected cases (Crow *et al* 1979). However the specificity of even this biochemical abnormality is open to question since the antipsychotic drugs themselves alter the levels of brain dopamine receptors and some research groups have reported normal binding in untreated cases. A defect in the opiod peptides in schizophrenia has been proposed more recently but significant changes in, for example, β-endorphin have not yet been demonstrated (Mackay 1981). One of the great difficulties in investigating the biochemistry of schizophrenia which is not encountered to the same extent in other diseases like Alzheimer's disease, Parkinson's disease, or Huntington's chorea, is the lack of precision in diagnoses and the probable existence of different sub-groups or types which may have to be examined separately. In the future, careful correlations between neurochemical data and clinical findings may help to identify specific abnormalities in particular subgroups.

Affective psychoses

Morphological investigations

The affective psychoses — depression and mania — have not generally been associated with specific morphological abnormalities in the brain, although isolated cases showing manic symptomatology have been associated with hypothalamic lesions (Corsellis 1976b). If structural changes do exist in these disorders, it is likely that they will require more subtle or sophisticated techniques for their demonstration than have hitherto been employed. Whilst there is clinical evidence of an association between physical illness and depression in the elderly (see, for example, Roth & Kay 1956, Kay *et al* 1964), there is no neuropathological evidence of a direct relationship between depression of either endogenous or neurotic type and senile degenerative change or ischaemic brain lesions. Thus, in contrast to a suggested clinical association between depression and cerebrovascular disease in the elderly (Post 1962, Roth 1955), the neuropathological investigations of Corsellis (1962) and Tomlinson *et al* (1968) did not show an increase in the incidence of cerebrovascular disease in depressed elderly patients.

A recent report of CT findings in affective disorders in the elderly (Jacoby & Levy 1980b) may possibly have identified a subpopulation of late-onset depressed patients with enlarged cerebral ventricles. If this finding is confirmed, it will be of considerable interest to determine the cause of the ventricular dilatation.

Chemical aspects

Although not yet proven, it seems likely that these psychiatric disorders are primarily associated with chemical rather than morphological abnormalities. Neurochemically, the most popular concept regarding the bio-chemistry of depression relates to the suggested abnormality in either or both of the monamine systems — noradrenaline and serotonin. As in schizo-phrenia, this concept arose primarily from a knowledge of the mode of action of drugs which are often effective in depression. Thus antidepressant drugs tend to alter the function of these particular transmitter systems in normal animal brains. The literature on the biochemistry of postmortem human brain in depression is surprisingly sparse, although there are reports of reductions in serotonin in the brains of suicide cases (Shaw *et al* 1967, Lloyd *et al* 1974). Recent postmortem biochemical studies in the cerebral cortex of elderly depressed patients have not revealed obvious abnor-malities in the cholinergic, noradrenergic, or γ-aminobutyric acid classical transmitter systems (Perry *et al* 1977, Cross *et al* 1981), nor in the levels of several neuropeptides, such as cholecystokinin octapeptide and vasoactive intestinal polypeptide (Perry *et al* 1981b). The involvement of certain 'veg-etative' functions in depression (including, for example, loss of appetite and libido) has stimulated a search for disturbances in hypothalamic–pitui-tary–endocrine organ inter-relationships. In dynamic neuroendocrino-logical studies in living subjects some abnormalities in the control of cortico-steroids, growth hormone, and thyroid releasing hormone levels have been identified. Until the respective hormone or peptide systems, including their receptors, are examined in the hypothalamus and other brain areas it may be difficult to assess the precise involvement of these particular chemicals in the aetiology of depression.

Anxiety neuroses

Anxiety or obsessional neuroses are common and often debilitating disor-ders amongst elderly people. There is, however, practically no information on either the morphological condition or chemical state of the brain in these disorders. Like schizophrenia and the affective psychoses, the symptoms of anxiety may be transient and amenable to various forms of therapy, which suggests that degenerative or other structural changes do not occur in the brain. There is, nevertheless, obvious scope for testing such an assumption in future studies. Disorders of this kind may present the clinician with the problem of differentiating an actual disease process from extremes of per-sonality; perhaps even different personality types may ultimately be disting-uished on some morphological or neurochemical basis.

Acute confusional and delirious states

Few neuropathological investigations have been conducted into the state of acute confusion (delirium) which commonly develops in association with physical illness such as cardiovascular or respiratory disease. This lack of pathological information is due in part to the assumption that such mental states result from systemic metabolic disturbances rather than as a consequence of morphological changes in the brain. There are also considerable difficulties in mounting such a neuropathological investigation which demands close clinical collaboration, accurate psychometric testing, and a knowledge of age-related neuropathological changes if elderly patients are involved. While it is accepted that confusional studies largely reflect systemic metabolic disturbances, a central question regarding such delirious conditions is whether they develop more readily in patients with pre-existing brain damage due to cerebrovascular degeneration or Alzheimer-type degeneration. Two separate investigations, conducted in Newcastle, have partially resolved this issue.

In the investigation of Tomlinson *et al* (1968) 13 out of 28 patients who died on a general medical ward were known to be in a state of terminal confusion. All 28 patients had been psychometrically assessed for intellectual normality and an absence of established dementia. There was no neuropathological evidence in this series of a direct relationship between terminal confusion and the extent of Alzheimer-type senile degeneration or cerebral infarction in the brain. In a later clinical study, Bergmann & Easthman (1974) assessed 100, elderly, consecutive admissions to a medical ward. Sixteen patients with a confusional state were identified and in four (25%) there were clinical features to suggest early organic brain disease. In a proportion of the remaining twelve patients, these authors presented evidence to show that previous psychiatric illness may have contributed to the confused state. The general conclusion which can be drawn from both of these studies is that in normal elderly people the presence of senile degenerative change or cerebrovascular disease is unlikely to predispose to the development of a mentally confused state. Individuals who may have early dementia tend, however, to develop delirium more readily than their unimpaired counterparts.

CONCLUSION

It seems likely that the major neuropathological features associated with normal ageing and organic psychiatric disease have been characterised, at least as far as macroscopic and light microscopic level appearances are concerned. In the numerous pathological studies, which have spanned nearly a century, investigators have identified and described the appearances and distributions of age-related changes and, more recently, clarified their association with behavioural or cognitive abnormalities in particular diseases. Beyond this descriptive level, however, our understanding of the precise nature and aetiology of many of the structural abnormalities has advanced very little. It is impossible at this stage to predict which of many approaches will provide an understanding of these fundamental aspects. Light and electron microscopic observations are likely to be further advanced by recently developed immunocytochemical techniques, while microchemical analysis in conjunction with conventional neurohistology will aid the localisation of specific chemicals within the nervous system. The characterisation of brain proteins and peptides should extend beyond simple extraction, isolation and analytical procedures, to in vitro protein synthesis using RNA extracted from human brain in conjunction with tissue or bacterial culture techniques. In the more conventional fields of neurotransmitter and neuropeptide analysis, the search for disease-specific alteration will be enhanced by synaptosomal release studies utilising material prepared from frozen tissue. The investigation of more realistic animal models, such as the ageing primate brain, and the extension of neurochemical studies with the new technique of positron emission tomography will improve our understanding of the psychiatric disease and the ageing process. With the latter technique, further advances are likely to be of particular interest to the clinician since they ultimately promise to be of diagnostic value. Positron emission tomography will in due course enable the distributions and functional activities of specific neuronal pathways to be examined in the living brain and so provide new vistas for both clinician and pathologist and, hopefully, a common meeting ground for both.

Over recent years, an interesting concept which has emerged in relation to morphological changes in the ageing brain is the apparent existence of a functional 'threshold' in the brain. Thus the ageing brain may, for example, contain a certain density of cortical senile plaques and hippocampal neurofibrillary tangles or a certain volume of ischaemic tissue without any obvious impairment of mental function. Then, beyond this level, which may well vary in different individuals, further morphological involvement is inevitably associated with impairment of mental function and the onset of psychiatric diseases such as dementia. This observation suggests that the brain, or at least major areas such as the cerebral cortex, is less sensitive to structural damage than might be imagined and that there may be a degree of redundancy or even a limited capacity for regeneration or compensatory hypertrophy of neuronal processes. It is not yet clear whether all individuals, given an extended life-span, would inevitably cross the 'threshold' and cease to function normally, although a significant number of elderly people can undoubtedly reach the tenth decade of life without any obvious impairment of intellectual ability. However, as far as can be ascertained, when the 'threshold' is crossed, degeneration is progressive and the disease process irreversible. Whether useful treatments or even preventative steps will be found in the so-called organic psychiatric diseases of old age is not known. The current situation with respect to therapy in the organic diseases is in sharp contrast to that in diseases of functional type, where progressive degenerative changes of the brain have not been established and where the disorder is often, in some cases, not only treatable but may actually remit. It would be unduly pessimistic however to infer from this comparison that there is no prospect of help for the patient with progressive degenerative brain disease. The classical example of Parkinson's disease (p. 47) has encouraged many people to believe that continued research in this area is worthwhile.

ACKNOWLEDGEMENTS

The advice and encouragement of Bernard E. Tomlinson and Garry Blessed, the photographic work of Dorothy Irving, and secretarial assistance of Isobel Campbell are all gratefully acknowledged.

REFERENCES

ADAMS R.C., FISHER C., HAKIM S. *et al* (1965) Symptomatic occult hydrocephalus with 'normal' cerebrospinal fluid pressure: A treatable syndrome. *New England Journal of Medicine* **273**, 117–26.

ADOLFSSON R., GOTTFRIES C.G., ORELAND L. *et al* (1978) reduced levels of catecholamines in the brain and increased activity of monoamine oxidase in platelets in Alzheimer's disease: therapeutic implications. In *Alzheimer's Disease: Senile Dementia and Related Disorders,* eds R. Katzman, R.D. Terry and K.L. Bick. Raven Press, New York.

ALLEN J. H., MARTIN T.J. & MCLACIN L.W. (1979) Computed tomography in cerebellar atrophic processes. *Radiology* **130**, 397–82.

ALZHEIMER A. (1907) Über eine eigenartige Erkrankung der Hirnrinde. *Allgemeine Zeitschrift für Psychiatrie und Psychisch — Gerich Hiche Medizin* **64**, 146–8.

ANTUONO P., SORBI S., BRACCO L. *et al* (1980) A discrete sampling technique in senile dementia of the Alzheimer type and Alcoholic dementia: Study of the cholinergic system. In *Aging of the Brain and Dementia,* eds L. Amaducci, A.N. Davison and P. Antuono. Raven Press, New York.

ASANO N. (1967) Pneumoencephalographic study of schizophrenia. In *Clinical Genetics in Psychiatry,* ed H. Mitsuda. Igaku-Shoin, Tokyo.

BALL M.J. (1976) Neurofibrillary tangles and the pathogenesis of dementia: a quantitative study. *Neuropathology and Applied Neurobiology* **2**, 395–10.

BERGMANN K. & EASTHAM E.T. (1974) Psychogeriatric ascertainment and assessment for treatment in an acute medical ward setting. *Age and Ageing* **3**, 174–88.

BIRD E.D. & IVERSEN L.L. (1974) Huntington's chorea — postmortem measurement of glutamic acid decarboxylase, choline acetyltransferase and dopamine in basal ganglia. *Brain* **97**, 457–72.

BLACK P.M. (1980) Idiopathic normal-pressure hydrocephalus. *Journal of Neurosurgery* **52**, 371–7.

BLACKWOOD W., HALLPIKE J.F., KOCEN R.S. *et al* (1969) Atheromatous disease of the carotid arterial system and embolism from the heart in cerebral infarction: A morbid anatomical study. *Brain* **92,** 897–10.

BLESSED G. (1980) Clinical aspects of the senile dementias. In *Biochemistry of Dementia,* ed P.J. Roberts. John Wiley, New York.

BLINKOV S.M. & GLEZER I.I. (1968) *The Human Brain in Figures and Tables.* Plenum Press, New York.

BOLLER F., MIZUTANI T., ROESSMANN U. *et al* (1979) Parkinson disease, dementia and Alzheimer disease: clinicopathological correlations. *Annals of Neurology* **7,** 329–35.

BONDAREFF W., MOUNTJOY C.Q. & ROTH M. (1981) Selective loss of neurones of origin of adrenergic projection to cerebral cortex (nucleus locus coeruleus) in senile dementia. *Lancet* i, 783–4.

BOWEN D.M. & DAVISON A.N. (1980) Biochemistry of Alzheimer's disease. In *The Biochemistry of Psychiatric Disturbances,* ed G. Curzon. John Willey, New York.

BREWER C. & PERRETT L. (1971) Brain damage due to alcohol consumption: an air-encephalographic psychometric and electroencephalographic study. *British Journal of Addiction* **66,** 170–82.

BRITISH MEDICAL JOURNAL (1981) Minor Brain Damage and Alcoholism. Editorial **283,** 455–6.

BRODY H. (1955) Organization of the cerebral cortex. III A study of aging in the human cerebral cortex. *Journal of Comparative Neurology* **102,** 511–56.

BRODY H. (1970) Structural changes in the aging nervous system. *Interdisciplinary Topics in Gerontology,* vol. 7, 9–21. Karger, Basel.

BRODY H. (1978) Cell counts in cerebral cortex and brain stem. In *Alzheimer's disease, Senile Dementia and Related Disorders,* R. Katzmann, R.D. Terry and K.L. Bick. Raven Press, New York.

BROSER K. (1949) Hirngewicht und Himprozess bei Schizophrenia. Archiv für Psychiatrie und Nerven Krankheiten, vereinigt mit Zeitschrift für die gesamte. *Neurolgie und Psychiatrie* **182,** 439–49.

CALA L.A., JONES B., MASTAGLIA F. *et al* (1978) Brain atrophy and intellectual impairment in heavy drinkers — a clinical, psychometric and computerized tomography study. *Australian and New Zealand Medical Journal* **8,** 147–53.

CANDY J.M., OAKLEY A.E., PERRY E.K. *et al* (1981a) Existence *in vitro* of fibrillary aggregates of substance P, cholecystokinin octapeptide, somatostatin and related molecules. *Journal of Physiology* **320,** 112P.

CANDY J.M., PERRY R.H., PERRY E.K. *et al* (1981b) Distribution of putative cholinergic cell bodies and various neuropeptides in the substantia innominata of the human brain. *Journal of Anatomy* **133,** 124–5.

CARLEN P.L., WILKINSON D.A., WORTZMAN G. *et al* (1981) Cerebral atrophy and functional deficits in alcoholics without clinically apparent liver disease. *Neurology* **31,** 377–85.

CARTER C.J. (1981) Loss of glutamine synthetase activity in the brain in Huntington's disease. *Lancet* i 782–3.

CELESIA G.G. & WANAMAKER W.M. (1972) Psychiatric disturbance in Parkinson's disease. *Disease of the Nervous System* **33,** 577–83.

COLON E.J. (1972) The elderly brain. A quantitative analysis of the cerebral cortex in two cases. *Psychiatria, Neurologia and Neurochirurgia* (*Amst.*) **75,** 261–70.

CONSTANTINIDIS J. (1978) Is Alzheimer's disease a major form of senile dementia? Clinical, Anatomical and Genetic Data. In *Alzheimer's Disease: Senile Dementia and Related Disorders,* eds, R. Katzman, R.D. Terry and K.L. Bick. Raven Press, New York.

CORSELLIS J.A.N. (1962) *Mental Illness and the Aging Brain.* Oxford University Press.

CORSELLIS J.A.N. (1976a) Ageing and the Dementias. In *Greenfield's Neuropathology,* 3rd ed, eds W. Blackwood and J.A.N. Corsellis. Edward Arnold, London.

CORSELLIS J.A.N. (1976b) Psychoses of Obscure Pathology. In *Greenfield's Neuropathology,* 3rd ed, eds W. Blackwood and J.A.N. Corsellis. Edward Arnold, London.

CORSELLIS J.A.N. (1978) Post traumatic Dementia. In *Alzheimer's Disease: Senile Dementia and Related Disorders,* eds R. Katzman, R.D. Terry and K.L. Bick. Raven Press, New York.

COURVILLE C. (1966) *The Effects of Alcohol on the Nervous System of Man.* San Lucas Press, Los Angeles.

CROSS A.J., CROW T.J., PERRY E.K. *et al* (1981) Reduced dopamine-beta-hydroxylase activity in Alzheimer's disease. *British Medical Journal* **282,** 93–4.

CROW T.J., JOHNSTONE E.C. & OWEN F. (1979) Research on Schizophrenia. In *Recent Advances in Clinical Psychiatry 3,* ed K. Granville-Grossman. Churchill Livingstone, Edinburgh.

DASTUR D.K. (1959) The pathology of schizophrenia. *Archives of Neurology and Psychiatry* **81,** 601–14.

DAVIES P. (1978) Studies on the neurochemistry of central cholinergic systems in Alzheimer's disease. In *Alzheimer's Disease: Senile Dementia and Related Disorders,* eds R. Katzman, R.D. Terry and K.L. Bick. Raven Press, New York.

DAVIES P., KATZMAN R. & TERRY R.D. (1980) Reduced somatostatin-like immunoreactivity in cerebral cortex from cases of Alzheimer's disease and Alzheimer senile dementia. *Nature* (London) **288,** 279–80.

DAVIS P.M.J. & WRIGHT E.A. (1977) A new method for measuring cranial cavity volume and its application to the assessment of cerebral atrophy at autopsy. *Neuropathology and Applied Neurobiology* **3,** 341–58.

DAVISON K. & BAGLEY C.R. (1969) Schizophrenic-like psychoses associated with organic disorders of the central nervous system. In *Current Problems in Neuropsychiatry,* ed R.N. Herrington. Headley Bros., Ashford.

DE BONI U. & CRAPPER D.R. (1978) Paired helical filaments of the Alzheimer type in cultured neurons. *Nature* **271,** 566–8.

DEKABAN A.S. & SADOWSKY D. (1978) Changes in brain weights during the span of human life. Relation of brain weights to body heights and body weights. *Annals of Neurology* **4,** 346–56.

DYAN A.D. (1970a) Quantitative histological studies on the aged human brain. 1. Senile Plaques and Neurofibrillary Tangles in 'Normal' Patients. *Acta Neuropathologica* **16,** 85–94.

DYAN A.N. (1970b) Quantitative histological studies on the aged human brain. II. *Acta Neuropathologica* **16,** 95–102.

ELLIS R.S. (1920) Norms for some structural changes in the human cerebellum from birth to old age. *Journal of Comparative Neurology* **32,** 1–32.

EPSTEIN P.S., PISANI V.D. & FAWCETT J.A. (1977) Alcoholism and cerebral atrophy: alcoholism. *Clinical and Experimental Research* **1,** 61–5.

FISHER C.M. (1951) Occlusion of the internal carotid artery. *Archives Neurology and Psychiatry* **65,** 346–77.

FORNO L.S. (1966) The pathology of parkinsonism. *Journal of Neurosurgey* **24,** (suppl. 2), 266–71.

FORNO L.S. (1978) The locus coeruleus in Alzheimer's disease. *Journal of Neuro-*

pathology and Experimental Neurology **37,** 614.

FOX J.H., RAMSAY R.G., HUCKMAN M.S. *et al* (1976) Cerebral ventricular enlargement: chronic alcoholics examined by computerized tomography. *Journal of the American Medical Association* **236,** 365–8.

FRIEDE R.L. (1965) Enzyme histochemical studies of senile plaques. *Journal of Neuropathology and Experimental Neurology* **24,** 477–91.

GAJDUSEK D.C. & GIBBS C.J.Jr. (1971) Transmission of two subacute spongiform encephalopathies of man (Kuru and Creutzfeldt–Jacob disease). *Nature* **230,** 588–91.

GAMBETTI P., VELASCO M.E., DAHL D. *et al* (1980) In *Aging of the Brain and Dementia,* eds L. Amaducci, A.N. Davison and P. Antuono. Raven Press, New York.

GIBSON P. & TOMLINSON B.E. (1977) The numbers of Hirano bodies in the hippocampus of normal and demented subjects with Alzheimer's disease. *Journal of the Neurological Sciences* **33,** 199–06.

GLENNER G.G. (1980A) Amyloid deposits and amyloidosis. The beta-Fibrilloses. *New England Journal of Medicine* **392,** 1283–92.

GLENNER G.G. (1980B) Amyloid deposits and amyloidosis. The beta-Fibrilloses. *New England Journal of Medicine* **302,** 1333–43.

GLENNER G.G. (1978) Current knowledge of amyloid deposits as applied to senile plaques and congophillic angiopathy. In *Alzheimer's Disease: Senile Dementia and Related Disorders* eds R. Katzman, R.D. Terry and K.L. Bick. Raven Press, New York.

GLENNER G.G., EIN D. & TERRY W.D. (1972) The immunoglobulin origin of amyloid. *American Journal of Medicine* **52,** 141–7.

GLENNER G.G., TERRY W., HARADA M. *et al* (1971) Amyloid fibril proteins: Proof of homology with light chains by sequence analysis. *Science* **172,** 1150–1.

GOLDEN C.J., MOSES J.A., ZELAZOWSKI R. *et al* (1980) Cerebral ventricular size and neuropsychological impairment in young chronic schizophrenics. *Archives of General Psychiatry* **37,** 619–23.

GONATAS N.K., ANDERSON W. & EVANGELISTICA I. (1967) The contribution of altered synapses in the senile plaque: an electron microscopic study in Alzheimer's dementia. *Journal of Neuropathology and Experimental Neurology* **26,** 25–39.

GONZALEZ C.F., LANTIERI R.L. & NATHAN R.J. (1978) The CT scan appearance of the brain in the normal elderly population: a correlative study. *Neuroradiology* **16,** 120–2.

GOULD R.P. (1978) The APUD cell system. In *Recent Advances in Histopathology,* eds P.P. Anthony and N. Woolf. Churchill–Livingstone, Edinburgh.

GRUNDE–IQBAL I., JOHNSON A.B., WIŚNIEWSKI H.M. *et al* (1979) Evidence that Alzheimer neurofibrillary tangles originate from neurotubules. *Lancet* i, 578–80.

GUSTAFSON L. & HAGBERG B. (1978) Recovery in hydrocephalic dementia after shunt operation. *Journal of Neurology, Neurosurgery and Psychiatry* **41,** 940–7.

HACHINSKI V.C., LASSEN N.A. & MARSHALL J. (1974) Multi-infarct Dementia. A cause of mental deterioration in the elderly. *Lancet* i 207–10.

HAKIM S. – ADAMS R.C. (1965) The special clinical problem of symptomatic hydrocephalus with normal cerebrospinal fluid pressure: Observations on cerebrospinal fluid hydrodynamics. *Journal of the Neurological Sciences* **2,** 307–27.

HALL T.C., MILLER A.K.H. & CORSELLIS J.A.N. (1975) Variations in the human Purkinje cell population according to age and sex. *Neuropathology and Applied*

Neurobiology **1**, 267–92.

HAUGH J.O. (1962) Pneumoencephalographic studies in mental disease. *Acta Psychiatrica Scandinavica* **38**, (suppl. 165).

HAUGH J.O. (1968) Pneumoencephalographic evidence of brain damage in chronic alcoholics. *Acta Psychiatrica Scandinavia* (suppl. 203) 135–43.

HENDERSON G., TOMLINSON B.E. & GIBSON P.H. (1980) Cell counts in human cerebral cortex in normal adults throughout life using an image analysing computer. *Journal of the Neurological Sciences* **4**, 113–36.

HILLBOM E. (1951) Schizophrenic-like psychoses after brain trauma. *Acta Psychiatrica et Neurologica Scandinavica* (suppl 60), 36–47.

HIRANO A. (1965) Neuropathology of amyotrophic lateral sclerosis and Parkinsonism–Dementia complex on Guam. *Exerpta Medica International Congress Series No. 100.*

HIRANO A., DEMBITZER H.M., KURLAND L.T. *et al* (1968) The fine structure of some intraganglionic alterations. *Journal of Neuropathology and Experimental Neurology* **26**, 167–82.

HOCH–LIGETI C. (1963) Effects of aging on the central nervous system. *Journal of the American Geriatric Society* **11**, 403–8.

HORVATH T.B. (1975) Clinical spectrum and epidemiological features of alcoholic dementia. In *Alcohol, Drugs and Brain Damage* ed J.G. Rankin. Addiction Research Foundation of Ontario, Toronto.

HOREL J.A. (1978) The neuroanatomy of amnesia. *Brain* **101**, 403–45.

HUBBARD B.M. & ANDERSON J.M. (1981) A quantitative study of cerebral atrophy in old age and senile dementia. *Journal if the Neurological Sciences* **50**, 135-45.

HUBER G. (1958) Endogene Psychosen und himatrophischen Befund. *Fortschritte Neurologie Psychiatrie* **26**, 354–71.

HUBER G. (1961) Klinische und neuroradiologische Untersuchungen an Chronisch Schizophrenan. *Nervenarst* **32**, 7–15.

HUTCHINSON E.C. & YATES P.O. (1957) Carotico-vertebral stenosis. *Lancet* i, 2–8.

IQBAL K., GRUNDKE–IQBAL I., WIŚNIEWSKI H.M. *et al* (1975) Chemical pathology of neurofibrils: Neurofibrillary tangles of Alzheimer's presenile–senile dementia. *Journal of Histochemistry and Cytochemistry* **23**, 563–9.

IQBAL K., GRUNDKE–IQBAL I., WIŚNIEWSKI H.M. *et al* (1978) Chemical relationship of the paired helical filaments of Alzheimer's dementia to human normal neurofilaments and neurotubules. *Brain Research* **142**, 321–32.

IQBAL K., WIŚNIEWSKI H.M., SHELANSKI M.L. 2et al (1974) Protein changes in senile dementia. *Brain Research* **77**, 337–43.

ISHII T. & HAGA S. (1976) Immuno-electron microscopic localization of immunoglobulin in amyloid fibrils of senile plaques. *Acta Neuropathologica* **36**, 243–9.

JACOB H. (1952) Senility. In *Proceedings 1st International Congress in Neuropathology (Rome)* **2**, 422.

JACOBY R.J. & LEVY R. (1980a) Computed tomography in the elderly, 2: senile dementia: diagnosis and functional impairment. *British Journal of Psychiatry* **136**, 256–69.

JACOBY R.J. & LEVY R. (1980b) Computed tomography in the elderly, 3: affective disorders. *British Journal of Psychiatry* **136**, 270–5.

JACOBY R.J., LEVY R. & DAWSON J.M. (1980) Computed tomography in the elderly, 1: the normal population. *British Journal of Psychiatry* **136**, 249–55.

JOHNSTONE E.C., CROW T.J., FRITH C.D. *et al* (1978) The dementia of dementia praecox. *Acta Psychiatrica Scandinavica* **57**, 305–24.

JORGENSON L. & TORVIK A. (1969) Ischaemic cerebrovascular diseases in an autopsy series. Part 2 Prevalence, location, pathogenesis and clinical course of cerebral infarcts. *Journal of the Neurological Sciences* **9**, 285–300.

JOSEPHY H. (1949) Acid phosphatase in the senile brain. *Archives of Neurology and Psychiatry* **61**, 164–9.

KAY D.W.K., BEAMISH P. & ROTH M. (1964) Old age mental disorders in Newcastle upon Tyne. Part 1. A study of prevalence. *British Journal of Psychiatry* **110**, 146–58.

KIDD M. (1963) Paired helical filaments in electron microscopy in Alzheimer's disease. *Nature* (London) **197**, 192–3.

KIDD M. (1964) Alzheimer's disease — an electron microscopic study. *Brain* **87**, 307–21.

KONIGSMARK B.W. (1969) Neuronal population of the ventral cochlear nucleus in man. *Anatomical Record* **163**, 212–13.

LHERMITTE F., GAUTIER J.C. & DEROUESNÉ C. (1970) Nature of occulsions of the middle cerebral artery. *Neurology* **20**, 82–8.

LLOYD K.G., FARLEY I.J., DOCK J.H.N. *et al* (1974) Serotonin and 5-hydroxyindol acetic acid in discrete areas of the brain stem of suicide victims and control patients. *Advances in Biochemical Psychopharmacology* **11**, 387–97.

MACKAY A.V.P. (1981) Endorphins and the Psychiatrist. *Trends in Neuroscience* **4**, iv–xi.

MALECI O. (1934) Contributo all conoscenza delle variazioni quantitative delle cellule nervose nelle senescenza. *Archivo Italiano Anatomio* **33**, 883.

MANN D.M.A., LINCOLN J., YATES P.O. *et al* (1980) Changes in the monoamine containing neurons of the human central nervous system in senile dementia. *British Journal of Psychiatry* **136**, 533–41.

MANN D.M.A. & SINCLAIR K.G.A. (1978) The quantitative assessment of lipofuscin pigment, cytoplasmic RNA and nucleolar volume in senile dementia. *Neuropathology and Applied Neurobiology* **4**, 129–35.

MARCHIAFAVA E. & BIGNAMI A. (1903) Sopra un alterozione del Corpo Calloso Osservata in Soggetti Alcoolisti. *Rivista di Patologia Nervosa e Mentale* **8**, 544–9.

MARSDEN C.G. & HARRISON M.J.G. (1972) Outcome of investigation of patients with presenile dementia. *British Medical Journal* ii, 249.

MARTTILA R.J. & RINNE U.K. (1976) Dementia in Parkinson's disease. *Acta Neurologica Scandinavia* **54**, 431–41.

McGEER E.G. & McGEER P.L. (1976) Neurotransmitter metabolism in the aging brain. In *Aging*, vol. 13, eds R.D. Terry and S. Gershan. Raven Press, New York.

MESSERT B., WANNAMAKER B.B. & DUDLEY A.W. (1972) Re-evaluation of the size of the lateral ventricle of the brain. *Neurology* (Minneapolis) **22**, 941–51.

MILLER A.K.H., ALSTON R.L. & CORSELLIS J.A.N. (1980) Variation with age in the volumes of grey and white matter in the cerebral hemispheres of man: measurements with an image analyser. *Neuropathology and Applied Neurobiology* **6**, 119–32.

MONAGLE R.D. & BRODY H. (1974) The effect of age upon the main nucleus of the inferior olive in the human brain. *Journal of Comparative Neurology* **155**, 61–6.

MOOSY J. (1971) Cerebral Atherosclerosis: Intracranial and extracranial lesions. In *Pathology of the Nervous System*, vol. 2, ed J. Minkler. McGraw-Hill, New York.

NAESER M.A., GEBHARDT C. & LEVINE H.L. (1980) Decreased computerized tomography numbers in patients with senile dementia. *Archives of Neurology* **37**, 401–9.

NASRALLAH H.A., JACOBY C.G. & McCALLEY-WHITTERS M. (1981) Cerebellar atrophy in schizophrenia and mania. *Lancet* i, 1102.

64   *Robert & Elaine Perry*

NEITO D. & ESCOBAR A. (1972) Major Psychoses. In *Pathology of the Nervous System*, vol. 3, ed J. Minkler. McGraw-Hill, New York.

NEUMANN M.A. & COHN R. (1953) Incidence of Alzheimer's disease in a large mental Hospital: relation to senile psychosis and psychosis with cerebral arteriosclerosis. *Archives of Neurology and Psychiatry* **69**, 615–36.

NORDBERG A., ADOLFSSON R., AQUILONUIS S.M. *et al* (1980) Brain enzymes and acetycholine receptors in dementia of Alzheimer type and chronic alcohol abuse. In *Aging of the Brain and Dementia*, eds L. Amaducci, A.N. Davison and P. Antuono. Raven Press, New York.

OGATA J., BUDZILOVICH G.N. & CRAVIOTO H. (1972) A study of rod-like structures (Hirano bodies) in 240 normal and pathological brains. *Acta Neuropathologica* **21**, 61–7.

PANTELAKIS S. (1954) Un type particulier d'angiopathie sénile du système nerveux central: l'angiopathie congophile. Topographie et fréquence. *Monatsschrift für Psychiatrie und Neurologie* **128,** 219–56.

PEARSE A.G.E. (1972) In *Histochemistry: Theoretical and Applied*, 3rd edn, vol. 2. Churchill-Livingstone, Edinburgh.

PEARCE J. (1974) Mental change in parkinsonism. *British Medical Journal* ii 445.

PERRY E.K., BLESSED G., TOMLINSON B.E. *et al* (1982) Neurochemical activities in human temporal lobe related to aging and Alzheimer-type changes. *Neurobiology of Aging.* **2**, 251–6.

PERRY E.K., OAKLEY A.E., CANDY J.M. *et al* (1981a) Properties and possible significance of substance P and insulin fibrils. *Neuroscience Letters* **25,** 3212–5.

PERRY E.K. & PERRY R.H. (1980) The cholinergic system in Alzheimer's disease. In *Biochemistry of Dementia* ed P.J. Roberts. John Wiley, New York.

PERRY E.K., PERRY R.H., GIBSON P.H. *et al* (1977) A cholinergic connection between normal aging and senile dementia in the human hippocampus. *Neuroscience Letters* **6,** 85–9.

PERRY E.K., TOMLINSON B.E., BLESSED G. *et al* (1978) Correlation of cholinergic abnormalities with senile plaques and mental test scores in senile dementia. *British Medical Journal* ii, 1457–9.

PERRY R.H., DOCKRAY G.J., DIMALINE R. *et al* (1981b) Neuropeptides in Alzheimer's disease, depression and schizophrenia. A postmortem analysis of vasoactive intestinal peptide and cholecystokinin in cerebral cortex. *Journal of the Neurological Sciences* **51**, 465–72.

PERRY R.H., BLESSED G., PERRY E.K. (1980) Histochemical observations on cholinesterase activities in the brains of elderly normal and demented (Alzheimer-type) patients. *Age and Ageing* **9**, 9–16.

PERRY T.L., HANSEN S. & KLOSTER M. (1973) Huntington's chorea: deficiency of γ-aminobutyric acid in brain. *New England Journal of Medicine* **288**, 337–42.

POST F. (1962) *The Significance of Affective Symptoms in Old Age*. Oxford University Press.

ROBINSON D.S., DAVIS J.M., NIES A. (1972) Aging, monamines and monoamine-oxidase levels. *Lancet* i, 290–1.

RON M.A., ACKER W., & LISHMAN W.A. (1980) Morphological Abnormalities in the Brains of Chronic Alcoholics. A Clinical, Psychological and Computerised Axial Tomography Study. *Acta Psychiatrica Scandinavica* **62**, (suppl. 286), 51–56.

ROSEN W.G., TERRY R.D., FULD P.A. *et al* (1979) Pathaligical verification of ischaemic score in differentiation of dementias. *Annals of Neurology* **7**, 486–8.

ROSENBERG G.A., KORNFIELD M., STOURING J. *et al* (1979) Subcortical arteriosclerotic encephalopathy (Binswanger): Computerized tomography. *Neurology*

29, 1102–6.

ROSENTHAL R. & BIGELOW L.B. (1972) Quantitive brain measurements in chronic schizophrenia. *British Journal of Psychiatry* **121,** 259–64.

ROSSOR M.N., EMSON P.C., MOUNTJOY C.Q. *et al* (1980) Reduced amounts of immunoreactive somatostatin in the temporal cortex in senile dementia of Alzheimer type. *Neuroscience Letters* **20,** 373–7.

ROTH M. (1955) The natural history of mental disorders in old age. *Journal of Mental Science* **101,** 281–301.

ROTH M. (1978) Aging of the brain and dementia: an overview. In *Aging of the Brain and Dementia,* Eds L. Amaducci, A.N. Davison and P. Antuono. Raven Press, New York.

ROTH M. & KAY D.W.K. (1956) Affective disorders arising in the senium, II Physical disability as an aetiological factor. *Journal of Mental Science* **102,** 141–50.

ROTH M. & MORRISSEY J.D. (1952) Problems in the diagnosis and classification of mental disorders in old age. *Journal of Mental Science* **98,** 66–80.

SALMON J.H. (1969) Senile and presenile dementia: ventriculoatrial shunt for symptomatic treatment. *Geriatrics* **24,** 67–72.

SANDOZ P. & MEIER-RUGE W. (1977) Age-related loss of nerve cells from human inferior olive and unchanged volume of its grey matter. *IRCS Medical Science* **5,** 376.

SCHEIBEL A.B. (1978) Structural aspects of the aging brain: spine systems and the dendritic arbor. In *Alzheimer's Disease: Senile Dementia and Related Disorders,* eds R. Katzman, R.D. Terry and K.L. Bick. Raven Press, New York.

SCHEIBEL M.E., LINDSAY R.D., TOMIYASU U. *et al* (1975) Progressive dendritic changes in aging human cortex. *Experimental Neurology* **47,** 392–403.

SCHWARTZ C.J. & MITCHELL J.R.A. (1961) Atheroma of the carotid and vertebral arterial systems. *British Medical Journal* **2,** 1057–63.

SCOVILLE W.B., & MILNER B. (1957) Loss of recent memory after bilateral hippocampal lesions. *Journal of Neurology, Neurosurgery and Psychiatry* **20,** 11–21.

SHAW D.M., CAMPS F.E. & ECCLESTON E.G. (1967) 5-hydroxytryptamine in the hind brain of depressive suicides. *British Journal of Psychiatry* **113,** 1407–11.

SHEFER V.G. (1973) Absolute number of neurons and thickness of cerebral cortex during aging, senile vascular dementia and Pick's and Alzheimer's disease. *Neuroscience and Behavioural Physiology* **6,** 319–24.

SIMCHOWITZ T. (1910) Histologische Studien über die senile Demenz. *Histologische and Histopathogische Arbeiten über die Grosshirnrinde* **4,** 267–444.

SCHOCHET S.S., LAMPERT P.W. & EARLE K.M. (1968) Neuronal changes induced by intrathecal vincristine sulfate. *Journal of Neuropathology and Experimental Neurology* **27,** 645–58.

SLATER E., BEARD A.W. & GLITHERS E. (1963) The schizophrenia-like psychoses of epilepsy. *British Journal of Psychiatry* **109,** 95–150.

STOREY P.B. (1966) Lumbar air encephalography in chronic schizophrenia: a controlled experiment. *British Journal of Psychiatry* **112,** 135–144.

TANAKA Y., HAZAMA H., KAWAHARA R. (1981) Computerized tomography of the brain in schizophrenic patients. *Acta Psychiatrica Scandinavica* **63,** 191–7.

TAYLOR D.C. (1975) Factors influencing the occurrence of schizophrenic-like psychosis in patients with temporal lobe epilepsy. *Psychological Medicine* **5,** 249–54.

TERRY R.D. (1963) The fine structure of neurofibrillary tangles in Alzheimer's disease. *Journal of Neuropathology and Experimental Neurology* **22,** 629–42.

TERRY R.D., FITZGERALD C., PECK A. (1977) Cortical cell counts in senile dementia (abstr.), *Journal of Neuropathology and Experimental Neurology* **36**, 663.

TERRY R.D., GONATAS N.K. & WEISS M. (1964) Ultrastructural studies in Alzheimer's presenile dementia. *American Journal of Pathology* **44**, 267–97.

TERRY R.D., PECK A., DeTERESA R. *et al* (1981) Some morphometric aspects of the brain in senile dementia of the Alzheimer type. *Journal of Neuropathology and Experimental Neurology* **30**, (abstr.), 314.

TERRY R.D. & WIŚNIEWSKI H. (1970) The ultrastructure of the neurofibrillary tangle and the senile plaque. In *Alzheimer's Disease and Related Conditions*, eds G.E.W. Wolstenholme and M. O'Connor. A. Ciba Foundation Symposium. J. & A. Churchill, London.

THÖRNER G.W., LANGE H.W. & HOPF A. (1977) Quantitative Untersuchungen der Basalganglien des Menschen bei extrapyramidal-motorischen Erkrankurgen. *Verhandlunger der Anatomischen Gesellschaft* **71**, 99–101.

TOMLINSON B.E. (1972) Morphological brain changes in non demented old people. In *Aging of the Central Nervous System*, eds H.M. von Praag and A.F. Kalverboer. De Ervon F. Bohn, New York.

TOMLINSON B.E. (1979) The Aging Brain. In *Recent Advances in Neuropathology*, no. 1, eds W. Thomas Smith and J.B. Cavanagh. Churchill Livingstone, Edinburgh.

TOMLINSON B.E. (1980) The structural and quantitative aspects of the dementias. In *The Biochemistry of Dementia*, ed P.J. Roberts. John Wiley, New York.

TOMLINSON B.E., BLESSED G. & ROTH M. (1968) Observations on the brains of non-demented old people. *Journal of the Neurological Sciences* **7**, 331–56.

TOMLINSON B.E., BLESSED G. & ROTH M. (1970) Observations on the brains of demented old people. *Journal of the Neurological Sciences* **11**, 205–42.

TOMLINSON B.E. & IRVING D. (1977) The numbers of limb motor neurons in the human lumbosacral cord throughout life. *Journal of the Neurological Sciences* **34**, 213–9.

TOMLINSON B.E., IRVING D. & BLESSED G. (1981) Cell loss in the locus coeruleus in senile dementia of Alzheimer type. *Journal of the Neurological Sciences* **49**, 419–28.

VICTOR M., & BANKER B.Q. (1978) Alcohol and Dementia. In *Alzheimer's Disease: Senile and Dementia and Related Disorders*, eds R. Katzman, R.D. Terry and K.L. Bick. Raven Press, New York.

VICTOR M., ADAMS R.D. & COLLINS G.H. (1971) *The Wernicke-Korsakoff Syndrome: A Clinical and Pathological Study of 245 patients, 82 with Postmortem Examinations.* Davis, Philadelphia.

VIJAYASHANKAR N. & BRODY H. (1971) Neuronal population of the human abducens nucleus. *Anatomical Record* **169**, 447.

VIJAYASHANKAR N. & BRODY H. (1973) The Neuronal population of the nuclei of the trochlear nerve and the locus coeruleus in the human. *Anatomical Record* **172**, 421–2.

WERNICKE C. (1881) *Lehrbuch der Gehimkrankheiten*, vol. 2. Theodor Fischer Kassel und Berlin.

WESTERMARK P., GRIMELIUS L. & POLAK J.M. (1977) Amyloid in polypeptide hormone-producing tumours. *Laboratory Investigation* **37**, 212–5.

WHITE P., HILEY C.R., GOODHARDT M.J. *et al* (1977) Neocortical cholingergic neurons in elderly people. *Lancet* i, 668–70.

WIŚNIEWSKI K., JERVIS G.A., MORETZ R.C. *et al* (1979) Alzheimer neurofibrillary tangles in diseases other than senile and presenile dementia. *Annals of Neurology* **5**, 288–94.

WOODARD J.S. (1962) Clinico-pathological significance of granulovacuolar degeneration in Alzheimer's disease. *Journal of Neuropathology and Experimental Neurology* **21,** 85–91.

WRIGHT J.R., CALKINS E., BREEN W.T. *et al* (1969) Relationship of amyloid to aging. Review of the literature and a systematic study of 83 patients derived from a general hospital population. *Medicine* **48,** 39–60.

YATES C.M., SIMPSON J., MALONEY A.F.S. *et al* (1980) Neurochemical observations in a case of Pick's disease. *Journal of the Neurological Sciences* **48,** 257–63.

YAGISHITA Y., ITOH N., AMANO N. *et al* (1980) The fine structure of neurofibrillary tangles in a case of atypical presenile dementia. *Journal of the Neurological Sciences* **48,** 325–32.

The Psychology of Ageing: assessment of defects and their management

Robert Woods

This chapter focusses on some psychological aspects of both assessment and management of elderly psychiatric patients. However, it will not simply describe the work of a clinical psychologist with the elderly. In recent years the number of psychologists interested and working in this field has increased dramatically, but this specialty remains relatively unpopular, and psychogeriatric units in many areas continue to have little or no psychological service. This chapter aims to develop psychological dimensions relevant to all disciplines working in old age psychiatry.

To date there has been far more research and literature on psychological assessment than on psychological treatment of elderly patients. In this chapter equal weight will be given to both aspects, to reflect the potential importance of the treatment area and the changing emphasis of current psychological practice and research. No discussion of assessment or treatment of elderly people showing abnormalities of functioning would be possible without some consideration of psychological changes in normal elderly people. These provide the context for the assessment of abnormal deficits and may set limits to the goals of any treatment procedures. Without knowledge of them, those working with the elderly are left to rely on the often misleading mythology about growing old.

The chapter comprises three sections: firstly, a discussion of important aspects of psychological functioning in 'normal' old age; secondly, a review of the nature of psychological deficits in elderly psychiatric patients and their assessment; finally, a description of psychological treatment and management approaches and an evaluation of their effectiveness, with priorities for future development highlighted.

NORMAL AGEING

It is impossible in a few pages to cover every aspect of the psychology of ageing. A comprehensive treatment of this whole area is given by Birren & Schaie's (1977) multi-author text. The intention here is to draw attention to some relevant key issues and to illustrate some of the methodological problems that affect interpretation of results in this field.

Cognitive decline in old age — myth or fact?

It may appear counter-intuitive to suggest that cognitive powers do not decline in old age, and data such as those shown in Fig. 2.1 appear to lend empirical support to the traditional view. Fall-off seems to start in early adult-hood, and to accelerate at the age of 60 or so. These results are not in dispute, but their validity and implications have led to much controversy; the reasons for this will be summarised here.

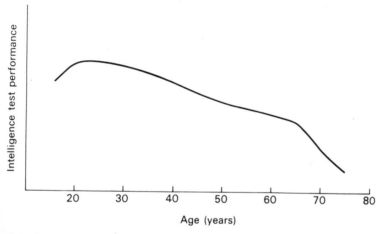

Fig. 2.1 Decline in intellectual test performance with age — cross-sectional data. (Derived from Wechsler 1955.)

Multi-dimensional changes

Different aspects of intelligence show different rates of decline. Fig. 2.2 shows this for verbal and performance levels, although by the age of 65 rates of decline are approximately parallel. Similarly 'crystallised' abilities (e.g. well learned, consolidated, verbal skills) tend to show less decline than 'fluid' abilities (flexible and novel reasoning capacity) (see Horn & Donald-son 1976). It has been suggested that a loss of speed could account for the differential decline — performance and fluid tests are more likely to emphasise speed of response. However Botwinick (1977) points out that allowing unlimited time on these tests does *not* bring scores to the level of younger subjects.

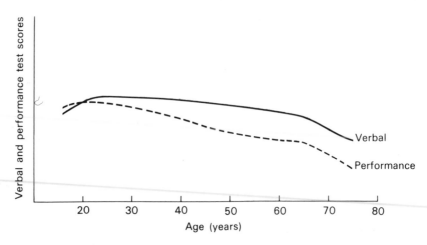

Fig. 2.2   Differential decline in verbal and performance abilities with age. (Derived from Wechsler's (1955) WAIS data.)

Design of studies (Table 2.1)

The data shown in Fig 2.1 are cross-sectional— at one point in time people of different age-cohorts are assessed so that people born, for example, in 1910 are compared with those born in 1960, with all the differences in opportunities and life experiences this must entail (see Table 2.1). Longitudinal studies— repeated measures on the same individuals— were thought to be preferable, but there are flaws here also. Schaie and colleagues have suc-

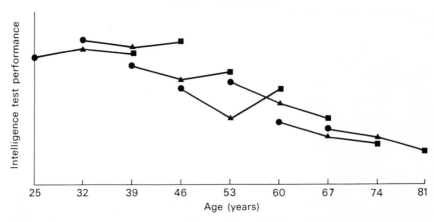

Fig. 2.3   Notional results illustrating cross-sequential findings (Schaie *et al*). ● indicates initial test scores; ▲ scores seven years later; ■ scores 14 years after initial test. The points connected indicate the longitudinal component; joining any of the three sets of symbols would give a cross-sectional pattern.

Table 2.1 Age changes in cognitive abilities — methodologies, results and drawbacks.

Design	Studies	Results	Problems
Cross-sectional: subjects of all ages assessed at one point in time	Wechsler (1955) (see Fig. 2.1) — WAIS; many others!	Decline beginning in early adulthood	Cohorts differ in education, nutrition, early medical care, occupational opportunities, etc.
Longitudinal: repeated measures on same subjects	Owens (1966) — Army Alpha Test	General Improvement 19–49; little loss to age 61	Selective drop-out; subjects available for re-test tend to have higher initial scores (Botwinick 1977)
	Eisdorfer & Wilkie (1973) —WAIS	60–69 year olds —performance loss over 10 years and four tests	Practice effects — familiarity with test and test situation
	Jarvik et al (1962)	8 year period—decline on performance tasks; initial mean age 67.5	Timing of re-test critical — if too frequent, greater loss of subjects Results confounded with cultural changes over the study period, changes in societal influences and expectations, changes in social environment
	Blum et al (1972)	Subjects from Jarvik et al retested after 20 years; overall decline	
	Savage et al (1973) —WAIS	7 year period; decline in verbal, increase in performance scores; four tests, initial mean age 71; only 1/6th remained in study	
Cross-sequential: all age-groups assessed 1956; if available reassessed in 1963 and 1970 (see Fig. 2.3). *New* subjects of all ages also assessed in 1963 and 1970	Schaie et al reviewed by Botwinick (1977) Primary Mental Abilities Test	Some clear decline in older age groups. Independent measures show more decline than repeated measures — but less than cross-sectional; cohort differences relatively large; pattern of decline as previously	Statistical treatment of results open to criticism— Horn & Donaldson (1976, 1977). Each method of analysis confounds some variables (Botwinick 1978, pp. 372ff)

ceeded in superimposing the two designs; a cross-sectional study was carried out and then individuals were reassessed 7 and 14 years later — a 'cross-sequential' methodology. An additional refinement at re-test was also to assess new subjects from the same population as in the original cross-sectional study. Much controversy has surrounded this complex work, reflected in an exchange of articles between Horn & Donaldson (1976, 1977) and Baltes & Schaie (1976) (Schaie & Baltes 1977). There does seem to be agreement that, in older age groups (50+, 60+, 70+ according to function), there is evidence of intellectual decline, on average. Cross-sectional methods show most decline, longitudinal least, with independent samples occupying an intermediate position. Cohort differences can be as large as age differences over much of the life-span.

Plasticity

Baltes & Willis (1979) argue that cognitive functioning in individuals is not fixed or static. They suggest that individuals vary greatly in their patterns of development, hence there are large observed individual differences in the rate of change of intellectual abilities. They describe this as long-term plasticity. Its existence means that generalisations about the 'ageing process' may have limited applicability to the individual case.

Short-term plasticity is also thought possible. This is supported by studies showing that the intellectual performance of elderly people can be improved by various experimental interventions (Patterson & Jackson 1980, Baltes & Barton 1977). A number of environmental and situational factors have been shown to have a specific adverse effect on the performance of the elderly. These include fatigue (Furry & Baltes 1973), negative self-evaluations (Bellucci & Hoyer 1975), and cautiousness (Birkhill & Schaie 1975). However, Labouvie-Vief *et al* (1974) are probably overstating their case in saying that deficits in the elderly reflect *only* a lack of exposure to or practice in the type of tasks used. For instance, Hoyer *et al* (1978) showed *greater* improvement in younger subjects in one of the few intervention studies to include a younger control group. Clearly many elderly people do not perform to their full potential in the cognitive test situation, but how much wider the gap is between performance and competence in the elderly has not been established.

Intelligence tests

Intelligence tests were originally designed for the assessment of children and adolescents; they are validated against the construct of what intelligence means in these age groups; they predict academic attainments and work performance well. Are they then relevant to older people and to what it means to be an intelligent older person? Some years ago Demming & Pressey (1957) developed a test more appropriate for the life-style and culture of older people — a test of practical information. They found scores *increased* with age!

Models of intellectual change

Horn & Donaldson's (1976) fluid-versus-crystallised model was mentioned above. They argue that results on a particular task will depend on the mix of the two elements in that task. The formulation emphasises probabilities, and does not say that decrement is inevitable in all people, or even that it is an intrinsic part of the ageing process; rather that fluid ability is likely to decrease with age and crystallised ability to increase with age. Labouvie-Vief *et al* (1974) present an operant analysis, focussing on environmental deficiencies, as mentioned above, with intellectual behaviour being seldom prompted or reinforced in older people. Schaie (1977–78) points to changing cognitive styles over the life-span, reflecting different demands made on cognition. Cognition at first is acquisitive then, in turn, achieving, responsible, executive, and finally reintegrative. Existing tests tap only the first two types; a decline in these with age may then be accompanied by an increase in other functions not yet assessed. The reintegrative stage has close links with the concept of wisdom being a perogative of the elderly. More recently a 'multi-causal and interactive model of influences on ageing' has been developed by Baltes & Willis (1979). This is set out in Table 2.2. Whichever model is preferred — and each has its insights — we can conclude that, on average, there is some decline in old age. The myths to be exploded are that decline begins early in life, that all aspects of intelligence are affected, and that

Table 2.2 Multi-causal and interactive model of influences on ageing. (Derived from Baltes & Willis 1979).

Type of influence	Definition	Examples
Normative age-graded influences	Includes biological and environmental factors that are highly age-related, and are experienced by most individuals within particular ageing cohorts	Education, biological maturation
Normative history-graded influences	Includes biological and environmental factors correlated with historical change. Most individuals within particular cohorts would experience these; different cohorts might be differentially affected	Wars, economic depressions
Non-normative critical life events	Those which do not occur for most individuals in an age- or history-related manner	Divorce, cerebrovascular accident, change of job

Table 2.3 Factors shown to affect cognitive functioning; they are likely to be present in any sample of older people, and could contribute to the observed average decline and inter-individual variability.

Factor		Evidence for effects on cognitive performance
Health: general	Botwinick & Birren (1963)	Optimally healthy older people had higher WAIS scores than those with mild — though generally asymptomatic — medical abnormality
raised blood pressure	Wilkie & Eisdorfer (1971)	Subjects (60–69 years) with raised diastolic blood pressure showed more decline on WAIS than those with normal blood pressure over a 10 year period
hearing loss	Granick *et al* (1976)	Hearing loss related to worse cognitive performance; most deficits on verbal tests
Terminal drop	Birren (1968), Jarvik & Falek (1963), Savage *et al* (1973)	In the period before death (up to four years in latter study) lower cognitive performance observed
Mental illness	Savage *et al* (1973)	A representative sample of elderly could include 25% of cases of dementia and depression — both associated with cognitive deficits

decline applies universally and inevitably to all elderly people. The causes of this decline are many and varied. Botwinick (1978) points out that age cannot be a causal variable; it is simply a crude index of other events and processes occurring in time. Some of these factors are detailed in Table 2.3; they fall within Baltes & Willis (1979) 'non-normative critical life-events' category.

Changes in other cognitive functions

Speed

Slowing of performance is often described and it is true that reaction time in 60-year olds, is on average, 20% slower than in 20-year olds (Birren *et al* 1979). This difference is related to central decision-making processes rather than to peripheral motor or sensory systems (Botwinick 1978); older people seem to have difficulty in maintaining readiness for a fast response while younger people show greater psychophysiological anticipatory changes in the 'preparatory interval', when the subject is warned that a stimulus is about to appear (Thompson & Nowlin 1973). Welford (1977) suggested that old people take longer to monitor the outcome of the previous response, so they are more impaired when a fast rate of responding is required. They tend, when possible, to opt for accuracy rather than speed, and will take longer than necessary over their response to ensure it is correct. If the task requires a complex recoding between stimulus and response there is greater impairment, perhaps because of diminished ability to manipulate items in short-term storage. Raised blood pressure, cerebrovascular and cardiovascular disorders, and low levels of activity have all been related to slower reaction time (Birren *et al* 1979). There is a great deal of overlap between older and younger subjects (Botwinick 1978).

Problem solving

Generally, older people are less successful at solving complex problems. Possible contributing factors are lower intelligence, reduced memory, slower information-processing and greater rigidity and concreteness in thought (Botwinick 1978, Rabbitt 1977). Reducing memory load and setting the logical operations in a concrete context do help. Older people do have difficulty in using organisational strategies, e.g. note-taking, and are at a disadvantage with irrelevant or redundant information (Rabbitt 1965).

Rabbitt (1977) points out that the level of task difficulty is often very high. Random, unsystematic, and inappropriate strategies may thus be ways of coping with an impossible task and not simply the results of inflexible problem-solving strategies. Slowness may increase memory load, sometimes to the extent of rendering the task insoluble. Older people show no greater cautiousness in choice of alternative courses of action as long as no 'safe', completely predictable option is allowed. If it were, this would be preferred, despite being unrewarding (Botwinick 1969).

Several studies have sought to train old people in problem-solving skills. Some positive results have been obtained (see Botwinick 1978) but it is not clear that old people are differentially aided.

Memory

Differences in memory performance between young and old have been often demonstrated (Schaie & Zelinski 1979); most studies have been cross-sectional. We will consider here the differential changes in various aspects of memory, and conditions which aid and hinder memory performance.

Many suggestions for sub-dividing memory have been made. The most influential is shown in Fig. 2.4, together with a refined version emphasising memory as a continuous, rather than a sequential, process.

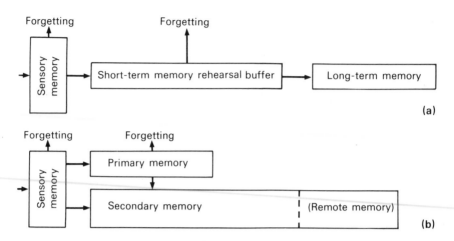

Fig. 2.4 (a) A multi-stage model of memory; information is passed sequentially from each stage to the next. (b) More recent models emphasise that information can pass directly into secondary memory. Primary memory is seen as a temporary holding and organising system; sensory memory is a pre-perceptual store of extremely short duration (less than 1 second).

Sensory memory. A pre-perceptual store of extremely short duration which can be difficult to measure in older subjects; there is some evidence suggestive of an age-decrement (Botwinick 1978).

Primary memory. As measured by the number of digits recalled in correct order, shows little change. If the stimulus material has to be re-organised (e.g. if recall in reverse order is required), or attention is divided, the age difference is greater (Craik 1977).

Secondary memory. The extent of impairment of secondary memory depends upon acquisition and retrieval conditions. Self-paced learning and the creation of a supportive atmosphere partially reduce the deficit. Leech & Witte (1971) rewarded *any* response and showed that performance then increased. The frequency of 'don't know' responses fell, suggesting that the older person needed additional incentive to make a response when uncertain. In studies of recognition memory, using a signal detection analysis that allows separation of memory and decision strategy components, older subjects have *not* generally been shown to be more cautious (e.g. Harkins *et al* 1979). The presence of a 'safe' option may, once more, lead to a greater apparent caution.

Older people show less spontaneous use of memory facilitating mediational and organisational techniques. If a sorting task is used to aid the subject in organising the material, the age differences in subsequent recall are reduced. Self-generated mediators appear to be more helpful than those provided by the experimenter, and older people seem to prefer verbal mediation to the visual imagery which tends to be the choice of younger subjects (see Botwinick 1978).

Assessing learning by recognition, rather than recall measures, reveals less deficit. Impairment can be shown, particularly if guessing rates are taken into account (e.g. Harkins *et al* 1979), including re-test after a week or a month's delay (Botwinick 1978). Recall involves an extra process, namely retrieving the item from storage, rather than simply matching it to the re-presented item. Additional evidence for a retrieval difficulty in the elderly is their benefit from cues which aid retrieval (e.g. Laurence 1967, Hultsch 1975). Recognition could, however, simply be a less sensitive memory test. Perhaps items do not need to be so well learned to be recognised as they do to be recalled. Acquisition and storage may also be impaired; there is some deficit on recognition and Drachman & Leavitt (1972) failed to show *differential* benefit for older people with retrieval cues.

Craik (1977) integrates the possible retrieval and acquisition deficits; he suggests that older people fail to engage spontaneously in deeper levels of processing when presented with an item to be learned or a minimal retrieval cue. He has argued generally that a memory's durability depends on the depth of processing carried out on it. Shallow encoding might be in terms of physical characteristics (e.g. is word in capitals or lower case?) while deep levels relate to the item's meaning (semantic encoding). There is some evidence, reviewed by Craik (1977), that younger subjects are superior to older people at deeper levels of processing on incidental learning tasks. This is where a recall task is given unexpectedly following the subject carrying out a non-memory task on the material involved. On a recognition task, Rankin & Kausler (1979) found evidence for semantic encoding by elderly subjects, but this seemed to be insufficiently elaborated to efficiently discriminate words that were to have been learned from new words with similar meanings.

Remote memory. Although Craik (1977) argues that secondary memory operates in the same manner after 30 seconds as after 30 years, a fourth type of memory — remote (or tertiary) memory — may usefully be distinguished. This applies to material learned some time ago, rather than in a recent experimental situation. Botwinick & Storandt (1980), using events going back 60 years, found generally good memory for famous past events for all age groups, with no clear deficit in old age. However, neither is there evidence for old people being *superior* in recall of past events or well known faces (Warrington & Sanders 1971).

The major memory loss in the elderly is in secondary memory, particularly when recall measures are used. Older people's difficulty in using imagery, mediation, organisational strategies, and deep processing spontaneously to facilitate memory are important, not least in their implications for minimising these deficits.

Personality and adjustment

The cognition versus personality distinction is somewhat artificial; personality variables (e.g. cautiousness) affect cognitive performance and vice versa. Personality assessment of elderly people is problematic: questionnaires often contain items which are more appropriate for students than senior citizens; while the validity of projective techniques (e.g. the Rorschach test) (see Savage 1973) is questionable. Neugarten (1977) comments that the disarray in the general field of personality is inevitably reflected in the ageing literature.

Some consistent themes have emerged: age changes are relatively small (Schaie & Parham 1976), the most consistently reported change is towards greater introversion and withdrawal from others and activity (Neugarten 1977).

Cumming & Henry (1961) concluded that disengagement was not simply imposed by society forcing retirement, restricting useful roles, and so on. Rather, it was a mutual process meeting the older person's psychological needs, as well as those of society. Disengagement was seen as a normal process essential for good adjustment. Against this was the view that keeping active, maintaining interests or developing new ones, made for good adjustment. Neither view seems to be universally applicable (Neugarten 1977). Most old people are either happy and active or unhappy and inactive, but for about 25% the predictions of disengagement theory do apply — with happy, inactive and unhappy active people being identified. These are, however, crude categorisations — 'happiness' is difficult to define, as is the quality of activity. Having a confidant (Lowenthal & Haven 1968) or attachment bonds (Bergmann 1978) may lead to activities that are helpful in coping with the changing demands of ageing.

Health, social, and economic factors are critical to adjustment; they prevent some who would enjoy activity from participating. Neugarten (1977) stresses that, given identical conditions, it is then life-long personality patterns which are important in determining adaptation in late life. Various typologies of personality in groups of older people have been identified (Reichard *et al* 1962, Neugarten *et al* 1968, Savage *et al* 1977), which emphasise a 'mature' type showing almost 'super-adjustment', as well as more disturbed groups.

In view of the observed continuity of personality and large individual differences, the biographical approach may be worth pursuing (Bromley 1978, Johnson 1976). Indirect methods are replaced by direct 'testimony' from those who know the subject well. This method has the potential to reveal much more of how psychosocial crises are dealt with by different individuals at various points in their life-span.

Conclusions on normal ageing

On average, age-related decrements are small while inter-individual variability is large. Continuity in functioning is the rule, other factors being equal. Miller (1977a) argues that other factors are so common in old age they might be viewed as part of the 'normal' ageing process, and not as incidental features. It is important for these not to be lost within the compass of an overall 'ageing' process, if our understanding of elderly individuals is to develop. is to develop.

It has been suggested that, in contrast to the orderly progression of development, old age is an erratic disintegration with various parts of the organism decaying at different rates. Nevertheless, there have been attempts to conceptualise old age as a period of psychological growth: notably, Erikson's (1963) eight stages of man which has a final stage of 'ego-integrity'. The developmental task is self-acceptance of what has been and what is to come. This is paralleled in Butler's work on reminiscence and life-review (e.g. Butler & Lewis 1973), where reminiscence is seen as a natural way of achieving this self-acceptance. If achievements, regrets, feelings of guilt, and sadness cannot be accepted in the context of the person's life-span, despair may result — despair of a life seen as valueless, wasted, or mis-directed, or of approaching death. Similarly, in the cognitive sphere, Schaie (1977–78) sees a reintegrative function emerging in old age.

A great many elderly people do make something of old age; their adaptive capacity is often underestimated. A stereotyped view of normal ageing omits the diversity and breadth of the final part of the life-span.

PSYCHOLOGICAL CHANGES IN ELDERLY PSYCHIATRIC PATIENTS — THEIR NATURE AND ASSESSMENT

Dementia

Cognitive changes

By definition cognitive changes in dementia are not in doubt; what is important is their form and their susceptibility to experimental manipulation. Can conditions for optimal performance of demented patients be specified? Are particular areas relatively preserved? Rational psychological management of dementia requires answers to such questions. Most of the research has focussed on senile dementia or pre-senile dementia of the Alzheimer type.

Dements show below average IQ: verbal IQ is higher than performance IQ on both the Wechsler Adult Intelligence Scale (WAIS) and the Ravens Matrices/Mill Hill Vocabulary Scale combination (Savage *et al* 1973, Miller 1977a). The fluid-versus-crystallised intelligence distinction is again relevant: dements are more impaired in novel situations requiring flexibility of thought, although deficits in speed and perceptual organisation may also contribute to the poorer performance.

All WAIS subtest scores were significantly lower than normals in the study by Savage *et al* (1973) and these results, together with those of Miller (1977a) and Whitehead (1973a), show a similar (although more extensive) pattern of decline to that in normal ageing — vocabulary scores highest, followed by digit span and other overlearned verbal tasks; performance tasks score lowest with picture completion (spotting a missing part of a drawing) being the best of these since it has a more crystallised component. The verbal decline leads others (e.g. Botwinick 1978) to conclude that the normal ageing and dementia patterns are qualitatively different.

Sensory memory

Perhaps because they are often seen as a central feature in the early stages of dementia, memory changes have been extensively investigated. Sensory memory may prove difficult to elucidate since most paradigms for its measurement involve other basic control processes that may also be impaired. Miller (1977b) used a backward masking technique to obtain evidence of impairment in presenile dements, which suggested a deficit from the very first point in the memory system.

Primary memory (PM)

Digit span reflects primary memory. Savage *et al* (1973) showed this ability to be impaired compared with normals — although it remains relatively well preserved. Kaszniak *et al* (1979) also showed reduced span in patients suspected of having dementia with atrophy which was confirmed by CT scan, and a reduced word-span has been found in preseniles (Miller 1977a).

Evidence from serial position curve tests also supports the theory of a deficit; Miller (1977a) has demonstrated relatively impaired recall of the most recent words in a list as well as of those at the beginning of the list. These deficits are thought to involve primary and secondary memory respectively.

Acoustic encoding is thought to be the major system in PM. Since controls were much more affected by acoustic similarity between words to be learned, Miller (1977a) has postulated inefficient acoustic encoding in dementia.

The dichotic listening technique has been extensively used (e.g. Inglis & Sanderson 1961). Different strings of digits are presented simultaneously to each ear and the subject recalls first from one ear then the other. For lists up to three digits, recall from the first ear is remarkably similar in normals and dements, but the second (and thus slightly delayed ear) shows impairment.

This has been viewed as a PM deficit, but Craik (1977) points out difficulties in interpreting results on this task, which may reflect more a difficulty in divided attention than PM per se.

Secondary memory (SM)

Deficits of secondary memory are well documented. In presenile dementia, Miller's serial position curve results have been mentioned above; the deficit in SM was not attributable to poor PM since a slower rate of presentation — allowing more time for words to go into SM — aided only the controls. Learning, over repeated trials, of lists, one, two or three items above the individual's span was poorer also. In older dements, learning of paired-associates is impaired both on recall and recognition tests. Identical word pairs are not subsequently re-learned more quickly, suggesting an acquisition problem (Inglis 1957). Miller's (1977a) demonstration that partial informa-tion — giving the initial letters of the word as a retrieval cue — led to near normal performance in presenile dements also implicates retrieval. This phenomenon of poor recall and recognition but good partial information has parallels in amnesia (Warrington & Weiskrantz 1970). Miller (1977a) examines two possible explanations: he finds no evidence for distorted encoding (although Larner (1977) did report encoding breakdown with older dements) and contradictory evidence for the notion that the patient is unable to inhibit the recall of incorrect responses. Thus dements, in free recall, do not produce a greater number of incorrect responses and words from previous lists; however, they are differentially impaired when the number of response alternatives in a recognition task is increased from two to eight, providing more competing responses to inhibit. Partial information may simply be a test that requires only partial learning for correct recall; Miller (1979) again draws the parallel with amnesia research, where Woods & Piercy (1974) have shown a similar effect in normals when the memory trace is weak.

Whitehead (1975) reports better performance in dements when the recognition task involves the choice of one of two stimuli, rather than a separate decision being made for each of the stimuli. The forced-choice procedure seemed to elicit responses when the subject was uncertain. However results from signal detection analyses of recognition tasks do not suggest a greater degree of caution in dements' responses. Their decision strategies have been described as 'liberal' (Larner 1977), showing little concern for accuracy (Miller & Lewis 1977), and 'more or less random' (Heller 1979).

Non-verbal memory

Several studies have showed deficits using pictorial material (e.g. Kendrick *et al* 1979), but material that is difficult to code verbally has rarely been used.

Complex pictures, thought difficult to verbalise, were used by Whitehead (1975) but deficits were as marked as with familiar words, in contrast to studies of normal performance. Facial recognition was examined by Ferris *et al* (1980). A signal detection analysis was used which showed that elderly normals and dements did *not* differ on recognition performance, false alarm rate or decision strategy. Both elderly groups performed worse than a younger group at a range of delay intervals (from 0.5 to 40 minutes), having a higher rate of false alarms and, if anything, taking more risks. Verbal memory tasks showed the familiar differences between elderly normals and dements, so these unexpected and potentially important results cannot be attributed to the groups being entirely atypical.

Conditioning

Although classical conditioning is slower in dementia (e.g. Solyom & Barik 1965), operant conditioning has been shown to be relatively normal if rewards appropriate for the particular patient are used (Ankus & Quarrington 1972). Dements showed some sensitivity to the relationship of rewards to the operant response (pulling a lever): males preferred fluids, while female patients responded better for monetary reward, which they had greater opportunity to spend. There may then be some residual learning ability under appropriate conditions.

Speed

Demented patients are slower than normals on a number of tasks. These include digit-copying (Kendrick *et al* 1979), naming common objects, especially when less common (Lawson & Barker 1968), identifying tachistoscopically presented pictures (Neville & Folstein 1979), and transferring pegs from one set of holes to another (Miller 1977a). In the latter study, a five-choice reaction time procedure was also used; in contrast with normal ageing, presenile dements seemed to be more impaired on the time taken to execute the movement, rather than in time spent deciding where to move. With older demented subjects and a slightly different task, Ferris *et al* (1976) concluded that the additional cognitive load where a choice was involved (rather than a simple reaction time situation, where there is only one stimulus and one response) differentially impaired dements. Woods' (1981) preliminary data from a card-sorting task of continuous choice reaction time suggest that both movement and decision times are impaired and more variable in dementia. Demented patients appear to be particularly affected by increases in the information load of the task (i.e. the number of choices).

Language

Although clear dysphasic symptoms are occasionally seen, language deficits in dementia are generally subtle. Rochford (1971) compared dements' and dysphasics' naming ability, and concluded that dements had difficulty more in recognition (despite adequate vision) than naming. Facilitating recognition by using very familiar objects (body parts) dramatically improved dements', but not dysphasics', naming performance. Miller & Hague (1975) were unable to show 'poverty of speech', i.e. restricted vocabulary and expression, in presenile dements; they were slower to produce words, but were not more restricted in the range of words used in speech.

Personality

Personality assessment in dementia is problematic since the validity of personality tests with dements is dubious. Anecdotally, personality changes are evident — occasionally a reversal but more often an exaggeration of previous traits. Some show catastrophic reactions to failure — breaking down completely — others are undisturbed. A biographical approach is needed, together with observation of the individual in a variety of natural situations. Relatives' accounts should be considered carefully, as insidious changes arising from the dementia may not be well discriminated from life-long styles of functioning.

Behaviour

The loss of self-care ability and appearance of socially unacceptable behaviour are well known. Unfortunately, there have been few attempts to monitor these changes longitudinally, to explore which skills are lost first and which patterns of impairment are most common at different stages.

Table 2.4 Rank order of loss of eleven areas of behaviour, from nurse-ratings of 136 elderly psychiatric patients (mostly dementias).

1	Hobbies	5	Orientation in space	9	Control of bowels
2	Participation	6=	Recognition of persons	10	Ability to move
3	Ability to wash	6=	Ability to communicate	11	Ability to eat
4	Ability to dress	8	Control of bladder		

Ferm's (1974) cross-sectional data are shown in Table 2.4. The pattern of loss was similar in groups categorised as 'mild', 'moderate' and 'grave' dementia on a brief cognitive test. Although behavioural and cognitive scores are relatively well correlated, other factors are important. One is immobility — which has a relatively small correlation with severity of dementia, another is institutional variables — the extent to which independent behaviour is encouraged, even if it takes longer and could disrupt the routine. Ferm's conclusion that 'things learned late in life disappear first and those learned early are the last to disappear' is attractive, but probably premature.

Factor analysis of rating scale data from the CAPE (see below) on demented patients produced three factors listed in Table 2.5 (Pattie & Gilleard 1979). The distinction between dependency and disruption — on

Table 2.5 Factor structure of Behaviour Rating Scale (from Clifton Assessment Procedures for the Elderly — CAPE — Pattie & Gilleard 1979) in patients with dementia.

Factor I	Physical disability/communication disability
Factor II	Apathy
Factor III	Social disturbance

which dimensions the patient may be at quite different levels — has important implications for management and placement. Gilleard & Pattie (1980) have attempted to derive Guttmann scales on these factors; these are scales showing unidimensional cumulative change (see Table 2.6). Longitudinal follow-up of demented patients over a two-year period showed a linear trend in this factor, whereas social disturbance did not show a linear trend, change being related to initial level. The apathy factor increases and reaches a maximum (on this scale at least) relatively early in dementia; it resembles Ferm's lack of hobbies and poor participation and the observation by McFadyen *et al* (1980) of lower levels of activity engagement in cognitively impaired elderly people. It can be concluded that behavioural change should be viewed as multi-dimensional.

Conclusions

It is difficult to present a satisfactory psychological model of dementia from the available evidence. Discounting attempts to show psychological factors

Table 2.6 Guttmann scale of Factor I — physical disability/communication disability. May be viewed as one dimension of progressive deterioration. (Derived from Gilleard & Pattie 1980.)

1 Shown signs of confusion
2 Requires assistance bathing and dressing
3 Incontinent
4 Loss of ability to care for personal appearance
5 Almost always confused
6 Difficulties in communication
7 Loss of ability to understand others' communications
8 Unresponsive to communication

causing dementia (Miller 1977a), there have been several attempts to integrate some of the disparate findings into more general relationships. These include the theory that dementia represents an accelerated ageing of the nervous system. Evidence for and against this is reviewed by Miller (1977a). Studies showing qualitative differences between normal ageing and dementia (e.g. Kaszniak *et al* 1979) make this theory unlikely as a complete model of dementia. A model based on lower arousal has been postulated by Kendrick (1972); this has some psychophysiological support (Hemsi *et al* 1968, Davies *et al* 1977) and explains well results from the original Kendrick Battery. Findings from the revised Battery have led to the additional consideration of the effects of medication and activity (Kendrick & Moyes 1979). Other workers have implicated sensory deprivation, interacting with and exacerbating early memory loss to produce confused behaviour (Inglis 1962, Bower 1967), by analogy with the effects of sensory deprivation on young volunteers. The chronic sensory deprivation of the elderly patient — from loss of sensory acuity, unstimulating surroundings, or voluntary withdrawal — is a very different process from the acute deprivation that produces disturbed behaviour in younger people, although it is clear that memory loss must render a person more vulnerable to these effects. As yet, none of these models have much systematic unequivocal support and, generally, our psychological understanding of dementia remains primitive. Too little is known of the changes in ability over time, although Whitehead's (1977) demonstration of increasing cognitive impairment over a one-year period is an exception. Cross-sequential studies of patients with different severity of dementia are needed, with more emphasis on conditions that facilitate dements' performance.

Dementing patients have been treated as a homogenous group, even though McDonald (1969) identified two distinct groups — with and without parietal lobe symptoms (apraxia, right–left disorientation, etc.), and with different ages and prognoses (parietal lobe group, younger and worse prognosis) — suggesting this is an oversimplification. More account needs to be taken of the variability of breakdown of different aspects of function. This variability — both between and within subjects — may reflect a system under severe pressure, trying to maintain some function, even though in imminent danger of collapse. Different patients may adopt different strategies (denial, bland refusal to participate, use of aggression or social chit-chat to avoid situations seen as difficult, etc.). The system is easily overloaded and information processing ability may generally be slowed and impaired (c.f. Hibbard *et al* 1975). In short, mechanisms that normally come into play when the system is severely pressured, overloaded or faced with a near impossible task, may be relevant to the functioning of the demented person.

Depression

Cognitive changes in depression

The existence of cognitive changes in depression has long been recognised, and 'depressive pseudodementia' has been described, where the patient gives the impression of impaired awareness, orientation, and memory. Miller (1975) reviews psychological deficits in depression in younger patients; here an attempt will be made to outline the extent and nature of deficits in elderly patients.

Hospitalised affective patients have been shown to have lower WAIS scores — both performance and verbal — than normals (Savage *et al* 1973). Only comprehension, digit symbol, block design, and object assembly subtests failed to show significant impairment. In a community sample of 'neurotics' which included many subjects with diagnosis of reactive depression, Nunn *et al* (1974) also found lower WAIS scores than in a normal group. This study presents evidence suggesting that this is related to elderly people with less intellectual resources being more susceptible to neurosis. The deficit does not seem to be the precursor of an organic brain syndrome, nor related to test anxiety, poor motivation, nor to some common intervening variable such as physical illness or social class. Examining the pattern of subtest scores in depressed patients, Whitehead (1973a) concluded that the pattern of deficits was the same in normal ageing, depression, and dementia. Her early dements overall scored lower than the depressives, whereas WAIS differences between the larger organic and affective groups of Savage *et al* (1973) were more patchy, being largely apparent on performance subtests; although the affective group's verbal level was — as with normals — higher than their performance level. In three further assessments over a seven-year period, the survivors of this group showed a tendency to increased performance and slightly reduced verbal functioning.

It is on memory and learning tests, however, that the deficits have been thought to be most apparent and it is this area which has stimulated most research. Regarding primary memory, Whitehead (1973b) argues that digit span is not impaired in depression, although this is by comparison with dements and well depressives, no normal group being included. This contrasts with the finding of Savage *et al* (1973) who noted impaired digit span from WAIS data; however, it may reflect differences in samples or the relatively greater difficulty of the WAIS subtest (which, in addition, involves recall of digits in reverse order).

In the same study, Whitehead (1973b) used a number of other memory and learning tasks. On the basis that scores improved after remission of the depressive illness, she identified two verbal learning tasks — the Synonym Learning Test (SLT) and the Serial Learning Test — as being impaired in depression. Other verbal memory tasks (immediate or delayed recall of memory passages, paired associate learning, a recognition task) did not show improvement. The finding of a lack of impairment in depression on paired associate learning is supported by Irving *et al* (1970) who used a normal control group, but not Savage *et al* (1973) whose affective and dementia groups did not differ significantly in performance on the same test. On the Modified Word Learning Test (the forerunner of the SLT) affectives did do better than dements but were still at a lower level than normals. A further complication is the failure of Davies *et al* (1978) to replicate significant psychological test improvements after remission of depression. They used a normal control group and found the depressed group to be impaired on paired associate and serial learning (the SLT was not given to controls). However the controls and depressives also differed on verbal intelligence and may not have been well matched in terms of social class and life-long intellectual level. Neville & Folstein (1979) showed normals and depressives to have similar scores on a relatively undemanding pictorial free recall task, but Kendrick *et al* (1979) have shown a clear deficit on their Object Learning Test (OLT) with a large normal comparison group, well matched for verbal IQ. It must be concluded that learning and memory deficits *can* occur in depression, but that the nature of samples and the tasks used may lead to no apparent deficit being observed. In many cases, the depressives occupy an intermediate position between normal and demented groups; the deficits here are less marked and universal than in dementia.

Several studies have examined the nature of the deficit. Whitehead (1974) found it was no less with familiar than with unfamiliar material. Analysis of errors between depressed and demented patients (Whitehead 1973b), holding learning level constant, showed dements to be prone to random errors, while depressives' errors included many more transpositions from other parts of the task. Both groups showed many omissions; remitted depressives significantly reduced this level of non-response. As noted above, signal detection analyses of recognition tasks allow separation of memory from response strategies, cautiousness, etc. Miller & Lewis (1977) showed depressive and normal groups to be similar in performance and significantly better than dements on the memory aspect, but the depressives used a much more conservative decision strategy than normals or dements. This was reflected in their lower false alarm rate, i.e. they were much more cautious about guessing. Similarly, Larner (1977) found depressives to be characterised by conservative performance, avoiding errors by only responding when more or less certain they had seen the word before. This distinction between memory and decision strategy may help account for the discrepant results on various tests of free recall noted above. Another factor is low intelligence which may be associated with neurotic disorders, as we have seen. Whitehead (1974) showed that patients with low verbal IQ s had lower learning scores, both when ill and remitted. Some of the tasks used may well be overdependent on intellectual capacity.

It might be anticipated there would be some slowing of functioning in depression, and this is borne out by Neville & Folstein (1979) who report slowness in crossing out target letters from an array of other letters. Several studies on speed of copying digits support this, e.g. Kendrick *et al* (1979), where speed was intermediate between normals and dements but significantly different from both. Similarly Davies *et al* (1978) found digit copying to be the only psychological test to improve with remission of depression (although this may be a practice effect; cf. Kendrick & Moyes (1979) who show normals also improve on re-test at a similar rate).

The impairment of cognition in depressed elderly patients may be summarised as indicating possibly reversible slowness in simple speeded tasks and a greater cautiousness and avoidance of risky responses, which may largely be responsible for the deficits often, but inconsistently, found in free-recall tasks. A susceptibility of those with lower intelligence to affective disorders and the confounding effects of low intelligence on some difficult learning tasks should also be noted. Given the severity of depressive preoccupation, anxiety, agitation, retardation, etc., it is perhaps surprising how *little* cognitive change they show in testing situations that always have some degree of stress and failure attached. Kendrick & Moyes (1979) point out that, in many studies, patients are receiving antidepressant and/or other medication; they have suggested that this may exacerbate the patients' reduced activity level arising from the depression. They present evidence consistent with both these factors affecting performance on certain cognitive tests, and postulate a 'drug-induced pseudodementia' where digit copying, but not object learning, is impaired. However, the possibility that it is the most severe cases of depression that both receive additional medication and show cognitive deficits needs to be taken into account before these effects are clearly established.

Diagnostic testing

Traditionally, psychological assessment has been used as a diagnostic aid, particularly in the differentiation of dementia and affective disorders. A great deal of research has been aimed at developing tests which discriminate more and more efficiently between them, or which are sensitive to 'brain damage'. A basic method has been to compare an estimate of the patient's premorbid level of intelligence with the currently assessed level in order to ascertain whether intellectual deterioration has occurred. Estimates have been based on verbal IQ level or vocabulary level, on the basis that these are least affected by deterioration — although the decline in them which has been noted above makes them imperfect predictors. Educational and occupational records have been used but a problem here is the large variability of IQ within occupational groups (e.g. many unskilled labourers have above-average IQ s). Another related approach is to compare WAIS subtests thought to show little deterioration ('hold' tests) with those thought to be most sensitive to dementia ('don't hold' tests). A number of 'deterioration quotients' have been suggested, most notably Wechsler's own DQ. Savage *et al* (1973) in both community and hospital samples show that, while on average the DQ in dements is higher than in other groups, the variability is so large that a high misclassification rate is unavoidable. They report similar misclassification problems with another commonly used index, the discrepancy between verbal and performance levels. A basic problem with these indices is the assumption that the normal person will score equally well on each component, which is untenable in the individual case.

Crookes (1974) has developed a WAIS deterioration index on the basis of differential performance of dements and depressives, and reports that it misclassifies few depressives; however, cross-validation of such findings on a fresh sample is needed. It has been suggested that word reading ability may give a better estimate of premorbid intellectual level (Nelson & McKenna 1975) and, while early results are encouraging, it would be naïve to expect near perfect prediction from this or any other measure.

A number of learning tasks have been developed primarily as diagnostic tests; many of these were mentioned above in the discussion of changes in depression. As Irving *et al* (1970) and Savage *et al* (1973) have demonstrated, the degree of misclassification for any one test may often be high. The acceptability to patients of some of the tests and their usefulness with patients of low IQ has also been questioned. Other diagnostic tests are based on drawing geometric designs, either by copying or from memory. Cowan *et al* (1975) suggested that a copying task (the Bender-Gestalt) was less consistent in discriminating dements and affectives than a learning task, but Crookes & McDonald (1972) obtained more promising results with the Benton Visual Retention Test, which is a recall task.

Most diagnostic tests have been validated on cases of dementia and depression where the diagnosis is clear cut; in practice they would rarely be used in such a situation. It has long been recognised (e.g. Post 1965) that, where the diagnosis is doubtful, the psychological test results are likely to be equivocal. The importance of the standardisation sample is illustrated by the Revised Kendrick Battery, which showed near perfect discrimination on clear-cut acute cases (Kendrick *et al* 1979) but misclassified nearly half of a sample of long-stay psychiatric patients (Gibson *et al* 1980). The consequences of the alternative diagnoses need to be taken into account. Ron *et al* (1979) reported a follow-up of cases of presenile dementia in which they judged the diagnosis not to be supported in 31% of the cases. They suggested that, where doubt exists, the label of dementia would be better not applied in view of its negative connotations. If dementia is present then, in time, it will become apparent. Diagnostic testing must also take into account the problem of base rates; the usefulness of the test depends on the relative proportions of the diagnostic groups in those who are tested. A large preponderance of one group means that the test will have to discriminate extremely well in order to add anything to the discrimination achieved by 'guessing' the more common diagnosis each time.

An alternative use of psychological assessment is primarily to *describe* rather than to *discriminate*; ' . . . to reveal patterns of ability and impairment without any necessary direct implication for psychiatric diagnosis' (Savage *et al* 1973); ' . . . in determining the degree of recovery [or] gauging by means of serial testing the rate of progress of dementia' (Post 1965). Diagnosis may still be aided, but the emphasis here is on considering psychological data alongside other information; Ron *et al* (1979) — retrospectively — showed this approach to increase diagnostic efficiency considerably. An important general point is that, while good performance on a task may be taken more or less at face value, poor performance should always lead to an examination of the possible reasons for the failure, which in most cases can be multi-determined.

Brief cognitive assessment

The majority of elderly patients should not be assessed by a psychologist; the cost and time involved, and the inadequacies of the tests are not compensated for by any gains (e.g. in predicting outcome, Kuriansky *et al* 1976). The psychologist could more usefully pursue other roles, particularly in relation to treatment. There is every indication though that each patient should be assessed on brief psychological tests. Memory and information tests — of which there are many — are particularly useful. Performance on these tests relates to pathological changes (Blessed *et al* 1968), to measures of atrophy on computed tomography (Jacoby & Levy 1980), and to outcome (Whitehead 1976). The information/orientation subtest of the Clifton Assessment Procedures for the Elderly (Pattie & Gilleard 1979) has been extensively researched, and is claimed to have comparable validity to other longer and more detailed tests with the psychogeriatric population. A parietal lobe test (McDonald 1969) should also be used routinely. These tests enable what would be collected as clinical data to be quantified in a more reliable, replicable, communicable form.

More detailed psychological assessment would be appropriate to explore more complex issues, where these are clinically relevant. For example, where someone is thought to have previously been very intelligent, the brief tests may not be sensitive enough to record the actual impairment; conversely, where the person is of life-long low intelligence, a misleadingly low score may be obtained — occasionally leading to a misdiagnosis of dementia (Bergmann *et al* 1971). Where a patient has apparently recovered from a confusional state, more detailed testing may be helpful in identifying whether there is residual impairment. Where a person's impairment seems patchy or brief tests are in conflict with other information (e.g. the person gets lost on the ward but scores well on a verbal orientation test), then it may be useful to map out areas of preservation and impairment. It is useful to consider before a psychological assessment is carried out what the results will contribute to the management of the case.

Detailed cognitive assessment

Clinical psychologists are as idiosyncratic in their choice of tests as they are in their attitudes to assessment. A large number of tests have been reviewed by Kramer & Jarvik (1979). We will mention here some tests in common use for examing a patient's pattern of abilities.

The WAIS is the intelligence test most widely used. Savage *et al* (1973) have shown that its standardisation holds up well on elderly people in the United Kingdom, and Britton & Savage (1966) have developed and standardised a useful short form of the test. Raven's Coloured Progressive Matrices and Mill Hill Vocabulary Scale similarly can be used to measure performance and verbal intellectual levels respectively; however they lack the variety of task performances demanded by the full WAIS. In their favour they are relatively simple and quick to administer.

Memory testing is more controversial, and no really satisfactory test is available. Kendrick's OLT is acceptable to patients and can be used descriptively (by calculation of the OLT quotient — comparable with IQ) as well as diagnostically. Williams' (1968) memory tasks include both verbal and non-verbal learning and a test of delayed cued recall, which is particularly useful (White *et al* 1969). The Wechsler Memory Scale (Wechsler 1945) has been much criticised, and certainly its use to provide a single 'memory quotient' cannot be recommended. Several workers have adapted the test so that there is a measure of delayed recall (e.g. Whitehead 1973b, Russell 1975) and, following on from Kear Colwell's (1973) work on providing a rational factorial basis for comparing different aspects of memory on this scale, Skilbeck & Woods (1980) have identified three factors in psychogeriatric samples: a verbal learning and current orientation factor, an attention/concentration factor, and a visual recall factor. Some normative data on elderly subjects are available from the studies of Hulicka (1966), Klonoff & Kennedy (1966), and Cauthen (1977). Visual memory is often assessed using the Benton Visual Retention test (p. 89).

Kendrick's *Digit Copying Test* is a useful measure of speeded performance on a simple task, which again yields a quotient for descriptive use. Other areas of function are more problematic to assess in a standard way. With regard to language, for example, a number of clinical tests are available to assess dysphasic problems, but these have been developed and used mainly with younger people. Particularly useful of these is the Token Test (De Renzi & Vignolo 1962) which tests comprehension of increasingly complex instructions. Many of the neuropsychological tests used with younger patients are unsuitable; for example, poor performance on some of the Halstead–Reitan Battery of tests has been shown with normal older people (Klisz 1978). In general only simple neuropsychological tests can be used, and the results of these must be interpreted with clinical judgement with regard to the overall pattern of abilities the person shows.

It has been suggested above that repeated psychological assessment would be useful in monitoring the progress of the disorder, response to treatment and so on. In view of practice effects and 'normal' variability in performance, it is preferable to use those tests on which there are re-test data. This is available for the Kendrick Battery (Kendrick *et al* 1979), for the short WAIS and some learning measures (Savage *et al* 1973), and the WAIS vocabulary, digit span forwards and some memory tasks (Whitehead 1977). The test chosen also has to be of appropriate difficulty so that the initial score is neither near perfect nor near zero, to allow scope for change in either direction.

Assessment of behaviour

In many situations, assessment of the person's behaviour will be more important than cognitive assessment, particularly in decisions about placement and so on. Here there are two main alternatives: the first is analogous to the cognitive test situation when the person is asked to perform certain tasks and performance on them is rated by the observer. The best example of this is the Performance Test of Activities of Daily Living (PADL), described by Kuriansky & Gurland (1976). The subject is rated on detailed scales on his performance of 16 tasks, ranging from drinking from a cup to making a telephone call, in a structured situation. The other alternative is for an informant (nurse, relative, etc.) to rate the person's functioning from their general observations of them over a period of time (e.g. the previous week). The Shortened Stockton Geriatric Rating Scale, which forms part of the CAPE (Pattie & Gilleard 1979), is a well-standardised and extensively validated brief example of the large number of scales that have been developed. The validation of this scale has been carried out in relation to placement, outcome, levels of adjustment, survival and number of personal social services received. A fuller psychogeriatric dependency rating scale has recently been described by Wilkinson & Graham-White (1980). Hall (1980) provides a useful review of behavioural assessment using rating scales in younger patients.

Personality assessment

Comments previously made on personality assessment in normal ageing and dementia indicate the limited clinical role of questionnaires. Certain self-report measures may be useful in monitoring change in selected capable patients, e.g. analogue scales of mood, etc. (Aitken 1969); the personal questionnaire (Shapiro 1961); life-satisfaction indices (see Lawton 1971); and depression rating scales (Beck 1961).

Assessment — conclusions

The psychological assessment techniques currently available for the elderly are open to criticism. They are often too difficult, too long, and too stressful —exposing the patient to many failures. They emphasise deficits rather than abilities, contain inappropriate material, and are too insensitive to change. Concentration on the dementia versus depression diagnostic issue has led to relative neglect of other groups of patients. Some welcome exceptions to this include Neville & Folstein's (1979) study which is comparatively unusual in that a group of elderly Korsakoff patients were included (differentiated from the other groups by having poor recall but very fast object recognition). The same workers' attempts to sub-divide the dementia category are also promising, as is Heller's (1979) preliminary analysis of memory deficits in Parkinson's disease. This showed a reduction in some aspects of memory performance and a more cautious decision strategy, although deficits were much less marked than in dementia. Paraphrenics and late recurrent schizophrenics were included in the study of Savage *et al* (1973); their results on intellectual and learning tests were remarkably similar to those of the hospitalised affective group. There are encouraging signs that consideration of the other factors that affect test performance, and a move towards tests of specific psychological functions derived from the experimental psychology (rather than the psychometry) tradition, will lead to some of these problems being overcome (Cohen & Eisdorfer, 1979). At present it is advisable to recall the comments of Kuriansky *et al* (1976) on assessing elderly patients: '. . . taking such patients through a Test Battery calls . . . for an immense amount of patience, sympathy and the ability to provide support and encouragement.'

TREATMENT AND MANAGEMENT

Psychological approaches to the treatment of affective disorders

Reviews of dynamic psychotherapy with elderly patients are provided by Rechtschaffen (1959), Gottesman *et al* (1973), and Bergmann (1978). Generally it is fair to say that this area has attracted little interest, following Freud's contention that elderly people were not suitable for psychoanalysis in view of their rigidity. There has also been a dearth of appropriate models. Bergmann (1978) usefully describes the major tasks faced by elderly people and the therapist's task in helping their achievement. In this section the emphasis will be on approaches emanating from the more recent behavioural tradition, but readers should bear in mind the common ground in practice, if not in theory, between the various approaches (see also Chapter 7).

There are few published reports of the use of behaviour therapy in the treatment of depressed or anxious elderly patients, particularly if, for the present, institutional residents are not considered. Cautela (1969) provides an early speculative account of the use of relaxation, de-sensitisation, and thought stopping to counteract feelings of rejection and fear of death. 'Learning to be mortal' was one of the aims of a behaviour modification programme described by Preston (1973), intended for elderly people generally and not specifically for psychiatric patients. Control of anxiety and development of relevant social skills were also included, with the emphasis on an educational model. A detailed procedure — 'Stress Management Training' (Garrison 1978) — also utilises an educational approach, teaching relaxation and other anxiety control techniques to anxious elderly patients. A case report is given, and the use of the procedure with groups as well as individuals is described. Several further case reports were included in Woods' (1978) description of psychological treatment of depression in the elderly and Burton & Spall (1981) report the successful use of operant procedures to reinstate self-feeding in a depressed patient.

Although most of the techniques used have been shown convincingly to have utility with younger patients the evidence with the elderly is only at an anecdotal level. In the absence of research specifically directed to older people, it is not contended here that psychological treatment is more effective than other methods. Experience suggests that, with elderly patients, it may be seen as complementary to other approaches, and patients vary in the extent to which specific behavioural analysis and intervention is appropriate. Some short case studies follow to illustrate the potential application and illustrate some of the procedures found useful. All patients were concurrently receiving medication, but improvements were not contingent entirely on this.

Probably the most familiar application of psychological therapy is where particular situations are avoided because they are seen as stressful, even though the patient is quite capable of coping physically. This may lead to depression if, as in Case 1, the avoidance prevents the person from receiving previously enjoyed reinforcement.

Case 1. Mrs G, age 73, became depressed over a period of a few months. She was too anxious to go out of the house or do housework. She had 'colonic hurry' and had soiled herself on a bus and at an over 60 s club prior to depression starting. She was taught anxiety management techniques and gradually exposed to household tasks as an inpatient. With her husband's co-operation, the housework programme continued at home, with graded exposure to going out taking place in a small group at the day-hospital. Her husband had to learn not to panic when she had a 'bad turn'. Gradual improvement continued over some months: she went on buses, went shopping regularly, did agreed housework consistently, and was eventually able to return to the over 60 s club, church, and to find pleasure in her activities once more.

Case 2. Mrs N, age 75, whose second husband had died eight months before, was referred to the psychogeriatric day hospital for depression and severe headaches. She had moved to her sister's home temporarily after her bereavement and could not now face returning to her own flat. Her headaches prevented her concentrating on any activities and she was unable to go out in view of leg pain. No physical basis for this or her headaches was established. Behavioural treatment proceeded on several fronts. Her numerous somatic complaints were ignored; she was taught to control anxiety using relaxation and to turn negative cognitions into positive coping statements. She was encouraged gradually to take up previous hobbies and thus to build up her concentration again. Her fear of going out was tackled using graded exposure at the clinic, with her practising at her sister's home. Despite a break-in at her flat whilst it was unoccupied, her return there was agreed between her sister and herself, and she became able to go out to the shops and to church from there. Her grief for her husband's death was discussed extensively, but her main concern was her ability to live as an independent person for the first time in her life; therefore, her achievements and self-esteem were systematically reinforced.

A number of behavioural models of depression have been formulated; in essence they all implicate a change in the behaviour-reinforcement relationship, although they differ in detail. Seligman's (1975) 'learned helplessness' theory has generated a great deal of interest and research: in it depression is seen as arising from a perceived loss of control over reinforcers, with the patient believing that nothing he does will make any difference, bring any pleasure or enjoyment. The patient may cease to do things he is quite capable of doing, having experienced repeated failure (or even success!) unrelated to his own actions. Treatment involves coaxing the person into a situation where they do succeed and do experience some pleasure. As in Beck's cognitive therapy for depression, negative cognitive distortions of the activity are corrected (Rush *et al* 1975) and the person reinforced for their success.

Case 3. Mrs W, age 71, had always been a fit, active, independent, capable lady. Told by her GP she had Parkinson's disease, she discussed this with friends and acquired more and more of the symptoms. Her family decided she should live with them so she lost her own home, friends, etc. and depression began when the forms had to be signed. After two months as an inpatient, she was still mute, inactive and had poor appetite; she viewed herself as useless now she had lost her perfect health, and fitness, and her home. Treatment began by discovering some of her previous interests; a particular magazine she liked was obtained and she was encouraged to look at it and to express some minimal enjoyment of it. With encouragement she went for a walk in a local park, and was helped to express enjoyment of the flowers, birds, etc. From these small successes she went on to be more active on the ward, helping in the kitchen, asking to go to the hairdressers — generally expressing her needs and choices. She became almost talkative! A family session to discuss how she could live independently and actively at home was important in maintaining her improvement.

Case 4. Mr R, age 80, was admitted for treatment of depression. Following a serious suicide attempt, drug therapy brought a remission to a plateau before behavioural treatment was begun. His major complaint was of a throbbing pain in his ear (for which there was probably an untreatable physical cause). He monitored this constantly and felt unable to carry on living if it continued; such thoughts had preceded his suicide attempt. Treatment emphasised his degree of control over the pain, using relaxation to reduce its perceived intensity and distracting activities (e.g. music, domestic tasks) to prevent him focussing on it. Positive self-statements about his control over the pain were encouraged. At follow-up four months after discharge, the pain is still present but he now says 'I'm the boss.'

Elderly people experience multiple losses—mobility, physical health, the family home, work, loved ones and so on. Bereavement may be seen as a special case: it is not uncommon to come across depressed patients who have not accepted their loss some years on. The features of grief described by Parkes (1972)—searching for the lost person, feelings of guilt or anger, and a tendency to idealise the dead person — are encountered in varying degrees. They provide a useful perspective as does Rachman's (1980) concept of 'emotional processing', the absorption of disturbing emotional experiences and the factors hindering and facilitating this process. Ramsay (1975, 1977) likens an unresolved grief reaction to a phobia: the person avoids the distressing emotional response that working through the grief would entail. They have lost a potent source of reinforcement in their partner and may respond helplessly, rather than doing those things that would ultimately be helpful. Gauthier & Marshall (1977) draw attention to the impact of the social environment; abnormal grief reactions are seen as arising either from a 'conspiracy of silence' (with family and friends colluding to avoid the grief reaction) or from the normal grief reaction being extended by family and friends continuing to pay attention to grieving for too long rather than encouraging the bereaved person towards adaptive patterns of behaviour. Both Ramsay and Gauthier & Marshall describe therapeutic success: both use prolonged exposure to grief-producing stimuli (thoughts about, pictures of, or reminders of the dead person) to produce the full emotional response until it subsides in the presence of the stimuli (a flooding procedure). The latter workers also instruct family and friends to encourage other alternative behaviour and to reduce the level of sympathy shown. The flooding technique as described demands a great deal from therapist and patient; some patients certainly would refuse to participate. In such circumstances it may be necessary to maintain a trusting, supportive therapeutic relationship and to adopt a more gradual approach until the patient is ready for the intensive work. In each case careful analysis of the problem is required.

Case 5. Mrs H, age 73, was referred through a voluntary agency; her husband had died six months previously. She was full of guilt: '. . . if only I hadn't made him walk so far he wouldn't have got cancer'; '. . .if only I'd seen him before he died', etc. She lived in a large isolated house and felt extremely nervous about being alone. She felt unable to mix with other people. She was allowed to express her guilt, but her cognitive distortions were gradually challenged. Her family began to encourage her to be more independent, she began to arrive early for consultations to chat with other elderly people in a lounge area. Eventually she brought in many momentoes of her husband and showed a response to them that soon subsided. Subsequently, she increased her activities and showed much less emotional response in discussing her husband.

Studies of depression in institutional settings have included evaluation of the effects of the person having a sense of control and choice over the environment. Thus Langer & Rodin (1976) showed that residents receiving a communication emphasising their responsibility for themselves improved their '. . . general sense of well-being' compared with residents to whom the staff's responsibility for them was emphasised. Similarly Reid *et al* (1977) have shown resident's sense of control over the environment to be positively related to their level of contentment and their positive self-concept. Simpson *et al* (1981) showed that depressed residents in an old people's home were not less active than non-depressed residents, but the latter participated relatively more in the activities they enjoyed. Thus some residents were inactive but quite happy, often they enjoyed reminiscing; others were active but unhappy as they were not involved in the activities that they enjoyed.

Clearly indiscriminate activity programmes are *not* the answer to depression in institutions — activities need to be meaningful to the individuals concerned. Power & McCarron (1975) seem to have achieved this by weekly half-hour individual personalised sessions with depressed residents. They first encouraged attention and a response by tactile and verbal contact, and then encouraged social interaction with other residents. Depressed residents improved significantly both on self-report and nurse-report depression rating scales compared with untreated depressed residents. The social interaction that was initiated in the sessions seemed to continue as further gains were apparent at six week follow-up. This relatively simple procedure seems worth exploring, but its effectiveness is likely to be related to the initial level of interaction in the particular setting.

In the institution and with community residents, patients cannot be viewed in isolation, and must be treated in the context of their social network. A behavioural problem-solving approach (Garrison & Howe 1976) has wide applicability and involves defining the problems specifically; listing alternative courses of action; discussing the pros and cons of each; reaching agreement on specific tasks each person is to carry out, and the criteria for whether they have been achieved. This is followed by evaluation of outcome and repeating the whole process if necessary.

If the person's sense of control is important then this should apply to treatment also with a clear contract being agreed, consisting of what the therapist offers and what is required of the patient; this should be revised when necessary. The therapeutic relationship is essentially then adult–adult, with the emphasis on inter-dependence.

Obviously no evaluation of these psychological approaches can be made as yet; the author's impression is that some specific techniques, like relaxation, are more difficult to use with elderly than younger patients, but that the limited goals which can be of clinical significance in the elderly are relatively often achieved.

Psychological approaches to the management of dementia

Despite the generally prevailing therapeutic pessimism with regard to dementia, there are now a large number of accounts of 'successful' programmes. Reviews of the early literature are available in Miller (1977c) and Woods & Britton (1977). The reader should note that various studies have utilised a wide range of subject populations in the USA and UK. In some studies details of diagnosis are lacking, in others patients are described as having an organic brain syndrome but have been hospitalised for over 20 years, suggesting they are a different population to a typical group of UK patients with dementia. Clearly differences in diagnostic criteria (Copeland 1978) are relevant here.

Although most people having dementia are not in an institution, most of the programme development and evaluation has been carried out in institutions — where the problems are more visible and resources (such as they are) are concentrated. Suggestions for community approaches will be discussed later. The aims of treatment should be clarified at the outset. There is no cure here for dementia; 'management' may be a more appropriate description. The aim is to help the demented person function as independently as possible, to live as 'normal' a life as possible, and to enjoy the maximum quality of life. If deterioration can be slowed down, halted for a while, or even slightly reversed this is to the good; but the programmes generally work on the environmental aspects of the person–environment interaction that is involved in all behaviour.

Four major categories of treatment approaches were identified by Woods & Britton (1977). Their categorisation is, as will become apparent, somewhat arbitrary, but provides a useful starting point.

Stimulation and activity programmes. These are based on the notion that the patient is understimulated, and perhaps undergoing sensory deprivation (see above). An early controlled study was reported by Cosin *et al* (1958), who increased stimulation using full occupational therapy and social and domestic activities. Their demented patients showed improvements in purposive, appropriate behaviour early in the programme, which were lost when the programme stopped. Longer-lasting improvements have been obtained in subsequent studies on a variety of measures, including cognitive functioning (see Woods & Britton 1977). The types of stimulation used are too varied and broadly defined to constitute a test of the sensory deprivation model. More restricted stimulation — in the form of physical exercise — does seem to improve some types of cognitive performance in both long-stay elderly (Powell 1974) and dementing patients (Diesfeldt & Diesfeldt-Groenendijk 1977).

Changes to the environment. These include changes in chair arrangements from around the walls to small groups so as to increase social interaction (Sommer & Ross 1958, Peterson *et al* 1977); changes in meal time arrangements so as to increase social interaction by creating a more normal social situation (Davies & Snaith 1980) and also to increase eating skills, allowing choice of food and size of portion with no time pressure (Gustafsson 1976); and changes to the whole structure and regime of the institution, as in group living where the ward or old people's home is broken down into small living units of 8–10 people, with more opportunities for self-help, choice, and relevant activity (Hitch & Simpson 1972, Marston & Gupta 1977). The emphasis has been on providing a physical environment which encourages appropriate independent behaviour, and a nursing regime that holds back from encouraging dependence (Harris *et al* 1977a, Lipman & Slater 1977).

Reality orientation (RO). A full review of RO is provided by Woods & Holden (1981). There are two major components: 24 hour RO where every interaction with the patient is used to convey current information, with confused talk not being reinforced; and RO sessions, where a group of three or four patients meet, usually daily for half-an-hour, and experience success and gain awareness of their current surroundings through structured discussion and activities. A number of controlled evaluations have been carried out, most recently by Woods (1979), Hanley *et al* (1981), Johnson *et al* (1981), Zepelin *et al* (1981), and Merchant & Saxby (1981). The small but significant effect of RO on measures of verbal orientation is well documented, but changes in general behaviour and functioning have been less consistently found. Hanley *et al* (1981) and Hanley (1981) report sustained improvements in dements' ability to find their way around a ward following a simple direct training in ward orientation, together with the provision of large clear signposts, although the latter were not as effective in isolation.

Behavioural approaches. The principles of this approach are outlined by Harris *et al* (1977b), and Patterson & Jackson (1980) comprehensively review the extensive literature. There have been studies on eating skills, mobility, social interaction, social skills, participation in activities, incontinence, screaming, smoking and oral hygiene, in addition to more general programmes. However, with a few notable exceptions, these studies tend to be of long-term institutionalised patients, with disorientated patients being excluded in some studies. Some recent reports may be illustrative: Lopez *et al* (1980) successfully taught 56 elderly inpatients the skill of 'starting a conversation' (there was also some generalisation to new situations). Those with severe organic impairment were excluded here. Three recent studies have examined participation in activities: Quattrochi-Tubin & Jason (1980) increased social activity and participation in physical activity contingent on the provision of refreshments, and Konarski *et al* (1980) used prompts and reinforcement to increase participation in an activities programme, with gains being maintained after ten weeks but not generalising to other activities. The third study was the only one specifically to use demented elderly patients. Burton (1980) demonstrated a situation-specific increase in patients' appropriate, materially directed behaviour in OT sessions (with a reduction in sleeping!) when OT staff consistently prompted patients to use materials and reinforced them for so doing— a similar finding to that of Jenkins *et al* (1977), again with some demented elderly people.

Hussian (1980), in an innovative study, was able to control inappropriate wandering, stereotyped responding, and inappropriate sexual responding in elderly patients with Alzheimer's disease using large, bright discriminative cues (previously paired with reinforcement in individual training sessions) which seemed to facilitate other behavioural techniques that were ineffec-

tive in themselves. The artificial 'supernormal' stimuli were, in some instances, reduced in size and then removed altogether, with the behavioural
improvement being maintained. If it proves possible to use these cues to
build up adaptive behaviour as well as reduce maladaptive responses, this
approach could be a major step forward in the management of dementia.

Overview

There is a great deal of common ground between these various treatments;
most approaches involve some activity and stimulation, which may, in turn,
involve reinforcement of appropriate behaviour. RO entails changes to the
physical environment — in the provision of signs, notice boards, calendars,
etc. — and to the overall regime, through 24 hour RO with its emphasis on
appropriate communication. RO may be seen as a behavioural re-learning
procedure, with learning taking the place of the verbal orientation and ward
orientation that is usually taught. A full behavioural approach includes
consideration of the antecedents of behaviour, and much environmental
change seeks to prompt appropriate behaviour. Woods & Holden (1981)
suggest that the approaches should be seen as complementary, with RO
serving as a model for how change can occur in areas that are specifically
taught. As yet, the behavioural literature is rather sparse on improving
self-care and social interaction in dementia per se, with the exception of
Parker's (1974) ancedotal report of a re-educational approach. Some attention has been given to incontinence, but results are discouraging for day-time
continence (e.g. Grosicki 1968, Pollock & Liberman 1974), although Collins
and Plaska (1975) had a little success with the 'bell and pad' method for
nocturnal incontinence. These poor results may be due to the complexity of
the sequence of behaviours involved. Turner (1980) indicates the necessity
for careful analysis of the problem, and the success of King's (1980) multi-
modal approach suggests a need for joint medical and psychological intervention to maximise the chances of success.

A strategy with much to recommend it in the practical situation is firstly to
develop an enriched environment for those in institutions—an environment to which it is worth being reorientated! A choice of meaningful
activities and stimulation should be provided, and residents encouraged and
prompted — but not coerced — to participate. Small groups and 'normal'
social settings encourage interaction and mutual help between residents; in
large groups 'rational' residents ignore 'confused' residents and shut them
out, whereas in a small group they are more likely to take some responsibility for them. Staff attitudes are all important. Davies & Snaith (1980)
suggest the ward sister's management style may be important; it needs to be
'patient-orientated' for a therapeutic environment to be possible rather than
orientated towards 'batch processing' of patients and the completion of
essential physical care tasks. Staff at all levels of the hierarchy need to be

consistent in their encouragement and reinforcement of appropriate behaviour and in their avoidance of creating dependency; they also need to be aware of the importance of communication with the patient. This is not easy with a demented patient and techniques from RO, together with encouragement of reminiscence (Kiernat 1979), can be helpful here. The environment should to some extent be prosthetic in the sense that it compensates for gaps in the person's functioning; additional signs and notices need to be provided and clearer signals given as to what is expected. The demented person's limited learning ability may be maximally used to learn to benefit from memory aids and reminders.

The next stage is to look at individual patients, to carefully assess their functioning in the context of biographical data — their assets as well as problems — and to draw up a plan for each geared to their needs, specifying goals and the agreed means of achieving them (Davies & Crisp 1980, Brody *et al* 1973). Not all treatments will be individual: many patients may require RO or physical exercise or dressing practice. For some patients their needs may be met by the current environment and the plan will be to do nothing! The important point is for staff to have a consistent agreed approach to each patient. Carestaff themselves need support, for if the aim is to slow down deterioration, then they will not have the reward of seeing people improving. Having a structure within which to work alongside other team members can help morale, as can recognition of the difficulties they face, adequate training in coping with them, and opportunities for mutual support and encouragement.

Community approaches

Despite the numerical superiority of demented patients in the community, psychological approaches are far less developed there. Among the few attempts to modify the elderly person's functioning are the studies by Greene *et al* (1979, 1980) in a Glasgow day hospital. The first study demonstrated changes in verbal orientation in three single-case studies of day patients attending two or three times a week, and having two structured 30-minute RO sessions on the days they attended. The second study followed a group of similar patients, and also included relatives' ratings. Results showed a dramatic improvement in verbal orientation following RO which was lost when RO was stopped. Relatives rated patients' behaviour at home as unchanged, as was the degree of stress they felt; however the relatives' mood did improve during the RO phase and deteriorated at follow-up. Thus, despite relatives being unaware of the phases of the project, RO in the day hospital may have some subtle effect on the supporter in the home. This needs exploring further, but the results do suggest some usefulness for RO in day settings. Attempts to teach relatives to use RO in the home setting are being made, but have not been evaluated as yet.

Attitudinal and relationship problems may be encountered here, as in institutions; Woods & Holden (1981) have urged that RO be used flexibly; it may — like other techniques — be misused if basic attitudes, allowing respect, dignity, individuality, and choice, are absent.

Elderly people living alone may benefit from memory aids and reminders in their home — perhaps kept up to date by home-help and other visitors. Problem areas should be identified and a practical problem-solving approach adopted, with careful recognition of the risks involved in the various options and of the elderly person's opinions and views. Training sessions can be carried out in the person's home — helping them to leave purses, diaries, etc. in a consistent place, so they are not so easily lost, and helping them follow a structured routine as far as possible.

For those who live with their families or have relatives close by, supporting the supporters is the prime aim — again adopting a practical approach to the problems experienced, whilst being sensitive to the emotional trauma of seeing a loved one deteriorate mentally in their presence. Sanford (1975) described some of the problems relatives find most difficult to tolerate and recent research (Gilhooly 1980) has explored the mechanisms used to cope with this difficult situation. One type of response was described as 'behavioural' — the relative organised help from friends, relatives, health and social services, as if the disability were almost a challenge to be overcome, a job to be done. These relatives had high morale. The other type of response was 'psychological' — it constituted an effort to change or control the meaning of the distressing experience. These mechanisms included seeing the present as an improvement over the past or as the precursor of a brighter future; seeing some good in the experience or seeing it as a moral virtue; and shrinking the significance of the problem by seeing other areas of life as more important. Relatives using neither of these mechanisms had very low morale. Several relatives simply ignored the demented person when the strain was too much. The influence of the supporters' relationship with the demented person needs further evaluation.

Psychological support is desirable at an early stage, before a crisis or a state of rejection is reached. Mutual support from other relatives in a similar position may be an extremely useful way of providing this help (e.g. Hausman 1979), and may provide a setting for giving and sharing information, modifying attitudes and beliefs, and agreeing on simple behavioural tasks and limits. The group setting can give 'approval' for taking more risks, for refusing unreasonable requests, and simply for sharing frustrations, resentments, and grief. As Bergmann *et al* (1978) have shown, families provide a great deal of support for demented people and receive little support themselves; such groups could help to ease the problems they face.

Psychological treatment — conclusions

The preceding sections have shown the considerable potential — but as yet little achievement — of psychological treatment approaches. Potential exists outside the areas of depression and dementia also; the large American literature on the treatment of long-stay chronic elderly patients, hospitalised for many years, ranges from encouragement of social interaction (Hoyer *et al* 1974) to the use of wine and token economies (Mishara & Kastenbaum 1973, 1974). There is potential application of psychological approaches, to stroke patients, e.g. biofeedback for neuromuscular re-education; anxiety management for patients with speech problems whose anxiety about their speech prevents them using preserved ability to the full (Damon *et al* 1979); and sign language training for aphasic patients (Wisocki & Mosher 1980).

Is the effort worthwhile in terms of the clinical results obtained? Certainly some of the changes reported have been rather small; however, the approach to dementia outlined above can be viewed as adding to an increased quality of life, even if the patient's functioning does not change at all. Small changes can be important: a reduction in frequency of incontinence from six times to once a day would not show up on some rating scales, but would ease the burden for supporters.

While the treatment of anxiety and depression needs more careful evaluation, the treatment of dementia now requires more experimental input on the conditions most favourable for demented patients, those variables that aid learning and retention, and those skills that are most preserved. Treatments for dementia could then be developed and refined, with the useful components of the various packages being identified and implemented in the light of experimental findings. Alongside this must be further examination of supporters' attitudes — whether they can be modified both in institutions and in the community, and finally of the conditions preventing and facilitating the development of a therapeutic environment in both settings.

REFERENCES

AITKEN R.C.B. (1969) Measurement of feelings using visual analogue scales. *Proceedings of the Royal Society of Medicine* **62,** 989–93.

ANKUS M. & QUARRINGTON B. (1972) Operant behaviour in the memory disordered. *Journal of Gerontology.* **27,** 500–10.

BALTES M.M. & BARTON C.M. (1977) New approaches toward aging: a case for the operant model. *Educational Gerontology.* **2,** 383–405.

BALTES P.B. & SCHAIE K.W. (1976) On the plasticity of intelligence in adulthood and old age: where Horn and Donaldson fail. *American Psychologist.* **31,** 720–5.

BALTES P.B. & WILLIS S.L. (1979) The critical importance of appropriate methodology in the study of aging: the sample case of psychometric intelligence. In *Brain function in old age,* ed F. Hoffmeister and C. Muller, 164–87. Springer-Verlag, Berlin.

BECK A.T. (1961) An inventory for measuring depression. *Archives of General Psychiatry.* **4,** 53–63.

BELLUCCI G. & HOYER W.J. (1975) Feedback effects on the performance and self-reinforcing behaviour of elderly and young adult women. *Journal of Gerontology.* **30,** 456–60.

BERGMANN K., KAY D.W.K., FOSTER E.M. *et al* (1971) A follow-up study of randomly selected community residents to assess the effects of chronic brain syndrome and cerebrovascular disease. *Proceedings of the 5th World Congress of Psychiatry,* Mexico.

BERGMANN K. (1978) Neurosis and personality disorder in old age. In *Studies in Geriatric Psychiatry,* ed A.D. Isaacs and F. Post, 41–76. Wiley, New York.

BERGMANN K., FOSTER E.M., JUSTICE A.W. *et al* (1978) Management of the demented elderly patient in the community. *British Journal of Psychiatry.* **132,** 441–9.

BIRREN J.E. (1968) Increment and decrement in the intellectual status of the aged. *Psychiatric Research Reports.* **23,** 207–14.

BIRREN J.E. & SCHAIE K.W. (1977) eds *Handbook of the psychology of aging.* Van Nostrand Reinhold, Cincinnati, Ohio.

BIRREN J.E., WOODS A.M. & WILLIAMS M.V. (1979) Speed of behaviour as an indicator of age changes and the integrity of the nervous system. In *Brain function in old age,* ed F. Hoffmeister and C. Muller, 10–44. Springer-Verlag, Berlin.

BIRKHILL W.R. & SCHAIE K.W. (1975) The effect of differential reinforcement of cautiousness in intellectual performance among the elderly. *Journal of Gerontology.* **30,** 578–83.

BLESSED G., TOMLINSON B.E. & ROTH M. (1968) The association between quantitative measures of dementia and of senile change in the cerebral grey matter of elderly subjects. *British Journal of Psychiatry.* **114,** 797–811.

BLUM J.E., FOSSHAGE J.L. & JARVIK L.F. (1972) Intellectual changes and sex differences in octogenarians: a twenty year longitudinal study of aging. *Developmental Psychology* **7,** 178–187.

BOTWINICK J. (1969) Disinclination to venture response versus cautiousness in responding: age differences. *Journal of Genetic Psychology* **115,** 55–62.

BOTWINICK J. (1977) Intellectual abilities. In *Handbook of the psychology of aging,* ed J.E. Birren and K.W. Schaie, 580–605. Van Nostrand Reinhold, Cincinnati, Ohio.

BOTWINICK J. (1978) *Aging and behaviour.* Springer, New York.

BOTWINICK J. & BIRREN J.E. (1963) Cognitive processes: Mental abilities and psychomotor responses in healthy aged men. In *Human aging: a biological and behavioural study,* ed J.E. Birren., R.N. Butler., S.W. Greenhouse., L. Sokoloff and M. Yarrow., 97–108. Govt. Printing Office, Washington D.C.

BOTWINICK J. & STORANDT M. (1980) Recall and recognition of old information in relation to age and sex. *Journal of Gerontology.* **35,** 70–6.

BOWER H.M. (1967) Sensory stimulation and the treatment of senile dementia. *Medical Journal of Australia.* **1,** 1113–9.

BRITTON P.G. & SAVAGE R.D. (1966) A short form of WAIS for use with the aged. *British Journal of Psychiatry.* **112,** 417–8.

BRODY E.M., COLE C. & MOSS M. (1973) Individualizing therapy for the mentally impaired aged. *Social Casework* 453–61.

BROMLEY D.B. (1978) Approaches to the study of personality changes in adult life and old age. In *Studies in geriatric psychiatry,* ed A.D. Isaacs and F. Post, 17–40. Wiley, New York.

BURTON M. (1980) Evaluation and change in a psychogeriatric ward through direct observation and feedback. *British Journal of Psychiatry.* **137**, 566–71.

BURTON M. & SPALL R. (1981) Contributions of the behavioural approach to nursing the elderly. *Nursing Times* **77**, 247–8.

BUTLER R.N. & LEWIS M.I. (1973) *Aging and mental health: positive psychosocial approaches.* Mosby, St. Louis.

CAUTELA J.R. (1969) A classical conditioning approach to the development and modification of behaviour in the aged. *Gerontologist* **9**, 109–13.

CAUTHEN N.R. (1977) Extension of the Wechsler Memory Scale norms to older age groups. *Journal of Clinical Psychology.* **33**, 208–11.

COHEN D. & EISDORFER C. (1979) Cognitive theory and the assessment of change in the elderly. In *Psychiatric symptoms and cognitive loss in the elderly,* ed A. Raskin and L.F. Jarvik, 273–82. Hemisphere, Washington D.C.

COLLINS R.W. & PLASKA T. (1975) Mowrer's conditioning treatment for enuresis applied to geriatric residents of a nursing home. *Behaviour Therapy* **6**, 632–8.

COPELAND J.R.M. (1978) Evaluation of diagnostic methods. In *Studies in geriatric psychiatry,* ed A.D. Isaacs and F. Post, 99–118. Wiley, New York.

COSIN L.Z., MORT M., POST F. *et al* (1958) Experimental treatment of persistent senile confusion. *International Journal of Social Psychiatry.* **4**, 24–42.

COWAN D.W., WRIGHT P.M., GOURLAY A.J. *et al* (1975) A comparative psychometric assessment of psychogeriatric and geriatric patients. *British Journal of Psychiatry.* **127**, 33–41.

CRAIK F.I.M. (1977) Age differences in human memory. In *Handbook of the psychology of aging* ed J.E. Birren and K.W. Schaie, 384–420. Van Nostrand Reinhold, Cincinnati, Ohio.

CROOKES T.K. (1974) Indices of early dementia on WAIS. *Psychological Reports.* **34**, 734.

CROOKES T.B. & MCDONALD K.G. (1972) Benton's visual retention test in the differentiation of depression and early dementia. *British Journal of Social and Clinical Psychology.* **11**, 66–9.

CUMMING E. & HENRY W.E. (1961) *Growing old: the process of disengagement.* Basic Books, New York.

DAMON S.G., LESSER R. & WOODS R.T. (1979) Behavioural treatment of social difficulties with an aphasic woman and a dysarthric man. *British Journal of Disorders of Communication.* **14**, 31–8.

DAVIES A.D.M. & CRISP A.G. (1980) Setting performance goals in geriatric nursing. *Journal of Advanced Nursing.* **5**, 381–8.

DAVIES A.D.M. & SNAITH P.A. (1980) The social behaviour of geriatric patients at mealtimes: an observational and an intervention study. *Age & Ageing* **9**, 93–9.

DAVIES G., HAMILTON S., HENDRICKSON D.E. *et al* (1977) The effect of cyclandelate in depressed and demented patients: a controlled study in psychogeriatric patients. *Age & Ageing* **6**, 156–62.

DAVIES G., HAMILTON S., HENDRICKSON D.E. *et al* (1978) Psychological test performance and sedation thresholds of elderly dements, depressives and depressives with incipient brain change. *Psychological Medicine* **8**, 103–9.

DEMMING J.A. & PRESSEY S.L. (1957) Tests 'indigenous' to the adult and older years. *Journal of Counselling Psychology.* **4**, 144–8.

DE RENZI E. & VIGNOLO L.A. (1962) The token test: a sensitive test to detect receptive disturbances in aphasias. *Brain* **85**, 665–78.

DIESFELDT H.F.A. & DIESFELDT-GROENENDIJK H. (1977) Improving cognitive performance in psychogeriatric patients: the influence of physical exercise. *Age & Ageing* **6**, 58–64.

DRACHMAN D.A. & LEAVITT J. (1972) Memory impairment in the aged: storage versus retrieval deficits. *Journal of Experimental Psychology.* **93**, 302–8.

EISDORFER C. & WILKIE F. (1973) Intellectual changes with advancing age. In *Intellectual functioning in adults,* eds L.F. Jarvik, C. Eisdorfer and J.E. Blum, 21–9. Springer, New York.

ERIKSON E.H. (1963) *Childhood and society.* Norton, New York.

FERM L. (1974) Behavioural activities in demented geriatric patients. *Gerontologica Clinica.* **16**, 185–94.

FERRIS S., CROOK T., SATHANANTHAN G. *et al* (1976) Reaction time as a diagnostic measure in senility. *Journal of the American Geriatrics Society.* **24**, 529–33.

FERRIS S.H., CROOK T., CLARKE E. *et al* (1980) Facial recognition memory deficits in normal aging and senile dementia. *Journal of Gerontology.* **35**, 707–14.

FURRY C.A. & BALTES P.B. (1973) The effect of age differences in ability extraneous performance variables on the assessment of intelligence in children, adults and the elderly. *Journal of Gerontology.* **28**, 73–80.

GARRISON J.E. (1978) Stress management training for the elderly: a psycho-educational approach. *Journal of the American Geriatrics Society.* **26**, 397–403.

GARRISON J.E. & HOWE J. (1976) Community intervention with the elderly: a social network approach. *Journal of the American Geriatrics Society.* **24**, 329–33.

GAUTHIER J. & MARSHALL W.L. (1977) Grief: a cognitive-behavioural analysis. *Cognitive Therapy & Research* **1**, 39–44.

GIBSON A.J., MOYES I.C.A. & KENDRICK D. (1980) Cognitive assessment of the elderly long-stay patient. *British Journal of Psychiatry.* **137**, 551-7

GILHOOLY M.L.M. (1980) The social dimensions of senile dementia. Paper presented at British Psychological Society Annual Conference, Aberdeen.

GILLEARD C.J. & PATTIE A.H. (1980) Dimensions of disability in the elderly: construct validity of rating scales for an elderly population. Paper presented at British Psychological Society Annual Conference, Aberdeen.

GOTTESMAN L.E., QUARTERMAN C.E. & COHN G.M. (1973) Psychosocial treatment of the aged. In *The psychology of adult development and aging,* eds C. Eisdorfer and M.P. Lawton, 378–427. American Psychological Association, Washington D.C.

GRANICK S., KLEBEN M.H. & WEISS A.D. (1976) Relationships between hearing loss and cognition in normally hearing aged persons. *Journal of Gerontology.* **31**, 434–440.

GREENE J.G., NICOL R. & JAMIESON H. (1979) Reality orientation with psychogeriatric patients. *Behaviour Research and Therapy.* **17**, 615–7.

GREENE J.G., SMITH R. & GARDINER M. (1980) Reality orientation with psychogeriatric day-hospital patients — an empirical evaluation. Paper presented at British Gerontological Society Annual Conference, Aberdeen.

GROSICKI J.P. (1968) Effects of operant conditioning of modification of incontinence in neuropsychiatric geriatric patients. *Nursing Research* **17**, 304–11.

GUSTAFSSON R. (1976) Milieu therapy in a ward for patients with senile dementia. *Scandinavian Journal of Behavioural Therapy.* **5**, 27–39.

HALL J. (1980) Ward rating scales for long stay patients: a review. *Psychological Medicine.* **10**, 277–88.

HANLEY I.G. (1981) The use of signposts and active training to modify ward disorientation in elderly patients. *Journal of Behaviour Therapy and Experimental Psychiatry.* **12**, 241–7.

HANLEY I.G., McGUIRE R.J. & BOYD W.D. (1981) Reality orientation and dementia: a controlled trial of two approaches. *British Journal of Psychiatry.* **138**, 10–14.

HARKINS S.W., CHAPMAN C.R. & EISDORFER C. (1979) Memory loss and response bias in senescence. *Journal of Gerontology.* **34**, 66–72.

HARRIS H., LIPMAN A. & SLATER R. (1977a) Architectural design: the spatial location and interactions of old people. *Gerontology* **23**, 390–400.

HARRIS S.L., SNYDER B.D., SNYDER R.L. *et al* (1977b) Behaviour modification therapy with elderly demented patients: implementation and ethical considerations. *Journal of Chronic Diseases.* **30**, 129–34.

HAUSMAN C.P. (1979) Short-term counselling groups for people with elderly parents. *Gerontologist* **19**, 102–7.

HELLER M. (1979) A psychometric and experimental investigation of memory functioning in Parkinson's disease. MSc thesis University of Newcastle-upon-Tyne.

HEMSI L.K., WHITEHEAD A. & POST F. (1968) Cognitive functioning and cerebral arousal in elderly depressives and dements. *Journal of Psychosomatic Research.* **12**, 145–56.

HIBBARD T.R., MIGLIACCIO J.N., GOLDSTONE S. *et al* (1975) Temporal information processing by young and senior adults and patients with senile dementia. *Journal of Gerontology.* **30**, 326–30.

HITCH D. & SIMPSON A. (1972) An attempt to assess a new design in residential homes for the elderly. *British Journal of Social Work.* **2**, 481–501.

HORN J.L. & DONALDSON G. (1976) On the myth of intellectual decline in adulthood. *American Psychologist.* **31**, 701–9.

HORN J.L. & DONALDSON G. (1977) Faith is not enough: a response to the Baltes–Schaie claim that intelligence does not wane. *American Psychologist.* **32**, 369–73.

HOYER F.W., HOYER W.J., TREAT N.J. *et al* (1978) Training response speed in young and elderly women. *International Journal of Aging and Human Development.* **9**, 247–54.

HOYER W.J., KAFER R.A., SIMPSON S.C. *et al* (1974) Reinstatement of verbal behaviour in elderly mental patients using operant procedures. *Gerontologist* **14**, 149–52.

HULICKA I.M. (1966) Age differences in Wechsler Memory Scale scores. *Journal of Genetic Psychology.* **109**, 135–45.

HULTSCH D. (1975) Adult age differences in retrieval: trace development and cue dependent forgetting. *Developmental Psychology* **11**, 197–201.

HUSSIAN R.A. (1980) Stimulus control in the modification of problematic behaviour in elderly institutionalized patients. Paper presented at Association for the Advancement of Behaviour Therapy convention, New York.

INGLIS J. (1957) An experimental study of learning and 'memory function' in elderly psychiatric patients. *Journal of Mental Science.* **103**, 796–803.

INGLIS J. (1962) Psychological practice in geriatric problems. *Journal of Mental Science.* **108**, 669–74.

INGLIS J. & SANDERSON R.F. (1961) Successive response to simultaneous stimulation in elderly patients with memory disorder. *Journal of Abnormal and Social Psychology.* **62**, 709–12.

IRVING G., ROBINSON R.A. & McADAM W. (1970) The validity of some cognitive tests in the diagnosis of dementia. *British Journal of Psychiatry.* **117**, 149–56.

JACOBY R.J. & LEVY R. (1980) Computed tomography in the elderly 2. Senile dementia: diagnosis and functional impairment. *British Journal of Psychiatry.* **136**, 256–9.

JARVIK L.F. & FALEK A. (1963) Intellectual stability and survival in the aged. *Journal of Gerontology.* **18**, 173–6.

JARVIK L.F., KALLMAN F.J. & FALEK A. (1962) Intellectual changes in aged twins. *Journal of Gerontology.* **17**, 289–94.

JENKINS J., FELCE D., LUNT B. *et al* (1977) Increasing engagement in activity of residents in old people's homes by providing recreational materials. *Behaviour Research and Therapy.* **15**, 429–34.

JOHNSON C.H., MCLAREN S.M. & MCPHERSON F.M. (1981) The comparative effectiveness of three versions of 'classroom' reality orientation. *Age & Ageing* **10**, 33–5.

JOHNSON M. (1976) That was your life: a biographical approach to later life. In *Dependency or interdependency in old age,* eds J.M.A. Munnichs and W.J.A Van den Heuvel, 148–61. Martinus Nijhoff, The Hague.

KASZNIAK A.W., GARRON D.C. & FOX J. (1979) Differential effects of age and cerebral atrophy upon span of immediate recall and paired-associate learning in older patients suspected of dementia. *Cortex* **15**, 285–95.

KEAR COLWELL J.J. (1973) The structure of the Wechsler Memory Scale and its relationship to 'brain damage'. *British Journal of Social and Clinical Psychology.* **12**, 384–92.

KENDRICK D.C. (1972) The Kendrick battery of tests; theoretical assumptions and clinical uses. *British Journal of Social and Clinical Psychology.* **4**, 63–71.

KENDRICK D.C., GIBSON A.J. & MOYES I.C.A. (1979) The revised Kendrick Battery: clinical studies. *British Journal of Social and Clinical Psychology.* **18**, 329–40.

KENDRICK D.C. & MOYES I.C.A. (1979) Activity, depression, medication and performance on the Revised Kendrick Battery. *British Journal of Social and Clinical Psychology.* **18**, 341–50.

KIERNAT J.M. (1979) The use of life-review activity with confused nursing home residents. *American Journal of Occupational Therapy.* **33**, 306–10.

KING M.R. (1980) Treatment of incontinence. *Nursing Times* **76**, 1006–10.

KLISZ D. (1978) Neuropsychological evaluation in older persons. In *The Clinical Psychology of Aging,* eds M. Storandt, I.C. Siegler and M.F. Elias, 71–96. Plenum Press, New York.

KLONOFF H. & KENNEDY M. (1966) A comparative study of cognitive functioning in old age. *Journal of Gerontology.* **21**, 239–43.

KONARSKI E.A., JOHNSON M.R. & WHITMAN T.L. (1980) A systematic investigation of resident participation in a nursing home activities program. *Journal of Behaviour Therapy and Experimental Psychiatry.* **11**, 249–57.

KRAMER N.A. & JARVIK L.F. (1979) Assessment of intellectual changes in the elderly. In *Psychiatric symptoms and cognitive loss in the elderly,* eds A. Raskin and L.F. Jarvik, 221–72. Hemisphere, Washington D.C.

KURIANSKY J. & GURLAND B. (1976) The performance test of activities of daily living. *International Journal of Aging and Human Development* **7**, 343–52.

KURIANSKY J., GURLAND B. & COWAN D. (1976) The usefulness of a psychological test battery. *International Journal of Aging and Human Development* **7**, 331–42.

LABOUVIE-VIEF G., HOYER W.J., BALTES M.M. *et al* (1974) Operant analysis of intellectual behaviour in old age. *Human Development* **17**, 259–72.

LANGER E.J. & RODIN J. (1976) The effects of choice and enhanced personal responsibility for the aged: a field experiment in an institutional setting. *Journal of Personality and Social Psychology.* **34**, 191–8.

LARNER S. (1977) Encoding in senile dementia and elderly depressives: a preliminary study. *British Journal of Social and Clinical Psychology.* **16**, 379–90.

LAURENCE M.W. (1967) Memory loss with age: a test of two strategies for its retardation. *Psychonomic Science* **9**, 209–10.

LAWSON J.S. & BARKER M.G. (1968) The assessment of nominal dysphasia in dementia: the use of reaction time measures. *British Journal of Medical Psychology.* **41**, 411–14.

LAWTON M.P. (1971) The functional assessment of elderly people. *Journal of the American Geriatrics Society.* **19**, 465–81.

LEECH S. & WITTE K.L. (1971) Paired-associate learning in elderly adults as related to pacing and incentive conditions. *Developmental Psychology* **5**, 180.

LIPMAN A. & SLATER R. (1977) Homes for old people: toward a positive environment. *Gerontologist* **17**, 146–56.

LOPEZ M.A., HOYER W.J., GOLDSTEIN A.P. *et al* (1980) Effects of overlearning and incentive on the acquisition and transfer of interpersonal skills with institutionalised elderly. *Journal of Gerontology.* **35**, 403–8.

LOWENTHAL M.F. & HAVEN C. (1968) Interaction and adaptation intimacy as a critical variable. *American Sociological Review* **33**, 20–30.

MCDONALD C. (1969) Clinical heterogeneity in senile dementia. *British Journal of Psychiatry.* **115**, 267–71.

MCFADYEN M., PRIOR T. & KINDNESS K. (1980) Engagement: an important variable in institutional care of the elderly. Paper presented at British Psychological Society Annual Conference, Aberdeen.

MARSTON N. & GUPTA H. (1977) Interesting the old. *Community Care* (Nov. 16th), 26–8.

MERCHANT M. & SAXBY P. (1981) Reality orientation: a way forward. *Nursing Times* **77**, (33), 1442–5.

MILLER E. (1977a) *Abnormal Ageing: the psychology of senile and presenile dementia* Wiley, New York.

MILLER E. (1977b) A note on visual information processing in presenile dementia. *British Journal of Social and Clinical Psychology.* **16**, 99–100.

MILLER E. (1977c) The management of dementia: a review of some possibilities. *British Journal of Social and Clinical Psychology.* **16**, 77–83.

MILLER E. (1979) Memory and ageing. In *Applied Problems in Memory,* eds M.M. Gruneberg and P.E. Morris, 127–49. Academic Press, New York.

MILLER E. & HAGUE F. (1975) Some statistical characteristics of speech in presenile dementia. *Psychological Medicine.* **5**, 255–9.

MILLER E. & LEWIS P. (1977) Recognition memory in elderly patients with depression and dementia: a signal detection analysis. *Journal of Abnormal Psychology.* **86**, 84–6.

MILLER W.R. (1975) Psychological deficit in depression. *Psychological Bulletin.* **82**, 238–60.

MISHARA B.L. & KASTENBAUM R. (1973) Self-injurious behaviour and environmental change in the institutionalized elderly. *International Journal of Aging and Human Development* **4**, 133–45.

MISHARA B.L. & KASTENBAUM R. (1974) Wine in the treatment of long-term geriatric patients in mental institutions. *Journal of the American Geriatrics Society.* **22**, 88–94.

NELSON H.E. & MCKENNA P. (1975) The use of current reading ability in the assessment of dementia. *British Journal of Social and Clinical Psychology.* **14**, 259–67.

NEUGARTEN B.L. (1977) Personality and aging. In *Handbook of the psychology of aging,* eds J.E. Birren and K.W. Schaie, 626–49. Van Nostrand Reinhold, Cincinnati, Ohio.

NEUGARTEN B.L., HAVIGHURST R.J. & TOBIN S.S. (1968) Personality and patterns of aging. In *Middle age and aging,* ed B.L. Neugarten, 173–7. University of Chicago Press, Chicago.

NEVILLE H.J. & FOLSTEIN M.F. (1979) Performance on three cognitive tasks by patient with dementia, depression or Korsakov's syndrome. *Gerontology* **25**, 285–90.

NUNN C., BERGMANN K., BRITTON P.G. *et al* (1974) Intelligence and neurosis in old age. *British Journal of Psychiatry.* **124**, 446–52.

OWENS W.A. (1966) Age and mental abilities: a second adult follow-up. *Journal of Educational Psychology*. **51**, 311–25.

PARKER F. (1974) Second childhood. *Times Educational Supplement* (9th August), London.

PARKES C.M. (1972) *Bereavement: studies of grief in adult life*. Tavistock Publications, London.

PATTERSON R.L. & JACKSON G.M. (1980) Behaviour modification with the elderly. *Progress in behaviour modification* **9**, 205–39.

PATTIE A.H. & GILLEARD C.J. (1979) *Manual of the Clifton assessment procedures for the elderly (CAPE)*. Hodder & Stoughton Educational, Sevenoaks.

PETERSON R.F., KNAPP T.J., ROSEN J.C. *et al* (1977) The effects of furniture arrangement on the behaviour of geriatric patients. *Behavior Therapy*. **8**, 464–7.

POLLOCK D.P. & LIBERMAN R.P. (1974) Behaviour therapy of incontinence in demented in-patients. *Gerontologist* **14**, 488–91.

POST F. (1965) *The clinical psychiatry of late life*. Pergamon Press, Oxford.

POWELL R.R. (1974) Psychological effects of exercise therapy upon institutionalized geriatric mental patients. *Gerontologist* **14**, 157–61.

POWER C.A. & McCARRON L.T. (1975) Treatment of depression in persons residing in homes for the aged. *Gerontologist* **15**, 132–5.

PRESTON C.E. (1973) Behaviour modification: therapeutic approach to aging and dying. *Postgraduate Medicine*. **54**, 64–8.

QUATTROCHI-TUBIN S. & JASON L.A. (1980) Enhancing social interactions and activity among the elderly through stimulus control. *Journal of Applied Behaviour Analysis*. **13**, 159–63.

RABBITT P. (1965) An age decrement in the ability to ignore irrelevant information. *Journal of Gerontology*. **20**, 233–8.

RABBITT P. (1977) Changes in problem solving ability in old age. In *Handbook of the psychology of aging*, eds J.E. Birren and K.W. Schaie, 606–25. Van Nostrand Reinhold, Cincinnati, Ohio.

RACHMAN S. (1980) Emotional processing. *Behaviour Research and Therapy*. **18**, 51–60.

RAMSAY R.W. (1975) Behaviour therapy and bereavement. In *Progress in behaviour therapy*, ed J. Brengelmann, 77–84. Springer, Berlin.

RAMSAY R.W. (1977) Behavioural approaches to bereavement. *Behaviour Research and Therapy*. **15**, 131–5.

RANKIN J.L. & KAUSLER D.H. (1979) Adult age differences in false recognitions. *Journal of Gerontology*. **34**, 58–65.

RECHTSCHAFFEN A. (1959) Psychotherapy with geriatric patients: a review of the literature. *Gerontology* **14**, 73–84.

REICHARD S., LIVSON F. & PETERSEN P.G. (1962) *Aging and personality*. Wiley, New York.

REID D.W., HAAS G. & HAWKINS D. (1977) Locus of desired control and positive self-concept of the elderly. *Journal of Gerontology*. **32**, 441–50.

ROCHFORD G. (1971) A study of naming errors in dysphasic and in demented patients. *Neuropsychologia* **9**, 437–43.

RON M.A., TOONE B.K., GARRALDA M.E. *et al* (1979) Diagnostic accuracy in presenile dementia. *British Journal of Psychiatry*. **13**, 161–8.

RUSH A.J., KHATAMI M. & BECK A.T. (1975) Cognitive and behaviour therapy in chronic depression. *Behavior Therapy*. **6**, 398–404.

RUSSELL E.W. (1975) A multiple scoring method for the assessment of complex memory functions. *Journal of Consulting and Clinical Psychology*. **43**, 800–9.

SANDFORD R.A. (1975) Tolerance of debility in elderly dependents by supporters at home: its significance for hospital practice. *British Medical Journal*. iii, 471–3.

SAVAGE R.D. (1973) Old age. In *Handbook of abnormal psychology*, ed H.J. Eysenck. Pitman, London.

SAVAGE R.D., BRITTON P.G., BOLTON N. *et al* (1973) *Intellectual functioning in the aged*. Methuen, London.

SAVAGE R.D., GABER L.B., BRITTON P.G. *et al* (1977) *Personality and adjustment in the aged*. Academic Press, London.

SCHAIE K.W. (1977–8) Toward a stage theory of adult cognitive development. *Journal of Ageing and Human Development* **8**, 129–38.

SCHAIE K.W. & BALTES P.B. (1977) Some faith helps to see the forest: a final comment on the Horn and Donaldson myth of the Baltes–Schaie position on adult intelligence. *American Psychologist*. **32**, 1118–20.

SCHAIE K.W. & PARHAM I.M. (1976) Stability of adult personality traits; fact or fable? *Journal of Personality and Social Psychology*. **34**, 146–58.

SCHAIE K.W. & ZELINSKI E. (1979) Psychometric assessment of dysfunction in learning and memory. In *Brain function in old age*, ed F. Hoffmeister and C. Muller, 134–50. Springer-Verlag, Berlin.

SELIGMAN M. (1975) *Helplessness: on depression, development and death*. W.H. Freeman, San Francisco.

SHAPIRO M.B. (1961) A method of measuring psychological changes specific to the individual psychiatric patient. *British Journal of Medical Psychology*. **34**, 151–5.

SIMPSON S., WOODS R.T. & BRITTON P.G. (1981) Depression and engagement in a residential home for the elderly. *Behaviour Research and Therapy*. **19**, 435–8.

SKILBECK C.E. & WOODS R.T. (1980) The factorial structure of the Wechsler Memory Scale in samples of neurological and psychogeriatric patients. *Journal of Clinical Neuropsychology*. **2**, 293–300.

SOLYOM L. & BARIK H.C. (1965) Conditioning in senescence and senility. *Journal of Gerontology*. **20**, 483–8.

SOMMER R. & ROSS H. (1958) Social interaction on a geriatric ward. *International Journal of Social Psychiatry*. **4**, 128–33.

THOMPSON L.W. & NOWLIN J.B. (1973) Relation of increased attention to central and autonomic nervous system states. In *Intellectual functioning in adults*, eds L.F. Jarvik, C. Eisdorfer and J.E. Blum, 107–24. Springer, New York.

TURNER R.K. (1980) A behavioural approach to the management of incontinence in the elderly. In *Incontinence and its management*, ed D. Mandelstam. Croom Helm, London.

WARRINGTON E.K. & SANDERS H.I. (1971) The fate of old memories. *Quarterly Journal of Experimental Psychology*. **24**, 432–42.

WARRINGTON E.K. & WEISKRANTZ L. (1970) Amnesic syndrome: consolidation or retrieval? *Nature* **228**, 628–30.

WECHSLER D. (1945) A standardised memory scale for clinical use. *Journal of Psychology*. **19**, 87–95.

WECHSLER D. (1955) *Manual for the Wechsler Adult Intelligence Scale*. The Psychological Corporation, New York.

WELFORD A.T. (1977) Motor performance. In *Handbook of the psychology of aging*, eds J.E. Birren and K.W. Schaie, 450–96. Van Nostrand Reinhold, Cincinnati, Ohio.

WHITE J.G., MERRICK M. & HARBISON J.J.M. (1969) Williams' scale for the measurement of memory: test reliability and validity in a psychiatric population. *British Journal of Social and Clinical Psychology*. **8**, 141–51.

WHITEHEAD A. (1973a) The pattern of WAIS performance in elderly psychiatric patients. *British Journal of Social and Clinical Psychology*. **12**, 435–36.

WHITEHEAD A. (1973b) Verbal learning and memory in elderly depressives. *British Journal of Psychiatry*. **123**, 203–8.

WHITEHEAD A. (1974) Factors in the learning deficit of elderly depressives. *British Journal of Social and Clinical Psychology.* **13,** 201–8.

WHITEHEAD A. (1975) Recognition memory in dementia. *British Journal of Social and Clinical Psychology.* **14,** 191–4.

WHITEHEAD A. (1976) The prediction of outcome in elderly psychiatric patients. *Psychological Medicine* **6,** 469–79.

WHITEHEAD A. (1977) Changes in cognitive functioning in elderly psychiatric patients. *British Journal of Psychiatry.* **130,** 605–8.

WILKIE F. & EISDORFER C. (1971) Intelligence and blood pressure in the aged. *Science* **172,** 959–62.

WILKINSON I.M. & WHITE J.G. (1980) Psychogeriatric dependency rating scales (PGDRS): a method of assessment for use by nurses. *British Journal of Psychiatry.* *137,* 558–65.

WILLIAMS M. (1968) The measurement of memory in clinical practice. *British Journal of Clinical Psychology.* **7,** 19–34.

WISOCKI P.A. & MOSHER P.M. (1980) Peer-facilitated sign language training for a geriatric stroke victim with chronic brain damage. *Journal of Geriatric Psychiatry.* **13,** 89–102.

WOODS R.T. (1978) The clinical psychologist's contribution to treatment of the elderly. Paper presented at British Psychological Society Conference, London.

WOODS R.T. (1979) Reality orientation and staff attention: a controlled study. *British Journal of Psychiatry.* **134,** 502–7.

WOODS R.T. (1981) Continuous reaction time in senile dementia. Paper presented at 12th International Conference of Gerontology, Hamburg.

WOODS R.T. & BRITTON P.G. (1977) Psychological approaches to the treatment of the elderly. *Age & Ageing* **6,** 104–12.

WOODS R.T. & HOLDEN U.P. (1981) Reality orientation. In *Recent advances in Geriatric Medicine,* 2, ed B. Isaacs. Churchill Livingstone, Edinburgh.

WOODS R.T. & PIERCY M. (1974) A similarity between amnesic memory and normal forgetting. *Neuropsychologia* **12,** 437–45.

ZEPELIN H., WOLFE C.S. & KLEINPLATZ F. (1981) Evaluation of a yearlong reality orientation program. *Journal of Gerontology.* **36,** 70–7.

CHAPTER 3

The Psychiatric Aspects of Physical Disease

John Grimley Evans

Human ageing, a progressive loss of adaptability in an individual over time, is due to a complex interplay between intrinsic (mainly genetic) and extrinsic (environmental) factors. Not all differences between young and old are due to ageing because in changing societies there will be cohort differences between successive generations. True ageing changes may also be aggravated by social factors that place greater stresses on older people than on younger — the poorer housing conditions of the elderly being a classical example. It is important to distinguish these separate factors that contribute to the overall age pattern of health and disability since they call for different types of response from different social agencies and scientific workers (Evans 1981).

In western societies the trend of nearly all these factors is to increase the prevalence of disease and disability with age. Incidence rates of cerebrovascular stroke, coronary heart disease and most cancers increase steeply with age. Other conditions such as chronic bronchitis may not increase in incidence in later life but the degree of disability caused in the individual may become greater. In the psychiatric sphere it is clear that the prevalence of senile dementia of Alzheimer's type, of other organic mental impairments, and of functional disorders, particularly depression, also increases steeply with age in later life (Kay *et al* 1970). Inevitably, by chance alone, physical and psychiatric disorders will co-exist more often in older patients than in younger and this factor alone would justify special training for psychiatrists and physicians with responsibility for the elderly.

Bergmann & Eastham (1974) studied a sample of elderly patients admitted to an acute medical unit. As might be expected they found a high prevalence of acute confusional states (16%); in addition they found prevalences of dementia (7%) and functional psychosyndromes (19%) similar to those in community studies (Kay *et al* 1970). But the relationship between physical and psychiatric disorder is more complex than simple concurrence. In a community study, Kay *et al* (1964) demonstrated a significant relation-

114

ship between physical and psychiatric disorders. Elderly people with functional psychiatric disorder showed higher morbidity and mortality rates than average for their age (Kay *et al* 1966) and greater use of institutional facilities including non-psychiatric hospital beds (Kay *et al* 1970).

Psychiatric disorder may present to the physician or surgeon in the guise of physical disease and physical disease may be the underlying cause of mental symptoms. Furthermore, even when mental and physical disorder occurring in the same individual are aetiologically independent, they will interact in the generation of symptoms and in the response to treatment. The interplay between physical and mental factors is one of the most pervasive and fascinating aspects of the practice of clinical medicine among the elderly.

PSYCHIATRIC DISORDER PRESENTING AS PHYSICAL DISEASE

The depressive symptom

Post (1965) drew attention to the masked depression as a characteristic form of the illness in the elderly. Patients with this condition may present to physicians with diffuse and non-specific physical symptoms often against a background of anorexia, weight loss, and lack of energy suggesting physical illness. All such cases require evaluation for physical disease but clues to the underlying primary depressive illness can often be found, particularly in sleep disturbance with anxious depressive rumination. Among depressed patients presenting to physicians, inability to get to sleep seems to be at least as common as the more classic symptoms of early morning waking, but this may reflect recognition of the latter as a depressive symptom by general practitioners leading to psychiatric rather than medical referral.

Greater difficulty arises with the elderly depressed patient who presents with a persistent and well defined physical symptom and who denies any other features suggesting a primary depressive illness. Indeed such patients may resent the suggestion that there might be a psychological element in their illness and angrily resist psychiatric referral. The commonest symptom to occur in this setting is pain. Atypical facial pain, particularly in women, is well known as a possible depressive symptom (Smith *et al* 1969). Although implicit in several clinical series (e.g. Kenyon 1964) it is less widely recognised that other types of pain and non-painful symptoms may play a similar role. The diagnostic problem may be a difficult one because many old people have organic pathology which could be causing their symptoms. Few elderly men presenting with low back pain will not have some degree of lumbosacral spondylosis. Thus, even when depression has been recognised, there remains the diagnostic dilemma of whether it is the primary condition or merely a secondary consequence of intractable physical discomfort. The apparent severity of the symptom is no help in the diagnosis: we have seen a patient becoming addicted to heroin prescribed for intractable leg pain which was assumed, wrongly, to be of malignant origin; in fact the problem was unequivocally a primary depressive one and responded swiftly and dramatically to appropriate treatment. A further facet of the problem is that even when the depression is clearly primary the pain or other symptom is rarely purely delusory. After the depression has been successfully treated the patient may still have the pain but it no longer causes him concern.

Apart from pain, other symptoms which may be presenting features of depression include tinnitus, myokymia, and pruritus. The severity of the symptoms may be described in florid terms but we have not encountered the bizarre interpretations of symptoms characteristic of monosymptomatic hypochondriacal psychosis (Munro 1980). The literature suggests that this syndrome is rare in later life but it is characteristic for diseases to be recognised in the young before they are detected among the old.

Psychotherapy has received less attention in the care of the elderly in Britain than in some other countries (Brink 1979, Roskos *et al* 1979). This should not excuse even the non-psychiatric doctor from attempting to gain some insight into a patient's state of mind and attitude to her symptoms. A major practical reason for this is to assess suicide risk. An elderly depressive must be assumed to be at high risk of suicide and in our judgement those who present with intractable physical symptoms are particularly so. Perhaps it is because they translate their affective distress into physical problems and look for physical solutions. We have an uncomfortable suspicion that some such patients may be precipitated into suicide by an initial, and from their point of view unsuccessful, contact with their doctor. In functional terms the medical consultation may represent the 'ordeal' and 'cry for help' elements of suicidal motivation. In parasuicidal behaviour in the young, these become elided into the self-harmful act itself rendering it ambiguous and so relatively safe compared with suicidal behaviour by the old.

Knowledge of the patient's personality and habits may be of diagnostic help. The presenting symptom may have clearly symbolic significance for the patient. It may mimic the first symptom of a loved (or hated) relative's fatal illness, or be a reputed typical symptom of a disease (usually cancer) which has a peculiar terror for the patient. The symptom may have particular relationship to the patient's valued activities: one elderly bachelor who had always been a physical fitness enthusiast presented with pain in the heel which prevented him walking his usual six miles a day. We speculate that, in psychogenic terms, the pain had become both the focus of inappropriate fears about his declining physical ability and an excuse for not continuing activities from which his depression had removed motivation.

Pain after stroke

One characteristic and frequently misunderstood setting for depressive pain is in the hemiplegic patient. Pain down the affected side of the body is a common and distressing consequence of stroke and is the result of at least three factors. One is damage to the central sensory pathways which presumably can usually only be assumed in those patients who had sensory symptoms or signs at some stage of their affliction. This damage affects central pain threshold, perhaps through disrupting a gate mechanism or shifting the balance between sensory stimuli and afferent pathways so that innocent stimuli are misinterpreted as painful (Melzack 1973). This is the basis of so-called 'thalamic' pain which, as a single and sufficient cause for post-hemiplegic pain, occurs much less frequently than it is diagnosed. The second factor is a peripheral painful stimulis in the affected limbs. Most commonly this arises in the hemiplegic shoulder. Adhesive capsulitis, rotator cuff degeneration, and subluxation (Fitgerald-Finch & Gibson 1975) are common, as is pain due to intense spasticity. Fibrotic shortening of muscles may be a late complication sometimes susceptible to surgical treatment. Causalgic pain with the vasomotor instability and osteoporosis of Sudeck's atrophy appears to be rarer now that most hemiplegic patients receive physiotherapy in the early stages of their illness, but simple disuse atrophy occurs in the hemiplegic limb and a fracture of the surgical neck of the humerus can both easily occur and easily be overlooked.

The third, and often dominant element in post-hemiplegic pain, is the affective one. Depression is well recognised as one of the commonest barriers to rehabilitation after stroke (Adams 1974) and one may indeed wonder why all patients with stroke do not become depressed. Intensive physical treatment to the peripheral painful stimulus together with appropriate antidepressant therapy will control most problems of pain after stroke. We tend to add a small dose of phenothiazine in the early stages of treatment to reduce anxiety and to interrupt an almost obsessive attention to the pain which many patients exhibit. Complete avoidance of analgesics in the first stages of treatment may be inhumane and risk losing the patient's confidence, but prescription should be timed to coincide with potentially painful physiotherapy and placebo can be substituted as the patient improves. The constructive and rational use of placebo is a highly valuable therapeutic tool but it requires careful co-ordination between doctor, nurse, and pharmacist to avoid the obvious possibility of disaster should the patient or relatives discover the nature of the medication and misjudge the motives of those prescribing it. It is possible that tricyclics may have a synergistic effect on analgesia independent of an antidepressant action. In some rare cases, episodic pain in the hemiplegic may be an epileptic phenomenon and there is a theoretical risk that tricyclics might make this situation worse or precipitate grand mal.

Depressive failure to cope with physical impairment

Many elderly people live for many years with physical impairments. Impairment may be transmitted into disability by a depressive illness. Unless a careful history is taken or there are other indications to show that the degree of physical impairment has not itself changed, the unwary doctor may attempt to treat the irrelevant physical disease and overlook the depression. Such patients often present to geriatric rehabilitation services or day hospitals where the problem is well known and routinely looked for. There is a risk, however, that some such sufferers may turn or be referred to the social services department and, in the absence of skilled medical evaluation, become unnecessary consumers of scarce resources. Foster *et al* (1976) in a community survey showed that, although old people diagnosed by a psychiatrist as having functional psychiatric disorder were not as a group heavy consumers of social services, 40% were judged by a social worker as being in need of services. As the authors suggest, a psychiatric screening instrument could have a valuable part to play in helping social workers, health visitors and general practitioners identify functional mental disorder in the elderly. In Newcastle, medical assessment of applicants for residential care, usually in geriatric day hospital setting, reveals a group of elderly people whose need for residential care is removed by identifying and treating depressive illness. Brocklehurst *et al* (1978) have reported on a similar scheme in Manchester.

It is not unusual to be presented with an elderly patient whose inability to cope with non-progressive impairment may arise because of depressive illness in the principal caring relative or friend rather than the patient herself. All geriatricians can recount anecdotes of domiciliary visits on which they realise that they have been referred the wrong patient and antidepressant therapy for the spouse is the key to the situation. This may be easy enough to recognise in the patient's home but is usually more difficult in outpatient clinic or surgery when the depressed carer does not accompany the alleged patient. Moreover the latter rarely has insight into what is happening usually because of being accustomed to the sick role and sometimes because of feelings of guilt and gratitude towards the carer. The maxim that the proper assessment of any elderly patient must include interviewing the principal carer stands up well in clinical experience.

Side-effects of drugs

As is well known the incidence of adverse reaction to drugs increases steeply with age (Wade 1972); also elderly people are given more drugs than are younger people (Jones *et al* 1980) and make frequent mistakes in taking them.

Drugs are a common cause of confusional states in the elderly and these will be considered in a later section. Here we are concerned with physical disorders which are side-effects of drugs being taken as a consequence of psychiatric illness. Where the drugs are being given for overt psychiatric disease, problems of diagnosis and management rarely arise especially if it is remembered that elderly patients may not be taking the drugs as prescribed and may be taking other things as well. Similarly the particular problems of faulty drug compliance in the demented patient can usually be recognised and should always be anticipated. Misuse of drugs by a patient with an unrecognised depression or a personality disorder may present as apparent physical disease. An example common in clinical practice is chronic benzo-diazepine intoxication which can mimic postural hypotension or non-specific physical disease (Evans & Jarvis 1972). Many elderly patients who crave and, alas, usually obtain continuous supplies of benzodiazepine sleeping tablets from their doctors are depressed and are seeking respite from the world in general and depressive nocturnal ruminations in particular. Chronic impairment from nightly benzodiazepines may be coloured by intermittent acute overdosage. These episodes are not necessarily overtly suicidal and can be passed off as accidental. However, clinical experience has made us sceptical of the 'barbiturate automatism' tradition in which patients confused by one dose of sleeping pills may inadvertently take another. We suspect that, although patients may not recall the multiple doses the following morning, at the time the majority know what they are doing. Under present prescribing practices in primary care it is all too easy for many patients regularly to collect four weeks' supply of sleeping tablets at fortnightly intervals and intermittent or chronic overdosage can pass unrecognised for long periods.

Bromides (Carney 1971) and barbiturates— potent causes of disorder to an earlier generation — are now rarely prescribed as hypnotics for the elderly, although the dogma that barbiturates produce confusion more often than any other hypnotic in the elderly does not appear to be soundly based (Hewick 1979). Nonetheless, because barbiturate overdosage has a higher fatality than poisoning with some other hypnotics, and because barbiturates induce hepatic microsomal enzymes and so increase the risk of osteomalacia, they should continue to be avoided.

Benzodiazepines and other tranquillisers prescribed for day time use are also frequently misused by the depressed elderly paient. The opportunity for this commonly arises because doctors have not appreciated the close relationship between anxiety and depression in the elderly. There also appear to be some doctors who believe that benzodiazepines are antidepressants. Analgesics are also commonly overused by the depressed elderly patient who may then present with dyspepsia, anaemia, gastrointestinal bleeding, or renal failure. These presentations may be sufficiently dramatic to distract physicians from wondering why the patient was taking the offending drug in the first place.

The more bizarre manipulative misuse of drugs sometimes seen in younger adults, diabetics for example, is not common among the elderly although ambiguous non-compliance occasionally raises the issue. Deliberate manipulative poisoning of elderly patients by their care attendants does occur however. Episodes of unexplained confusion, coma, postural hypotension, or loss of control of stably treated conditions such as heart failure, diabetes, or epilepsy in an elderly dependent patient in the community clearly raise the possibility of poor drug compliance. Where the drugs are supervised by a non-demented spouse or other caring relative, the possibility of deliberate misuse of medication has to be considered. Such misuse may represent a minor but perhaps dangerous manifestation of the frustration, anger, or hatred that underlie the physical violence against elderly people of 'granny battering' (Burston 1975). More commonly the motivation is to quieten an active or tiresome demented elderly person to provide some respite for the rest of the household. In some cases the intention is clearly to secure the admission to an acute medical ward of a demented patient that other forms of institutional care are refusing to admit. The underlying problem may be a depressive illness in a principal carer or simply that the burden falling on her (carers, of course, are usually female) is intolerably great. Bergmann *et al* (1978) found evidence that social services departments, in giving priority for domiciliary services to elderly people with no social contacts, may give inadequate support to caring relatives — a policy which is superficially rational but potentially disastrous. In many areas the limited feasibility of domiciliary care for demented elderly patients (Isaacs & Neville 1976) is insufficiently appreciated and, as a consequence, the provision of suitable institutional care is inadequate (Evans 1977). Darker forces may sometimes be at work: the bad husband, drunken and violent to his wife but in old age thrown on her care by a disabling stroke, may suffer not just her taunts and recriminations but also more physical forms of retribution including misuse of medication. Again, the doctor must know the carer as well as the patient.

Consequences of addiction

Apart from overuse of hypnotics, tranquillisers, and analgesics discussed in the previous section, the only common problem of addiction met among the elderly at present is alcoholism. Alcohol-related problems are commoner among the elderly than is generally recognised in Britain (James 1981), although the matter has received more attention in North America (Mayer 1979). The low income of pensioners compared with the population of working age makes the sacrifice necessary to fund an addiction to alcohol that much greater. Chronic subnutrition, inadequate clothing and warmth, and chronic restriction of lifestyle are characteristic markers of the elderly abuser of alcohol. In old men, the diagnosis may be easy enough since for cultural reasons they can drink openly and, since they no longer have to keep up appearances in order to retain employment, may give more honest answers to questions about their alcohol intake than will younger men. Alcohol dependence in elderly women is increasingly being recognised as a clinical problem and is often concealed. A home visit to check the contents of the dustbin for empty bottles or even to raise the occasional loose floorboard may be necessary to prove clinical suspicions. In many cases women start drinking heavily after their husbands die — when the pangs of loneliness, the loss of a sense of shared purpose in living, and the realisation that the future holds nothing to look forward to may prove intolerable. In the past it was not respectable for women to be seen purchasing alcohol in public houses but such social constraints are easing and the availability of alcohol in supermarkets may be contributing to alcoholism among elderly women — as it is also thought to be doing at younger ages.

Medical problems among the elderly which should raise the possibility of a contribution from alcohol dependence include the traditionally associated problems of cirrhosis, liver failure, and the various manifestations of thiamine deficiency — peripheral neuropathy, congestive heart failure, Wernicke's encephalopathy, and Korsakoff's psychosis. More commonly the presenting features are more subtly connected with alcohol. Recurrent falls or fractures, unexplained bruises, incontinence, episodic confusion or even coma, emotional instability and outbreaks of temper or violence, anorexia, weight loss and vomiting, haematemesis or melaena, folate deficient macrocytosis and anaemia, scurvy, gout, persistent non-compliance with prescribed medication, and defaulting from outpatients or day hospital attendances have all provided the primary clue to a previously undetected problem of alcohol dependence in elderly patients.

Very few elderly people with alcohol-related problems present the intense difficulty in management which is characteristic of the young alcoholic. Many, particularly women, have masked bereavement reactions, depressive illness, or social problems that sympathetic concern from a physician and social worker can resolve. Resolution of these problems or even opportunity to discuss them with friendly hearers may terminate the alcohol abuse. Skilled psychiatric treatment is necessary for a proportion of cases and some elderly women of respectable background are so ashamed when they realise their drinking has been detected that they are precipitated into an even deeper despair and require urgent psychiatric assessment. Often we have to recognise that an elderly person is having difficulties at levels of alcohol intake that would not be regarded as very high in society at large. This is partly because of age-associated increased susceptibility to the effects of alcohol, partly because of interaction with physical or mental impairments, and partly because of inadequate money to maintain good nutrition in addition to the alcohol intake.

Consequences of self-neglect

A familiar admission to medical wards is the socially isolated, self-neglected old lady who is admitted because she has become bedfast or incontinent and who may have bed sores and early contractures. Such patients may appear as Section 47 admissions in areas where such legislation is often used (Gray 1980) or may be hustled in with ambiguous consent after shocking the sensibilities of a social worker, neighbour, or relative. Medical investigation commonly reveals evidence of multiple nutritional deficiencies but it is often the bone pain, proximal myopathy and depression of osteomalacia that have precipitated the patient into the bedfast state. The patient's physical problems are clearly secondary to her mental state, and although dementia is one cause, it tends to be overdiagnosed. Paraphrenia may occasionally present in this way but is rare. Some patients in this group are found to be of low intelligence whose social competence in the past has been supported by a marriage partner. Following the death of the partner the unfortunate relict may be totally unable to cope and all her social connections have disappeared with her spouse. (These patients are usually female since, after loss of spouse, a woman is expected to cope better than a man. In the 1971 census the relative prevalence of being in residential care for widowed elderly compared with married (age-adjusted) persons was 5.1 for women but 9.6 for men (Evans 1978). That this sex difference largely reflects social competence and expectations rather than physical health is supported by the finding that the corresponding figures for being in non-psychiatric hospitals on census day were 1.7 and 2.0.)

Depression is a common cause of acquired social incompetence but various interesting personality disorders are also encountered among the non-coping elderly. The old psychopath, usually male with a history of broken marriage, alienated relatives, and poor work record (possibly with misuse of alcohol and minor domestic violence thrown in), is almost as familiar on medical wards as he is in Salvation Army hostels. Some may have been held in thrall by dominant wives and only emerge in their true colours after bereavement, but a history from often hostile and contemptuous children will reveal the long years of hidden personality inadequacy which went before.

Clark *et al* (1975) coined the term 'Diogenes syndrome' in describing a group of elderly patients who lived under conditions of astonishing self-neglect associated with the persistent hoarding of rubbish. These patients, some of whom have no definable psychiatric abnormality (Whitehead 1975) are discussed in Chapter 6. They may present with physical disease through subnutrition and self-neglect but also as victims of vandalism and criminal assault, possibly because of being identified with the archetype of the rich old miser.

PHYSICAL DISORDER
PRESENTING AS PSYCHIATRIC DISEASE

Dementia

Although it is proper to screen demented elderly patients for the recognised treatable causes of secondary dementia, the yield is disappointingly small. This subject is reviewed in Chapter 5.

Depression

Depression is a common reaction to physical disability. The fact that the depression is apparently 'reactive' does not mean that the patient may not benefit from appropriate antidepressant therapy in addition to treatment for the physical disorder. This is not a rationalisation of the 'pill for every ill' philosophy, however; as with all medical care of the elderly, compassionate judgement is necessary. This is particularly true of the depressive reaction to an acute disability. An elderly man who has had to have a leg amputated or an elderly women with a colostomy, particularly where the procedures have been carried out as emergencies and there has been no time for proper psychological preparation, may have to work through a bereavement reaction as intense and prolonged as that following the death of a spouse. The haphazard use of psychotropic drugs during this 'working through' may hinder what is essentially a healing process. If the process is clearly going wrong, skilled psychiatric advice should be part of the treatment; a common problem is arrest in the 'denial' phase in which the patient refuses to take any active role in the management of the impairment.

In addition to being a reaction to overt illness or disability, depression can be a sign or psychological consequence of covert illness. Depression can also be diagnosed because a doctor has misinterpreted a patient's complaint of feeling tired, run down, or generally unwell. Among the elderly, an occult malignancy is a common cause of depression but other more simply treated conditions can present in an identical manner. Tuberculosis particularly has to be remembered by a generation of doctors to whom it is a rare disease. Spinal and other forms of non-pulmonary tuberculosis may give rise to particular diagnostic difficulty among the elderly. Other chronic infections may present as depression with deceptively little in the way of more specific symptoms; pyelonephritis or osteomyelitis, suppurative arthritis (most commonly in a patient with established rheumatoid disease), and infective endocarditis occur often enough to merit special mention.

A physical disease commonly causing diagnostic difficulty by presenting predominantly as a depression in old age is giant-cell arteritis. This pathologically defined disease has been known for more than a decade to present as two characteristic clinical syndromes: cranial arteritis and polymyalgia rheumatica. A third syndrome is now recognised, comprising the anaemia and, usually, the high sedimentation rate, systemic disturbance, and depression common in the other two syndromes but without their specific physical symptoms. This so-called 'steroid-responsive anaemia of the elderly' is likely to be normocytic and normochromic in type, or less commonly of hypochromic microcytic type which is unresponsive to iron therapy. Either is liable to be misinterpreted initially as a manifestation of malignant disease. The response to steroids is dramatic, the depression vanishing as promptly as the other clinical features.

It is difficult to set any general rules about how intensively elderly persons presenting with depression should be investigated for possible physical disease. Undoubtedly where the severity is sufficient to warrant referral to hospital or consideration of moving into sheltered accommodation or residential care, blood count, serum electrolytes, urine analysis, and chest radiography would constitute proper minimal care. These investigations are also appropriate when minor degrees of depression being treated in general practice do not respond to therapy. However, many elderly patients whose depressions do not respond to treatment, do not return to their general practitioners to say so, and many general practitioners are too pre-occupied with other matters to notice. It is unfortunate that appointments systems in general practice have not been devised more for the benefit of patients and less for the convenience of doctors.

Acute confusional states

The abrupt onset of a syndrome comprising spatial and temporal disorientation, dysmnesis with global impairment of intellectual functioning, including difficulty in appropriate focussing and maintenance of attention, is one of the commoner presentations in geriatric medicine. The syndrome may be associated with drowsiness or with hyperactivity, and there may be illusions and delusions — often of persecutory type — leading to aggressive or fearful behaviour. Anxiety is usually present and may be extreme.

Terminology is a problem. It is convenient to use the term 'acute confusional state' as an empirical focussing designation for the clinical syndrome, equivalent, say, to 'acute abdominal pain'. Thus 'acute confusional state' is not a diagnostic but it is a defined syndrome; to use the term loosely may lead to diagnosis errors which are as important as categorising symptoms as acute abdominal pain which are actually in the lower chest. The cardinal feature of the acute confusional state is global cerebral dysfunction: two conditions which are sometimes mistaken for acute confusional states are transient global amnesia and aphasia, both of which represent localised cerebral dysfunction. In transient global amnesia, the patient shows an amnestic syndrome without other evidence of impaired intellect. Thus, although patients are apparently incapable of taking in and retrieving new information and may ask repetitive questions about present and recent events, they are able to carry out complex tasks of daily living which indicates preservation and accessibility of long-term memory, and show no loss of other intellectual functions or disturbance of consciousness. The condition probably reflects bilateral temporal lobe dysfunction, usually of vascular origin, but it may occasionally be epileptic. The state typically lasts a few hours and clears completely but, in the longer term, probably carries the same prognosis as any other form of transient cerebral ischaemia—an increased risk of stroke (Wandless 1981).

Patients who have suffered a dominant hemisphere cerebrovascular accident may show both aphasia and confusion but a jargon aphasia by itself may bear a superficial resemblance to a confusional state. In either case quiet observation and conversation with the patient will often reveal the diagnosis through characteristic dysphasic errors, such as neologisms, paralogisms and syntactic errors, without need for more formal testing. The focal nature of the patient's disability may be demonstrable by non-verbal tests of cognition but usually the striking feature is the preservation of attention and absence of the distractibility characteristic of the delirious patient.

The three groups of disorders commonly presenting to physician or psychiatrist as acute confusional states are functional psychosyndromes, decompensated dementia, and delirium.

Functional psychosyndromes

Many circumstances which are potent precipitants of delirium (see below), such as illness, trauma, or surgical operation, are psychologically as well as physiologically stressful so it is not surprising that functional psychiatric disorders may occasionally be precipitated and be mistaken for delirium in the old as in the young (Goldney & Lander 1979). Hypomania, however readily recognisable by psychiatrists, often presents difficulty to medical and nursing staff unfamiliar with its specific features; at younger ages the absence of slowing in the EEG may assist in the differential diagnosis from delirium but this has not been established as a criterion in the elderly and the practical difficulties in obtaining a satisfactory recording in an acutely confused elderly patient may be formidable. In the acute phase, the differential diagnosis may not be crucial since the symptomatic management of the two conditions is similar and in both conditions it is necessary to search for organic precipitants. Depressive reactions rarely give rise to diagnostic problems but may herald the onset of a delirium.

Other forms of functional psychosyndrome rarely present *de novo* in the elderly and rarely give a picture of acute confusional state as defined above; however they may occasionally give diagnostic difficulty if the history of previous episodes is unknown. A frequent error in the past, happily now less common, was to mistake mild or prodromal delirium for some kind of 'hysterical' reaction. This error can arise because the reaction of some patients to their awareness of intellectual impairment is to appear unconcerned and to attempt to 'laugh it off'. One extreme version of this tactic is to attempt to obscure the real impairment by overlaying it with such obvious deliberate errors as to produce a variant of the Ganser syndrome. In general, all elderly patients presenting with an acute syndrome of intellectual impairment, however 'functional' it may appear, should be assumed to have an underlying delirium and be investigated accordingly.

Decompensated dementia

Many elderly people with dementia adapt to their deterioration in intellect and memory by a progressive restriction of lifestyle so that they never venture outside a circumscribed, familiar and repetitive environment. If the sufferer is married or has a close family this process is usually supported by their providing the high informational redundancy necessary to maintain orientation and compensate for dysmnesis. In most cases, this family support represents a conscious and praiseworthy effort to care for a failing member. In some other instances, the most surprising degree of dementia may simply have passed unnoticed by other family members. This does not necessarily imply low levels of intelligence or perception; some families seem to have a lifelong convention that members, however close emotionally, never elevate their conversation with each other above the cliché and platitude — possibly as a means of avoiding all possibility of contention. In settings such as these, patients with dementia may subsist for long periods in a compensated state. Any disruption of the environment may cause an acute decompensation in which patients are unable to assimilate and adapt to new elements in their surroundings and may also lose confidence in familiar elements because of their altered context. Various crises of modern life in old age may precipitate such decompensation: removal of the spouse or other close supporting figure through death or admission to hospital, rehousing or simply having the decorators in, a well intentioned but ill advised holiday, or the patient's admission to hospital.

In the early stages it may be possible to recognise decompensated dementia for what it is but, after a time, a delirium often supervenes through factors such as lack of sleep, dehydration, and, typically, use of sedative drugs. Some authors believe that delirium can be induced in the demented directly by environmental change alone (Lipowski 1980). This view may possibly be correct but should not be allowed to prevent a search for organic mechanisms and precipitants of delirium in the demented since, as emphasised below, the two conditions commonly occur together. One situation in which the distinction between decompensated dementia and delirium is of great importance arises when the patient is seen in her own home. If the problem is one of decompensated dementia it might be possible to stabilise and manage the patient at home when admission to hospital— the appropriate procedure for many delirious states — would make the situation irretrievable by removing all recognisable and reassuring stimuli. In making the distinction between the two conditions, an accurate history to establish the absence or presence of pre-existing dementia, to identify appropriate decompensating factors, and to exclude possible precipitants of a delirium, is of crucial importance. Phenomenological differences between the two states are variable and quantitative rather than qualitative. The most consistent difference is in attention which, in all but the mildest degrees of delirium, is inconstant and hard to fix. Reduced alertness suggests delirium, as does a major degree of fluctuation in severity of disorientation, particularly if 'lucid intervals' are a feature. The assessment, of course, should include a full physical examination, including measurement of body temperature and examination of urine, since a manifest cause for delirium may be discovered. If doubt remains, the decision whether to admit the patient to hospital (with the risk of precipitating permanent institutionalisation) or to continue management, observation, and investigation at home (thereby risking delayed diagnosis of treatable physical disease) can only be made in full consultation between hospital and primary care teams and the patient's caring relatives or friends. The availability of suitable day hospital facilities undoubtedly contributes to the home care of some patients in this difficult group.

Delirium

Delirium is the commonest form of acute confusional state (as defined above) met with in the elderly and has recently been the subject of a compendious and scholarly review by Lipowski (1980). It is commoner in children and in the old than in young adults. Almost any physical illness or trauma in the elderly may cause or present as a delirium and its management calls for a combination of medical and psychiatric skills both in doctors and nurses. The majority of cases are of relatively abrupt onset, the main diagnostic difficulties arising when an accurate history is not available or, as discussed above, when acute confusion supervenes on a pre-existing dementia. Delirium may last at least as long as the causative factors are present and sometimes longer. This is particularly the case in delirium due to drugs which may continue for weeks or even years (Gilbert 1977).

Diagnostic difficulty may also arise if the delirium is mild or during a prolonged prodromal phase. Initially patients may experience difficulty only in thinking clearly and in concentrating; they may be anxious and irritable. As described earlier they may exhibit disturbed behaviour representing an attempt to deny or obscure their impairment. Sleep disturbance is usual with vivid and usually unpleasant dreams which, if the condition progresses, become increasingly difficult to distinguish directly or in memory from conscious experience. Dysmnesis and inability to maintain focussed attention lead to spatial and temporal disorientation. Misinterpretation of the environment is common — typically taking the form of false recognition. Delusions, particularly of persecutory type, are common but the frequency of true hallucinations probably varies with the cause of the delirium. Obvious anxiety and an appearance of bewilderment are characteristic features of the established delirium. At all stages delirium is usually worst at night and the elderly patient in hospital who becomes anxious and restless during the night should always be suspected of an incipient delirium.

Not every old person who develops an illness becomes delirious and surprisingly little is established about the pathogenesis of delirium. It appears to be the final common pathway of a number of different processes and is usually multifactorial in origin. It is useful to consider causative factors as precipitating or as predisposing and facilitating. First, however, we may consider the mechanism through which these causes produce delirium.

Mechanisms of delirium

Since there are such obvious similarities between the clinical features of delirium arising from widely different causes, there is an understandable desire to identify a singly underlying pathogenic mechanism through which all causes have their ultimate effect. Robinson (1956) postulated a failure of carbohydrate-dependent detoxification processes in the liver as the factor common to toxic deliriums of different causes. Kral (1975) sees delirium as a manifestation of the nervous system's age-associated loss of adaptability, particularly in the centrencephalic and neuroendocrine systems. Several workers, impressed by the dreamlike quality of experience during delirium, have postulated that the essential defect is in the organisation of consciousness, which allows, among other phenomena, the intrusion of dreams into the waking cycle. The evidence to support this view depends heavily on EEG changes in alcohol- and drug-withdrawal states and is not necessarily applicable to other forms of delirium in the elderly (Lipowski 1980). Levy & Gallagher (1978) have suggested that delirium is the result of specific failure in central nervous system inhibitory mechanisms.

Our working hypothesis of the mechanism of delirium is formulated in terms of neural noise and its increase by random or unbalanced neurotransmitter activity in critical pathways of the central nervous system. Gregory (1974) showed that some of the age-associated changes in perception are compatible with an increase in neural 'noise' in the informational sense, that is to say of random neural activity forming the background against which true signals have to be detected and decoded. In functional terms it is useful to view delirium as an exacerbation of neural noise so that environmental simuli are perceived against an increased hubbub of endogenous neural activity that both attenuates the input from the outside world and may be mistaken for it. This interference will affect memory and attention as much as perception and will lead both to an inability to recognise and suppress inappropriate associations and to distractibility. (Studies in the amnestic syndrome of dementia have shown that, in some circumstances at least, defective recall of remembered material is partly due to intrusion of incorrect material (Smith & Swash 1979).) The increased neural noise in delirium will be due ultimately to disorder of neurotransmitter activity. Anoxic or toxic effects on neurones may lead to inappropriate discharge or to failure of discharge secondary to leakage, failure of re-uptake or failure of synthesis of neurotransmitters. Substances modifying neurotransmitter activity produced or released elsewhere in the body may affect central nervous activity. These may include bacterial toxins, drugs, catecholamines, serotonin, and in some circumstances products of bacterial action in the gut. We may further postulate that two reasons why the elderly are more prone to delirium than are younger adults are, first, that neural noise is already increased and, second, that there is an age-associated impairment of the blood–brain barrier to some significant substances. Although the evidence is at present fragmentary, the latter factor could explain the increased central nervous system toxicity of some drugs (Castleden 1980). This increased toxicity has in the past been attributed, probably too readily, to an increased sensitivity of aged neurones to drugs.

While it must be supposed that any drug may sometimes cause delirium in the elderly, there is suggestive evidence that substances which affect particular aspects of neurotransmitter activity are specially significant. The cholinergic system has received most attention and is of interest because of its impairment in the global cerebral dysfunction of senile dementia of Alzhemier's type (Perry 1980, Perry *et al* 1980). Anticholinergic drugs that penetrate the central nervous system are potent precipitants of delirium, even when given as eye drops (Kounis 1974). Summers (1978) has produced evidence for anticholinergic drugs being more widely implicated than is generally recognised in the genesis of delirium after procedures such as cardiac surgery, electroconvulsive therapy, and cataract surgery. Anticholinergic delirium occurs also in the treatment of parkinsonism (Stephens 1967) and is apparently at least a partial explanation for the delirium caused by tricyclic antidepressant drugs (Heiser & Wilbert 1974) — although one must suspect that other neurotransmitter systems may also be involved. Phenothiazines have central anticholinergic properties which may explain their occasional production of delirium and the 'paradoxical' clinical reaction sometimes seen in elderly patients when phenothiazines in small or moderate doses increase rather than improve confusion and agitation.

Several studies have produced evidence that parenteral physostigmine, a cholinergic agent that readily crosses the blood–brain barrier, will rapidly if transiently ameliorate anticholinergic delirium (Duvoisin & Katz 1968) —

the delirium of cataract surgery (Summers & Reich 1979) and of anti-parkinsonism and tricyclic antidepressant therapy (Granacham & Baldessarini 1975) and some other drugs. As already noted, physostigmine has also been shown transiently to improve the dysmnesis of Alzheimer's disease (Smith & Swash 1979). This effect of physostigmine appears to be specific since it is reported to be ineffective in the treatment of delirium tremens (Lipowski 1980). Delirium tremens may be associated with disorders of catecholamine and serotonin systems rather than the cholinergic system. Giacobini *et al* (1960) reported increased noradrenaline excretion in the urine of patients with delirium tremens and, more recently, Banks & Vojnik (1978) found increased levels of 5-hydroxyindoleacetic acid in the cerebrospinal fluid and reduced levels of 5-hydroxytryptamine in the blood of patients with delirium tremens (and also in patients with clozapine-induced delirium). A basic methodological problem, obviously, is to distinguish the causes of delirium from its effects, but these data suggest that the mechanisms of dementia vary with the cause. Rabey *et al* (1977) report on the improvement of L-dopa-induced delirium by tryptophan. Petrie & Ban (1981) have reported rapid improvement in the delirium of some elderly patients by propranolol, a beta-adrenergic blocker which — being lipid-soluble — diffuses easily into the brain. Tyrer *et al* (1981) have also reported a beneficial effect of beta-adrenergic blockade on the severity of symptoms of benzodiazepine withdrawal. These findings suggest that some cases of delirium, perhaps particularly those associated with withdrawal of sedative drugs may be catecholamine mediated. It should be noted, however, that propranolol may on occasion cause delirium (Kuhr 1979), so again the beneficial effect of beta-blockade is specific to certain clinical situations.

It would be of great interest to know to what extent peripheral catecholamines released as an anxiety reaction can penetrate the elderly brain. At younger ages little penetration would be expected. Some neurotransmitters are also vasoactive substances and local release following ischaemic brain damage may interfere with cerebral function by causing changes in blood supply (Meyer *et al* 1976). It is possible that peripherally released catecholamines may have an effect on central nervous function by affecting cerebral blood flow (Loach & Benedict 1980).

Predisposing and facilitating factors

Special studies confirm clinical experience in demonstrating that organic brain damage, particularly the dementias, predisposes to delirium (Morse & Litin 1969, Hodkinson 1973). Hearing and visual defects are also important, both increasing the likelihood of misinterpretation of the environment by the patient and reducing accessibility to reassurance. Clinical experience also suggests that certain personality types are more prone to delirium than others. Kornfeld *et al* (1974) report that the incidence of post-cardiotomy delirium was positively correlated with a pre-operative assessment as a dominant (versus submissive) personality. One may speculate that dominant and obsessional personalities are most likely to experience anxiety at the circumstances of illness and mental obtundation with loss of control over external and mental environment. Bergmann (*Pers. Commun.*) has also suggested that it is the anxiety-prone personality that is most susceptible to delirium. An alternative hypothesis derives from the observations of Cartwright (1966) on the induction of phantasy and dreams by hallucinogenic drugs. This work supported the concept that some individuals are more field-dependent than others; that is to say their concept of reality is more determined by their immediate and current perceptions than that of field-independent subjects who maintain stable concepts of reality less susceptible to immediate perceptions. The first type is more likely to mistake phantasy, dream, or illusion for real experience than is the second.

Sleep disturbance predisposes to delirium, as well as being a feature of it, particularly when there are unresolved opposing influences of consciousness such as the use of hypnotic drugs in a setting not conducive to sleep (the average hospital ward for example). Sleep deprivation due to anxiety, pain, or noise are obvious and manageable problems: less obvious may be sleep disturbance and restlessness due to visceral stimuli from faecal impaction or bladder distension, for an elderly patient may not consciously identify a source of discomfort.

Environmental factors which can precipitate decompensation in dementia also predispose to and facilitate delirium. Unfamiliarity of the environment, inadequate and confusing sensory input, lack of adequate explanation and reassurance are factors of this type which are commonly encountered in hospital. Attempts at physical restraint, also not infrequent in a hospital ward, increase anxiety and feed delusions of persecution. These factors are particularly powerful at night when delirium is probably facilitated by physiological circadian rhythms as well as by the environment.

Precipitants of delirium

Any illness may precipitate a delirium in an appropriately predisposed elderly patient and the list of common causes in Table 3.1 is not comprehensive. Particularly potent are illnesses that, in younger patients, would cause fever. Obviously, this includes any form of infection with pneumonia being the most frequent, partly because it is a common infection and partly because toxins from infected lung tissue may pass directly into the systemic circulation. Urinary tract infection is also important, although there is doubt whether infection confined to the bladder causes delirium without having initiated a pyelonephritis. Asymptomatic urinary infections are so common in old age that one should not too readily assume that a positive urine culture has identified the cause of a delirium in an elderly patient.

Table 3.1   Causes of delirium in the elderly.

Infections	Pneumonia, pyelonephritis,* infective arthritis, peritonitis, infective endocarditis, tuberculosis, cholangitis,* cholecystitis, abscess, cellulitis, bedsores, intracranial (abscess meningitis encephalitis, empyema)
Neoplasms	Intracranial, extracranial
Cerebrovascular	Transient ischaemic attack,* thrombosis, haemorrhage, embolism,* subdural haematoma,* venous sinus thrombosis hyperviscosity syndromes, giant-cell arteritis
Cardio-respiratory	Myocardial infarction, cardiac arrhythmia,* cardiac failure,* pulmonary embolism,* respiratory failure*
Endocrine and metabolic	Ketotic and non-ketotic diabetic pre-coma, hypoglycaemia,* hepatic failure,* hypocalcaemia, hypercalcaemia, hypokalaemia, hyperkalaemia, uraemia, inappropriate ADH syndrome, hyperthyroidism, hypothyroidism, hypothermia,* hyperthermia, thiamine deficiency
Other	Cerebral: trauma, epilepsy.* Non-cerebral: gangrene, abdominal catastrophe
Drugs	See Table 3.2

* Causes of recurrent or relapsing delirium.

As is well known, infections in the elderly may be cryptic — causing few local signs and little systemic reaction apart from delirium. A further diagnostic difficulty is that delirium may precede the appearance of signs and specific symptoms; even in pneumonia this may be by as much as 48 hours. Pelvic sepsis (usually secondary to diverticulitis) and septic arthritis (usually in a patient with rheumatoid disease) are infective conditions worth looking for specifically and blood cultures may demonstrate a bacteraemia even when the source cannot be immediately identified. It is also pertinent to recall that the elderly are one of the higher risk groups for tuberculosis including non-pulmonary forms.

Myocardial infarction, perhaps with no history of pain and no specific physical sign is a well known but still often overlooked cause of delirium. The mechanism is assumed to be a fall in cardiac output and cerebral blood flow, perhaps with hypotension and high catecholamine secretion. An electrocardiogram and estimation of cardiac enymes are essential investigations of a delirium. Cardiac failure is also a cause of delirium, particularly at night, which may be disproportionate to the degree of failure estimated from the physical signs. Transient cardiac arrhythmias without infarction can be particularly difficult to diagnose without ambulatory electrocardiographic recording unless the patient is seen during an attack. Even without the persistent diffuse or border zone brain damage of prolonged ischaemia (Adams *et al* 1966), delirium due to a fall in cerebral perfusion may last some time after normal circulation has been restored. Arrhythmias — most commonly paroxysmal supraventricular tachycardia — are a cause of recurrent delirium and it is in this setting that ECG monitoring may be a justifiable investigation if more easily identified causes such as epilepsy, hypoglycaemia, and drug effects have been excluded. The yield of significant findings on 'blind' ECG monitoring after a single attack of delirium is very small and does not justify the expense of the investigation.

Epilepsy may also need to be considered in the single transient delirium but particularly in recurrent attacks. Although causes such as tumours, intracranial infection, or subdural haematoma may need to be excluded, most cases of epilepsy with onset in old age are vascular in origin and probably 15–20% of patients with stroke develop epilepsy if they survive two years (Fine 1967). Epilepsy may masquerade as recurrent stroke by causing residual neurological signs (Todd's paralysis) lasting up to 24 hours. Eye witness accounts of attacks will often give the diagnosis if they are available but they can mislead since some fits are due to cardiac arrythmias. More commonly no witness of the onset of the attack is available or the epilepsy does not produce grand mal or other typical manifestations. In these cases only the EEG or, in selected cases, a trial of therapy can help with the diagnosis. It is often technically difficult to carry out an EEG in acutely confused patients and the findings are often non-specific, but this investigation is probably more useful in distinguishing intracranial from extracranial causes of delirium than has been generally recognised (Obrecht *et al* 1979). The typical finding in delirium is of symmetrical slow wave activity and asymmetries or focal features suggest intracranial pathology.

Intracranial causes of delirium may give only minor neurological signs that may be difficult to elicit. Sizeable infarcts in the temporal or parietal lobes are easily missed if the specific neurological signs are not searched for and even cortical blindness may pass undiagnosed in an agitated delirious patient. (A syndrome of agitated delirium with visual field defect has been claimed as a specific entity (Medina *et al* 1977).) It is also clear that cerebral infarcts or haemorrhage may cause delirium without producing any localised neurological signs at all. This is one situation in which an EEG, CT scan, or other investigations may be of help. In some cases, probably associated with diffuse patchy ischaemia of the brain, all such investigations may yet be normal. The clinical examination of a confused patient typically requires many brief attempts over a period of hours but simple observation of the patient's behaviour often gives clues to visual field defects, sensory inattention, or agnosias with localising neurological significance. Infarction or haemorrhage are the commonest intracranial causes of confusional states but transient ischaemic attacks, tumours, subdural haematomata and intracranial infections fall within the differential diagnosis and may need specific treatment.

A high proportion of delirious states in elderly patients are caused by drugs. Overdosage may occur accidentally, because of suicidal intent, or through overadministration by others. Interaction between drugs and intercurrent illness may precipitate a reaction to a drug previously well tolerated; a decline in renal function causing digitalis toxicity is the classic example of this. Virtually any drug that has significant pharmacological reaction must be suspected as the possible precipitant of delirium but some of the more common offenders in current practice are listed in Table 3.2. A frequent problem in diagnosis is ascertaining accurately what drug the patient has actually been taking; general practitioner records are sometimes surprisingly misleading in this respect and a home visit and search may be necessary.

In hospital practice, delirium due to drug withdrawal on admission is a common hazard and may be difficult to diagnose particularly since, in the case of benzodiazepines, delirium may not develop until up to a week later (Fruensgaard 1976). Delirium tremens in old men admitted as emergencies to hospital was well recognised and often anticipated by previous generations of kindly clinicians, but the commonest problem now is withdrawal of benzodiazepine hypnotics and tranquillisers (Ayd 1979), although the occa-

Table 3.2 Drugs commonly causing delirium in the elderly (directly or through metabolic effects).

*Benzodiazepine hypnotics and tranquillisers
*Other sedatives and hypnotics
*Antidepressants
Antihistamines
Antispasmodics
Digitalis
Anti-parkinsonism anticholinergics
L-dopa
Hypoglycaemics
*Steroids
Cimetidine
Diuretics
Indomethacin and other non-steroidal anti-inflammatory drugs
*Alcohol
Phenothiazines
Quinidine
Beta-blockers
Anti-epileptics
Hypotensive agents

*Also cause withdrawal delirium.

sional elderly barbiturate addict is still to be encountered. Drug-withdrawal delirium, particularly when hypnotics are to blame, is often surprisingly persistent over two or three weeks or even longer. The simplest solution to such cases might seem to be reinstitution of the offending drug, but this is rarely in the patient's best interest and management of the delirium along conventional lines is to be preferred.

Several of the metabolic causes of delirium listed in Table 3.1 may be the consequences of drugs (Davies 1977). Examples include the various forms of diabetic crisis (with hyperosmolar non-ketotic coma being commoner than ketotic coma in the elderly) hypoglycaemia, hypo- and hyperkalaemia, hypercalcaemia and inappropriate antidiuretic hormone syndrome (Moses & Miller 1974). The last may also occur as a consequence of neoplasms or chest infection and is commoner among the elderly than has been recognised in the past; hyponatraemia usually gives the initial clue to the diagnosis.

Hypocalcaemia (most often due to osteomalacia) and hypercalcaemia (most often due to primary hyperparathyroidism) are not rare findings in the elderly. Hypocalcaemia is more often associated with depression than with delirium but may precipitate epilepsy. Hypercalcaemia due to hyperparathyroidism is most commonly mild and asymptomatic in old age, but hypercalcaemia due to malignancy or vitamin D intoxication may well be sufficiently severe to precipitate delirium. Patients with extensive Paget's disease of bone may become hypercalcaemic if confined to bed.

Thiamine deficiency may present as an acute delirium and the characteristic paralysis of external ocular movements of Wernicke's encephalopathy may appear later or not at all. The condition is more common in males and there is usually a history of alcohol addiction. Pellagra is a further possibility in such a patient but is apparently rare in Britain.

The prognosis of acute delirium, provided that secondary complications such as injury, infection, and dehydration do not occur, is essentially that of the underlying condition. Some such conditions, unfortunately, may turn out to be more serious than is at first supposed. Permanent brain damage may have followed an episode of hypotension due to shock or myocardial infarction (Adams *et al* 1966) and Bedford (1955) drew attention to the fact that postoperative delirium may herald the effects of permanent cerebral damage. Improvements in anaesthetic technique may have reduced the frequency of this complication of surgery in the elderly in recent years.

Principles of management

One of the more vexed questions in the management of elderly patients with delirium is where they should be looked after. There are two cardinal aims in management: the control of symptomatic distress and hyperactivity and the identification and treatment of precipitating organic disease. In some hospital settings these two aims will conflict. Every effort should be made to control the distress and the hyperactivity associated with confusion with as little use of drugs as possible. This will prove difficult if nursing staff are anxious about their ability to contain and control the patient. The necessary resources for physical diagnosis are usually only available in a medical ward or a district general hospital geriatric unit. However, it is not possible to carry out proper physical assessment and investigation of patients who have had to be rendered semi-comatose with drugs to stop them interfering with other seriously ill patients or wandering off the ward on to a busy street. The ideal ambience is a quiet, enclosed, but unrestrictive ward environment staffed by psychiatrically trained nurses in a general hospital and with physicians with expertise in geriatric medicine available to co-operate with psychiatrists in supervising the programme of investigation. This degree of co-operation between psychiatric and medical services may be difficult to attain in the absence of an appropriately orientated psychogeriatric assessment unit (Pitt & Silver 1980).

The principles of non-pharmacological control of delirium follow directly from knowledge of the predisposing and facilitating factors considered earlier. Anxiety is a crucial element and is fed by dysmnesis so that patients are continually in a state of not being sure where they are or what is happening to them. Natural fears that something sinister and dangerous has befallen them will be strengthened if they encounter obvious attempts at restraint or what may appear as physical or even sexual assault. Medical and nursing staff caring for confused patients need continually to try to appreciate what the patients perceive and are likely to deduce from the environment. Clearly they may also be experiencing hallucinations into which insight is impossible. Also one cannot share patients' past experiences which affect their interpretation of the present but one should start from the presumption that most of the patients' reactions and behaviour are reasonable in the context of the immediate environment as they perceive it through the veil of defective perception and dysmnesis.

On the basis of the model of increased neural noise derived from Gregory (1974), attempts should be made to improve patients' perception of the environment by such information–theory based mechanisms as increasing signal/noise ratio, increasing informational redundancy, and encouraging temporal summation. As Gilkes (1979) has emphasised, the aged eye requires higher light levels than are necessary for the young, and bright lighting without dazzle is the more necessary for the confused elderly patient. When approaching a confused patient, one should take care that one's face is fully illuminated and not cast into potentially sinister shadow. Deafness may be a crucial element in a confusional state and, although speaking slowly in a low pitched voice with clear lip movement may be sufficient, more intractable problems are common. Confused patients often have dread of mysterious equipment but intelligent use of specialised hearing aids can help in managing a deaf and confused patient. Just as one should speak slowly to a confused patient one should also move slowly, since haste may be perceived as aggression, or, since actions may be perceived only partially and without context, they may trigger non-specific alarm reactions.

The principle of maximising informational redundancy embraces several of the elements of Reality Orientation therapy which appears to benefit some demented elderly patients (Brook *et al* 1975, Holden & Sinebruchow 1978) but the full Reality Orientation regime is not applicable to acutely delirious patients. Constantly reminding the patient where she is and giving repetitive and reassuring explanations of what is happening is the most obvious way, but by no means the only one, in which informational redundancy can be provided. Clocks, calendars (large and easily read), and windows easily giving a view on the familiar outside world provide continuous cues to time and season. Staff approaching the patient should introduce themselves but should be clearly categorisable in other ways, a prominently carried stethoscope and a traditional bedside appearance and manner will help to identify the physician.

In providing such cues it is important to use signs and stereotypes that will be culturally familiar to the patient, bearing in mind that dysmnesis may have produced some temporal regression. The American literature on Reality Orientation therapy emphasises the use of Christian names in conversing with patients and this practice is increasingly prevalent among social workers and psychiatric nurses in Britain. This well intentioned gesture of friendliness may distress a confused elderly British patient. Owing to dysmnesis she may not remember introductions and to be addressed in such over-familiar fashion by strangers, particularly young strangers, may cause alarm and bewilderment. The patient is placed at a social disadvantage and may feel patronised and humiliated; a slightly more formal old world courtesy may be kinder.

It is important not to add to neural entropy by random or ambiguous stimuli in the environment. Background noise from radio or television, however comforting to ward maids and junior nurses, is bad for the confused patient. The visual environment should be as simple and comprehensible as possible, again bearing in mind the cultural background of elderly patients. When talking to patients every effort should be made to focus their attention; and holding their hand and making sure that other people are not talking or making distracting movements at the same time are aspects of good bedside technique.

Most important of all, people are at least as important as architecture in the environment of a delirious patient, and the presence of a familiar friend or relative can be a crucial therapeutic resource.

Drug therapy

The evidence reviewed earlier, on the special role of agents modifying neurotransmitter activity in the genesis and treatment of delirium, offers hope that specific therapy for delirious states with different underlying mechanisms may become available. At present this approach must be regarded as experimental until more accurate characterisation of the neuro-biochemical disturbances underlying delirium becomes possible. The major drug groups used in the control of delirium are the phenothiazines and the butyrophenone haloperidol. Because these drugs all have potentially serious side-effects, the aim of treatment is to use them as sparingly as necessary to control the patient's distress and non-adaptive behaviour. The delirious patient's anxiety appears to exacerbate the delirium; drugs can be used in smaller cumulative doses if they can be given prophylactically rather than after the delirium is fully established. A patient who regularly becomes delirious at night should be given the chosen therapeutic drug two hours before the symptoms are expected to appear. The patient who is seen at the height of a severe delirium, agitated and aggressive, should be given a large enough dose of a drug to 'switch off' the condition rather than a series of smaller doses which give only partial control and so allow the delirious state to be unnecessarily prolonged.

Phenothiazines have central cholinergic effects and this may partly explain the paradoxical reaction sometimes seen when small doses exacerbate a delirium. In larger doses they are associated with production of hypotension among other side-effects which may be particularly hazardous in the elderly. Haloperidol is probably more effective than chlorpromazine in doses which produce fewer serious side-effects (Ritter *et al* 1972). It can be given by injection, as tablets, or as drops which have little taste and can be included surreptitiously in food or drink if such a deception be considered ethical. A dose of 10 mg given intravenously will usually control the most serious delirium in an elderly patient and smaller oral doses will often suffice. This dose may be associated with dystonic side-effects which, in some circumstances, may need to be controlled with an anti-parkinsonian agent such as benztropine. Such agents are themselves potent producers of delirium and should be used only if the dystonic reaction is so severe as to threaten complication.

For mild forms of delirium, the phenothiazine thioridazine is still widely used in departments of geriatric medicine. In addition to the occasional paradoxical increase in delirium the drug may be insufficiently effective and may cause side-effects such as hypothermia. Its main use appears to be in controlling the sleep disturbance of an early delirium that has not yet produced other clinical features. In this situation chlormethiazole may be a satisfactory alternative.

Patients who have been treated with any of these agents require scrupulous nursing observation and care. This may amount to the full regime appropriate to an unconscious patient if the risks of hypotension, broncho-pneumonia, bedsores, contractures, dehydration, urinary and faecal retention, and the other hazards of the bedfast state in the elderly are to be avoided.

CONCLUSION

In concluding we return to a theme that has recurred in this chapter: proper care of the elderly requires skill and approaches from traditionally separated branches of medicine and nursing. The growing number of the elderly in Western populations requires a coherent response to the total needs of the elderly patient. This response must involve both appropriate degrees of co-operation between specialties and, perhaps more importantly, appropriate education of medical and nursing personnel with more interchange between psychiatric and non-psychiatric training.

REFERENCES

ADAMS G.F. (1974) *Cerebrovascular disability and the ageing brain.* Churchill Livingstone, Edinburgh.

ADAMS J.H., BRIERLEY J.B., CONNOR R.C.R. et al (1966) The effects of systemic hypotension upon the human brain. Clinical and neuropathological observations in 11 cases. *Brain* **89**, 235–68.

AYD F.J. (1979) Benzodiazipines: dependence and withdrawal. *Journal of the American Medical Association* **242**, 1401–2.

BANKS C.M. & VOJNIK M. (1978) Comparative simultaneous measurement of cerebrospinal fluid 5-hydroxyindoleacetic acid and blood serotonin levels in delirium tremens and clozaphine-induced delirious reaction. *Journal of Neurology, Neurosurgery and Psychiatry* **41**, 420–4.

BEDFORD P.D. (1955) Adverse cerebral effects of anaesthesia in old people. *Lancet* ii, 259–63.

BERGMANN K., & EASTHAM E.J. (1974) Psychogeriatric ascertainment and assessment for treatment in an acute medical ward setting. *Age and Ageing* **3**, 174–88.

BERGMANN K., FOSTER E.M., JUSTICE A.W. et al (1978) Management of the demented elderly patient in the community. *British Journal of Psychiatry* **132**, 441–9.

BRINK T.L. (1979) *Geriatric psychotherapy.* Human Sciences Press, London.

BROCKLEHURST J.C., CARTY M.H., LEEMING J.T. et al (1978) Care of the elderly: medical screening of old people accepted for residential care. *Lancet* ii, 141–2.

BROOK P., DEGUN G. & MATHER M. (1975) Reality orientation: a therapy for psychogeriatric patients: a controlled study. *British Journal of Psychiatry* **127**, 42–5.

BURSTON G.R. (1975) Granny-battering. *British Medical Journal* iii, 592.

CARNEY M.W.P. (1971) Five cases of bromism *Lancet* ii, 523–4.

CARTWRIGHT R. (1966) Dream and drug-induced fantasy behaviour. *Archives of General Psychiatry* **15**, 7–15.

CASTLEDEN C.M. (1980) Altered response to psychotropic drugs with ageing. In *The Ageing Brain: neurological and mental disturbances,* eds G. Barbagallo-

Sangiorgi and A.N. Exton-Smith. Plenum Press, New York.

CLARK A.N.G., MANKIKAR G.D. & GRAY I. (1975) Diogenes syndrome. A clinical study of gross neglect in old age. *Lancet* i, 366–8.

DAVIES D.M. (1977) *Textbook of adverse reactions to drugs.* Oxford University Press.

DUVOISIN R.C. & KATZ R.D. (1968) Reversal of central anticholinergic syndrome in man by physostigmine. *Journal of the American Medical Association* **290,** 1963–5.

EVANS J. Grimley (1977) Issues in institutional care in the United Kingdom. In *Care of the Elderly: meeting the challenge of dependency,* eds A.N. Exton-Smith and J. Grimley Evans. Academic Press, New York.

EVANS J. Grimley (1978) Demography and resources. *Medicine Series 3* no 1, 12–14.

EVANS J. Grimley (1981) The Biology of Human Ageing. In *Recent Advances in Medicine No. 18,* eds A.M. Dawson, N. Compston and G.M. Besser. Churchill Livingstone, Edinburgh.

EVANS J. Grimley & JARVIS E.H. (1972) Nitrazepam and the elderly. *British Medical Journal* iv, 487.

FINE W. (1967) Post-hemiplegic epilepsy in the elderly. *British Medical Journal* i, 199–201.

FITZGERALD-FINCH O.P. & GIBSON I.J.J. (1975) Subluxation of the shoulder in hemiplegia. *Age and Ageing* 4, 16–18.

FOSTER E.M., KAY D.W.K. & BERGMANN K. (1976) The characteristics of old people receiving and needing domiciliary services: the relevance of psychiatric diagnosis. *Age and Ageing* 5, 245–55.

FRUENSGAARD K. (1976) Withdrawal psychosis: a study of 30 consecutive cases. *Acta Psychiatrica Scandinavica* **53,** 105–18.

GIACOBINI E., IZIKOWITZ S. & WEGMANN A. (1960) Urinary norepinephrine and epinephrine excretion in delirium tremens. *Archives of General Psychiatry* **3,** 289–96.

GILBERT G.J. (1977) Quinidine dementia. *Journal of the American Medical Association* **237,** 2093–4.

GILKES M.J. (1979) Eyes on light. *British Medical Journal* i, 1681–3.

GOLDNEY R. & LANDER H. (1979) Pseudodelirium. *Medical Journal of Australia* i, 630.

GRANACHER R.P. & BALDESSARINI R.J. (1975) Physostigmine. Its use in acute anticholinergic syndrome with antidepressant and antiparkinson drugs. *Archives of General Psychiatry* **32,** 375–80.

GRAY J.A.M. (1980) Section 47. *Age and Ageing* **9,** 205–9.

GREGORY R.L. (1974) *Concepts and Mechanisms of Perception,* 167–227. Duckworth, London.

HEISER J.F. & WILBERT D.E. (1974) Reversal of delirium induced by tricyclic antidepressant drugs with physostigmine. *American Journal of Psychiatry* **131,** 1275–7.

HELLER S.S., KORNFIELD D.S., FRANK K.A. *et al* (1979) Postcardiotomy delirium and cardiac output. *American Journal of Psychiatry* **136,** 337–9.

HEWICK D.S. (1979) Barbiturate sensitivity in ageing and animals. In *Drugs and the Elderly,* eds J. Crooks and I.H. Stevenson, 211–19. Macmillan, London.

HOLDEN U.P. & SINEBRUCHOW A. (1978) Reality orientation therapy: a study investigating the value of this therapy in the rehabilitation of elderly people. *Age and Ageing* **7,** 83–90.

HODKINSON H.M. (1973) Mental impairment in the elderly. *Journal of the Royal College of Physicians of London* **7,** 305–17.

ISAACS B. & NEVILLE Y. (1976) The needs of old people. The 'interval' as a method of measurement. *British Journal of Preventive and Social Medicine* **30,** 79–85.

JAMES O.F.W. Alcoholism in the elderly. In *Alcohol-related problems — room for manoeuvre*, eds. N. Krasner, S. Madin & R. Walker. John Wiley, Chichester. In Press.

JONES D.A., SWEETNAM P.M. & ELWOOD P.C. (1980) Drug prescribing by GPs in Wales and in England. *Journal of Epidemiology and Community Health* **34**, 119–23.

KAY D.W.K., BEAMISH P. & ROTH M. (1964) Old age mental disorders in Newcastle-upon-Tyne. *British Journal of Psychiatry* **110**, 146–153.

KAY D.W.K., BERGMANN K., FOSTER E.M. *et al* (1966) A four-year follow up of a random sample of old people originally seen in their own homes. A physical social and psychiatric enquiry. *Excerpta Medica International Congress Series No. 150*, Proceedings of the Fourth World Congress of Psychiatry, 1668–70.

KAY D.W.K., BERGMANN K., FOSTER E.M. *et al* (1970) Mental illness and hospital usage in the elderly: a random sample followed up. *Comprehensive Psychiatry* **11**, 1–26.

KENYON F.E. (1964) Hypochondriasis: a clinical study. *British Journal of Psychiatry* **110**, 478–88.

KORNFIELD D.S., HELLER S.S., FRANK K.A. *et al* (1974) Personality and psychological factors in postcardiotomy delirium. *Archives of General Psychiatry* **31**, 249–53.

KOUNIS N.G. (1974) Atropine eye-drops delirium. *Canadian Medical Association Journal* **110**, 759.

KRAL V.A. (1975) Confusional states. In *Modern perspectives in the psychiatry of old age*, ed J.G. Howells, 356–62. Churchill Livingstone, Edinburgh.

KUHR B.M. (1979) Prolonged delirium with propanolol. *Journal of Clinical Psychiatry* **40**, 198–9.

LEVY L.L., & GALAGHER B.B. (1978) Toxic states delirium and epilepsy as expressions of disturbance of inhibitory mechanisms. *International Journal of Neurology* **11**, 356–70.

LIPOWSKI Z.J. (1980) *Delirium. Acute brain failure in man.* C.C. Thomas, Springfield, Illinois.

LOACH A.B. & BENEDICT C.R. (1980) Plasma catecholamine concentrations associated with cerebral vasospasm. *Journal of the Neurological Sciences* **45**, 261–71.

MAYER M.J. (1979) Alcohol and the Elderly: A Review. *Health and Social Work* **4**, 129–43.

MEDINA J.L., CHOKROVERTY S. & RUBINO F.A. (1977) Syndrome of agitated delirium and visual impairment: a manifestation of medial tempro-occipital infarction. *Journal of Neurology, Neurosurgery and Psychiatry* **40**, 861–4.

MELZACK R. (1973) *The puzzle of pain.* Penguin Education, Harmondsworth.

MEYER J.S., WELCH K.M.A., TITUS J.L. *et al* (1976) Neurotransmitter failure in cerebral infarction and dementia. In *Neurobiology of Ageing*, eds R.D. Terry and S. Gershon, 121–38. Raven Press, New York.

MORSE R.M. & LITIN E.M. (1969) Postoperative delirium: a study of etiologic factors. *American Journal of Psychiatry* **126**, 388–95.

MOSES A.M. & MILLER M. (1974) Drug-induced dilutional hyponatraemia. *New England Journal of Medicine* **291**, 1234–9.

MUNRO A. (1980) Monosymptomatic hypochondriacal psychosis. *British Journal of Hospital Medicine* **24**, 34–8.

OBRECHT R. OKHOMINA F.O.A. & SCOTT D.F. (1979) Value of EEG in acute confusional states. *Journal of Neurology, Neurosurgery and Psychiatry* **42**, 75–7.

PERRY E.K. (1980) The cholinergic system in old age and Alzheimer's disease. *Age and Ageing* **9**, 1–8.

PERRY R.H., BLESSED G., PERRY E.K. *et al* (1980) Histochemical observations on cholinesterase activity in the brains of elderly normal and demented (Alzheimer-type) patients. *Age and Ageing* **9,** 9–16.

PETRIE W.M. & BAN T.A. (1981) Propanolol in organic agitation. *Lancet* i, 324.

PITT B. & SILVER C.P. (1980) The combined approach to geriatrics and psychiatry: evaluation of a joint unit in a teaching hospital district. *Age and Ageing* **9,** 33–7.

POST F. (1965) *The clinical psychiatry of late life.* Pergamon, Oxford.

RABEY J.M., VARDI J., ASKENAZI J.J. *et al* (1977) L-tryptophan administration in L-dopa-induced hallucinations in elderly Parkinsonian patients. *Gerontology* **23,** 438–44.

RITTER R.M., DAVIDSON D.E., ROBINSON T.A. (1972) Comparison of injectable haloperidol and chlorpromazine. *American Journal of Psychiatry* **129,** 78–81.

ROBINSON G.W. (1956) Toxic delirious reactions of old age. In *Mental disturbances in later life,* ed O.J. Kaplan, 227–55. University Press, Stanford.

ROSKOS S.R., LERNER S., & KLINE B.E. (1979) The elderly patient in a therapeutic community. *Comprehensive Psychiatry* **20,** 359–69.

SMITH D.P., PILLING L.F., PEARSON J.S. *et al* (1969) A psychiatric study of atypical facial pain. *Canadian Medical Association Journal* **100,** 286–91.

SMITH C.M. & SWASH M. (1979) Possible biochemical basis of memory disorder in Alzheimer's disease. *Age and Ageing* **8,** 289–293.

STEPHENS D.A. (1967) Psychotoxic effects of benzhexol hydrochloride (Artane). *British Journal of Psychiatry* **113,** 213–8.

SUMMERS W.K. (1978) A clinical method of estimating risk of drug-induced delirium. *Life Sciences* **22,** 1511–6.

SUMMERS W.K. & REICH T.C. (1979) Delirium after cataract surgery: review of two cases. *American Journal of Psychiatry* **136,** 386–91.

TYRER P., RUTHERFORD D. & HUGGETT A. (1981) Benzodiazepine withdrawal symptoms and propanolol *Lancet* i, 520–2.

WADE O.L. (1972) Drug therapy in the elderly. *Age and Ageing* **1,** 65–73.

WANDLESS I. (1981) Transient Global Amnesia. *Gerontology.* **27,** 334–9.

WHITEHEAD A. (1975) Diogenes syndrome. *Lancet* i, 627–8.

CHAPTER 4

Psychopharmacology of Old Age

Malcolm Lader

The pharmacological treatment of the organic mental illnesses of old age is still at an experimental stage. Functional psychiatric conditions also tend to increase with rising age, and alongside other therapeutic approaches, their vigorous drug treatment is as necessary in the old as in the young since the cost in terms of personal, social, and societal distress is high. Furthermore, the treatment of these conditions by drugs is no different in principle from that in younger patients (Anderson 1974). It must form part of a general strategy combining drugs with psychotherapy, family counselling, and use of social resources. In addition, physical conditions which often aggravate or even precipitate the mental condition must be treated. Age, however, does modify the choice and use of psychotropic medication because drug actions, both pharmacokinetic and pharmacodynamic, are altered in the elderly. But care must be taken not to overtreat with drugs because of the dangers of drug-induced toxicity (Learoyd 1972).

This chapter discusses the principles of psychotropic drugs usage in the elderly (Bender 1964, 1967, Eisdorfer & Fann 1973, Hollister 1975, Sanathan *et al* 1977). The standard classes of psychotropic agents are outlined with reference to the special problems in old people (Eisdorfer 1975), and the compounds advocated to improve mental functioning in elderly people with failing faculties are examined, although the use of such compounds is not firmly established. This partly arises from the problems of clinical assessment in the elderly (Salzman *et al* 1972), and the problems of conducting adequately controlled clinical trials (Robinson 1967).

CLINICAL PHARMACOLOGY

With age, the body undergoes a wide range of physiological changes which alter the disposition and effects of drugs (Ramsay & Tucker 1981). These can be discussed under two headings: pharmacokinetics, the effect of the body on drugs, and pharmacodynamics, the effect of drugs on the body.

Pharmacokinetics

All four main aspects of pharmacokinetics are altered in old age (Crooks *et al* 1976, Friedel 1978). As gastric secretion declines, *absorption* of drugs from an acid medium is impaired. The disintegration of tablets and solution of capsules is sometimes slower or less complete in the elderly. Intestinal blood flow is decreased (Bender 1965) and absorption may thus be delayed; in itself this is not a disadvantage as drug levels may be less variable and peaked. However, absorption may be impaired (Bender 1968) or delayed to the point that it is incomplete.

Distribution is altered in the elderly. Plasma protein concentration lessens with age so that the amount of drug bound to protein diminishes (Wallace *et al* 1976). More drug is free in the plasma water and hence tissue concentrations will also be higher. Against this, the ratio of body fat to metabolically active tissue increases so a larger proportion of the drug in the body accumulates in the fat and is unavailable (Novak 1972). Psychotropic drugs are generally highly lipid-soluble (lipophilic) so this effect is most pertinent to them. Elderly people have less body mass in general than younger people. Consequently, a standard dose in absolute terms will be a high dose in the elderly in terms of dose per kg body weight—and even more so in terms of dose per kg metabolically active mass (Ritschel 1976).

Cerebral blood flow is decreased in the elderly, and grossly so in patients with cerebral arteriosclerosis. This tends to lessen the effects of drugs as brain perfusion is poor and distribution impaired.

Metabolism of drugs is mainly carried out by the liver microsomal enzymes. The different enzymes that metabolise drugs change in different ways with age. Hydroxylation and demethylation are common metabolic processes and are usually slower in the elderly, sometimes markedly so (e.g. Irvine *et al* 1974). By contrast, conjugating processes (e.g. with glucuronic acid) are little changed.

Finally, renal capacity steadily declines with age (Hansen *et al* 1970, Triggs *et al* 1975), resulting in diminished renal *clearance* of drugs, but it is unclear whether this is of clinical significance (Klotz *et al* 1975). The kidney also seems more susceptible to toxic effects.

Overall, ageing is associated with a definite prolongation of the action of most, but not all, psychotropic drugs. As a general rule, therefore, the action of a dose of a drug will be longer, sometimes several fold, in an aged person than in a young or middle-aged adult.

Pharmacodynamics

Much less is known of the mechanisms whereby elderly people respond differently than younger people to the same tissue concentration of drug

(Bender 1974). The responsitivity of tissue systems to drugs in general declines with old age (Reidenberg 1980). Whether this is related to a change in the number of receptors, in their affinity for the drug, or in the coupling between surface receptor and intracellular processes is unclear (Bender 1974). Perhaps several mechanisms operate.

Practical implications

Generally then, the elderly are more sensitive than the young to drugs (Salzman *et al* 1975), by a factor of up to about three. The dose of a drug, as well as having a more pronounced effect, also acts for longer, and consequently less drug is needed less often (Cole & Stotsky 1974). It is prudent to initiate treatment with 30–50% of the normal adult dose and to increase it gradually. Frail, thin, physically ill patients may respond to even lower proportional doses (Davies *et al* 1973). Some elderly patients, however, need and tolerate full doses. Clinical judgement is needed to arrive at the therapeutic dose without pushing the dose too rapidly and risking toxicity or edging the dose up too slowly and delaying the therapeutic response. The important factor is the half-life of the drug since it takes 4–5 times this period for steady-state kinetics to be reached. In the elderly, with prolonged drug half-lives, it may take a week in the case of amitriptyline or a month in the case of diazepam for this level to be achieved.

As a general rule, dosage should be more frequent in the elderly than in younger individuals. Thus, thrice-daily is preferable to twice-daily and twice-daily to once-daily. In this way, peaks in body levels will be less pronounced as the daily dose is divided up. However, the half-lives of many compounds are so prolonged in the elderly that smaller doses at *less* frequent intervals are justifiable. Once the body levels have built up, the increase following each dose is not proportionately large. In addition, the simpler the regimen, the better the compliance. Therefore, less frequent dosage should be aimed at. With drugs which have marked side-effects, such as the tricyclic antidepressants, single daily doses are feasible when given at night but not at other times. Even so, a once-nightly dosage may be hazardous in a physically frail or ill patient because of cardiotoxic effects following the absorption of a single large dose.

Sustained release preparations are the logical answer to providing a smooth, low-profile absorption curve — thereby avoiding toxicity in the elderly. However, such preparations require sophisticated formulation such as plastic matrices and the change in characteristics of these vehicles in the elderly has not been studied much.

Because of possibly impaired disintegration and absorption of tabletted drugs, liquid preparations (such as elixirs) are often to be preferred. Care should be taken in switching from one formulation to another lest the bio-availabilities differ significantly.

Drug interactions

Psychotropic drugs have many pharmacological actions, as best instanced by the antipsychotic drugs, the antidepressants, and lithium. They can therefore interact with some of the many other drugs — psychotropic and non-psychotropic — with which elderly people who tend to have multiple pathology (both physical and psychiatric) are commonly treated simultaneously (Learoyd 1972). However, the whole topic of drug interactions is uncertain: although many interactions, both pharmacokinetic and pharmacodynamic, can be demonstrated in animal preparations, it is much less clear which are important in clinical practice. The general rule must be the fewer drugs the better. There is no rationale for combining several drugs of the same class.

Questions about concomitant medication are particularly important in the elderly. If possible, close relatives or friends should be asked about drugs being taken and over-the-counter, patent medicines should also be enquired for. Where several drugs are being taken, hospital admission may be necessary to rationalise the treatment or to withdraw the patient from, say a barbiturate. Confusion in the elderly may be due to overmedication with psychotropic drugs and unsuspected drug interactions may elevate body levels of drug. The general metabolic state, such as salt depletion or thyroid insufficiency, may also alter drug effects and such metabolic alterations are commonest in the elderly.

ANTIDEPRESSANT DRUGS

Depression is the most common psychiatric disorder of late life up to the age of 75 (Blazer 1980) and both recurrences and first episodes occur frequently in the elderly. The presence of adverse personal and social circumstances should not mislead the doctor into making only half-hearted attempts to alleviate symptoms of depression in an elderly individual. What seems hopeless to a person when depressed, may seem tolerable when the mood reverts to normal. Response to medication is often particularly gratifying and rapid in older subjects.

Drug therapy, as always, must be a part of a coherent and flexible treatment schedule. Physical illness must be carefully sought as this may have led to the depressed state, or the symptoms of depression may mimic physical complaints (Dunn & Gross 1977, see also Chapter 3). The social and personal background of the patient should be assessed with respect to various strengths and weaknesses. Thus, the outlook for a depressed old man cared for by his wife is much better than for an isolated widower. Compliance is particularly poor in the elderly, probably because side-effects are more troublesome. Social support is not only helpful in a general way but also increases compliance.

Tricyclic antidepressants with sedative effects are generally preferred in the elderly because the clinical picture typically contains anxiety or agitation (Kantor & Glassman 1980). Amitriptyline is still very popular but has marked anticholinergic effects and some suspicion of cardiotoxicity. Imipramine is somewhat less sedative and doxepin is also recommended for the elderly. Of the newer drugs, mianserin is almost devoid of anticholinergic effects, is usefully sedative, and is much less cardiotoxic than its predecessors. A phenothiazine is often effective in agitated depression but usually as an adjunct to tricyclic antidepressants.

Because elderly people are generally sensitive to these drugs (as pointed out above), it is customary to start treatment with a third or a half of the usual dosage. Thus, for a frail old lady, 10 mg of amitriptyline or imipramine three times a day is appropriate. The dosage can then be increased cautiously but, in some cases, full dosage is eventually required. It is a mistake to assume that all elderly people will require a smaller dosage. The rate of increase is 25–50 mg per week for an outpatient, and faster for inpatients who are under close supervision. Dosage should be divided. The single dose at night which is preferred in some younger patients (Ayd 1974) is not advisable in the elderly because side-effects may be troublesome in the morning and, if the patient wakes at night, the side-effects (such as blurred vision, difficulty in micturition and dry mouth) may be excessive. Frightening dreams may also occur. Elderly patients find it difficult to remember to take thrice-daily dosage so the best compromise is to administer the drug night and morning in roughly equal proportions.

If the patient is not showing some improvement by the end of three weeks, or if side-effects are marked, monitoring of plasma concentrations of tricyclic antidepressants may give quite useful help. If the concentration is below the therapeutic level (roughly about 50 ng per ml), the dose of the drug should be increased. If the concentration is high (more than about 200 mg per ml), then the dosage should be lowered. However, this is only a guideline and some patients fail to respond whatever the concentration, while others respond to quite high levels.

Failure of response to tricyclics should lead to their gradual withdrawal over the course of a week before alternative treatment is substituted. Other drugs such as MAO inhibitors may be considered. However, these have a particular propensity for producing side-effects in the elderly, and postural hypotension may preclude attainment of adequate dosages for MAO inhibition. L-tryptophan is worth considering in doses of 3–6 g per day, either alone or with a tricyclic antidepressant. Its only appreciable side-effect is drowsiness so it is also indicated when side-effects to the tricyclic drug are too great. Evidence to-date suggests that L-tryptophan is fairly effective in mildly and moderately depressed patients but should not be used in the severely depressed, where ECT remains the treatment of choice.

Drug therapy is generally maintained for several months after response has occurred. Early withdrawal often results in relapse which, in the elderly patient, may occur suddenly and markedly. As the depression lifts, appropriate social measures may be instituted (Lippincott 1968). In particular, social isolation must be reversed by day hospital or day centre attendance, and membership of clubs. It is worth trying to persuade an elderly person to join an interest group which caters for all ages rather than an old age group. Some patients seem prone to relapse whenever drug therapy is withdrawn. They should be maintained on their drug but monitored over the years and the dosage adjusted as necessary. Some patients suffer fairly regular cyclical illnesses and the dosage should be increased at the expected time.

Side-effects with the tricyclic drugs are more marked in the elderly. Anticholinergic effects include toxic confusional psychosis, dry mouth, blurred vision, constipation, and urinary problems (Salzman *et al* 1975). Constipation may be particularly troublesome in the elderly and acute retention of urine may occur. The patient should be questioned about bowel habits and elderly males about existing symptoms of urinary hesitancy. Cautious dosage is required. Glaucoma is usually exacerbated by tricyclic antidepressants which are thus contraindicated. Mianserin is probably safe in this indication, as are nomifensine and trazodone, but cautious dosage should be used with expert monitoring.

Cardiovascular effects include ECG and myocardial changes (Cole & Stotsky 1974). A pretreatment ECG is a wise precaution to exclude arrhythmias which will tend to be worsened by tricyclic antidepressants. Either hypotension or hypertension may be induced. Hypotensive episodes can be quite severe and should be treated by bedrest and by reducing medication. The antihypertensive effects of such drugs as guanethidine, bethanidine, debrisoquine, and clonidine are attenuated by most tricyclic antidepressants. A diuretic or a beta-adrenoceptor blocking agent should be substituted as these do not interact with tricyclic antidepressants. Alternatively, or in addition, the patient's depression can be treated with mianserin or L-tryptophan — neither of which interact significantly with antihypertensive therapy.

Other side-effects may be troublesome. Manic swings or activation of schizophrenic symptoms may supervene. The dose should be reduced and antipsychotic medication added. Overdose is serious with most antidepressants and this should be borne in mind when choosing both the antidepressant and the size of the prescription. Mianserin, nomifensine, and L-tryptophan seem much safer.

Other treatments include antipsychotic medication combined with antidepressants to reduce severe agitation. Sedatives and hypnotics may be needed to lessen anxiety or induce sleep but should be used sparingly and for no more than three months; benzodiazepines are the sedative hypnotics of choice. Barbiturates should never be instituted in the elderly. Stimulant drugs such as amphetamine have no place in antidepressant therapy.

Lithium

Manic illnesses are not as uncommon in the elderly as used to be thought. Before the introduction of major tranquillisers and of lithium, the prognosis used to be poor, symptoms sometimes persisting and necessitating long-term institutionalisation. Lithium is being used increasingly in the aged as manic states are more frequently recognised and as the patient population maintained on lithium ages.

The half-life of lithium is prolonged 50–100% in the elderly mainly due to reduced renal clearance. Also, elderly patients seem more sensitive to lithium than are younger patients. Lithium should be started at a low-dose (250–400 mg/day of the carbonate in divided doses) and gradually increased. For the treatment of mania, serum concentrations of 0.8–1 mmol/l are usually sufficient. For the prevention of recurrent affective episodes, even lower concentrations may suffice.

The side-effects of lithium are many and generally, in the elderly, resemble those in younger patients; they include anorexia, vomiting, diarrhoea, and tremor as warning signs of incipient toxicity. The elderly are prone to develop memory disturbance and even confusion as a toxic effect of lithium which is thus another cause of pseudosenile dementia. Polyuria with polydipsia is another common side-effect and is a particular problem in the elderly who may complain of intolerable nocturia with many wakenings in the night to urinate. Hypothyroidism can also occur and may precipitate an elderly person with marginal thyroid function into frank myxoedema.

Electrolyte imbalance may result in lithium toxicity. The use of diuretics in the elderly must be very careful as must be any attempt to alter the diet of someone maintained on lithium. Renal disease, acute or of insidious onset, may also lead to lithium toxicity.

ANTIPSYCHOTIC DRUGS

The aged commonly suffer from psychotic illnesses. Schizophrenic disorders may occur as prolongations of earlier breakdowns or as paranoid states of late onset. Affective disorders may be severe and psychotic in intensity. Organic brain disorders may also result in psychosis. In all these instances, antipsychotic drugs are indicated for symptomatic relief of the condition (Tsuang *et al* 1971). In the late paranoid ('paraphrenic') states, response to antipsychotic medication may be very gratifying but in other conditions response may be modest (Birkett & Boltuch 1972).

The choice of antipsychotic medication is governed by two main considerations: the desirability of sedation and the pattern of side-effects tolerated by the individual patient (Davis *et al* 1973). Many antipsychotic drugs, such as chlorpromazine and thioridazine, are sedative (Altman *et al* 1973); this may be useful in an agitated patient but unnecessary or even unwanted in other patients, especially those characterised by inertia who may spend their day dozing and quickly lose touch.

The main side-effects are anticholinergic and extrapyramidal; these effects tend to counterbalance each other in that compounds with marked anticholinergic effects are generally less liable to induce extrapyramidal reactions than drugs with weak anticholinergic properties. Other side-effects which can be troublesome are hypotension and ECG changes. The extrapyramidal effects resemble those in younger individuals but dystonias are uncommon and akathisia infrequent. However, as agitation is frequent in the elderly, it is important to distinguish this from akathisia lest the dose of antipsychotic drug be mistakenly increased. The patient usually retains insight into akathisia, regarding it as foreign to himself, whereas he typically regards his agitation as justified by his predicament. Akinetic parkinsonism is the commonest extrapyramidal effect in the elderly; it begins within a few weeks of starting treatment but usually fades away after a few months. Unless the severity of the patient's clinical condition precludes this, it is best to treat the symptoms by lowering the dose of antipsychotic drug rather than by adding an antiparkinsonian drug. The latter course is liable, especially in the elderly, to lead to excessive anticholinergic effects with severe constipation, retention of urine, or toxic psychosis. There is also evidence that the effects of a number of antipsychotic drugs are negated by the addition of some antiparkinsonian agents, probably by an induction effect in the liver. Under no circumstances should an antiparkinsonian drug be prescribed routinely with an antipsychotic drug.

The most worrying extrapyramidal effect is tardive dyskinesia (Greenblatt *et al* 1968). This is found most commonly in the elderly, partly because they will have been longest on antipsychotic medication if they are chronically ill and partly because brain damage and degeneration may predispose to the disorder. There is a spontaneous prevalence of tardive dyskinesia in 1 or 2% of elderly people who have never taken antipsychotic drugs. The condition can occur after only a few months' treatment but is generally delayed for several years. It is commoner in patients treated with the injectable depot drugs than in those maintained on oral medication. Because of the high prevalence of this condition and the difficulty in treating it, it is imperative to review each patient's antipsychotic medication at regular intervals.

The anticholinergic activity of antipsychotic drugs produces a range of symptoms. Some, such as thioridazine, have powerful anticholinergic effects in moderate or high dosage approaching that of a standard dose of atropine. Dry mouth, blurring of vision, raised intra-ocular pressure, constipation, and urinary hesitancy are some of the symptoms. A central anticholinergic syndrome has been described which comprises memory impairment, disorientation, anxiety, restlessness and perceptual disturbances such as visual illusions and hallucinations. The danger of misdiagnosing this condition is greater in the elderly where psychotic conditions tend to be more pleomorphic than in younger patients. Treatment consists of lowering the dose of antipsychotic medication and withdrawing any antiparkinsonian medication.

Severe orthostatic hypotension can be a particular problem in the elderly. It may manifest itself as recurrent ischaemic attacks, cerebral or cardiac, or as confusion. Fainting can occur and may lead to falls and fractured limbs. Taking the blood pressure with the patient first recumbent and then standing may suggest the degree of alpha adrenergic block which underlies the condition and thus allow the clinician to warn the patient of possible problems. Treatment of the established condition comprises bed rest; sympathomimetic drugs are not indicated. In less severe states, the dose of antipsychotic medication can be slightly lowered. Haloperidol is less likely to produce hypotension than are the phenothiazines (Tobin *et al* 1970). Although haloperidol is more likely to produce extrapyramidal effects, these are often not a great problem in older subjects. Haloperidol is also available in parenteral form and can be invaluable in treating the acutely disturbed patient.

ECG abnormalities comprise prolongation of the QT interval, lowering and inversion of the T-wave and a variety of arrhythmias. They are particularly associated with thioridazine. Patients with pre-existing cardiac problems should be monitored by ECG as antipsychotic medication is instituted or the dosage is raised.

As with other drugs used in the elderly, dosage of antipsychotics should be initially modest and increment gradual (Ayd 1975). Oral medication is generally preferred to injections because of the reduced muscle mass in the elderly. Thioridazine is popular despite its anticholinergic effects as these seem better tolerated by the elderly than extrapyramidal effects. For patients with mild psychotic symptoms, agitation and restlessness, promazine is often effective, and is almost devoid of extrapyramidal effects.

ANTI-ANXIETY AND HYPNOTIC DRUGS

These are the most widely prescribed of all psychotropic drugs; indeed, by some yardsticks, they are the most widely prescribed of all drugs. However, their use is attended by some controversy and the ratio of benefits to dangers is least in the elderly (Dawson-Butterworth 1970, Gershon 1973).

The barbiturates were most used until the benzodiazepines ousted them a decade or so ago. The benzodiazepines are more effective, much safer in overdosage, less likely to induce dependence, and to interact with other drugs. The barbiturates are poorly tolerated by the elderly who may become sleepy and oversedated, or even ataxic, stumbling and confused (Gershon

1973); toxic delirious states have been reported. An insidious impairment of intellectual performance may occur and may lead to hospital admission under the mistaken idea that a dementing process is present. Despite these major drawbacks, barbiturates are still used and prescribing figures suggest that their usage is appreciable in the elderly. In most cases, the use of barbiturates has persisted for many years but careful review should be made and gradual withdrawal of the barbiturate considered.

Although the benzodiazepines have largely replaced the barbiturates, their widespread use in the elderly cannot be advocated (Linnoila & Vinkari 1976, Hall 1973). Many of the side-effects of the barbiturates are produced by benzodiazepines as well — ataxia and confusion being most notable. The use of benzodiazepines in the elderly should therefore be restricted to patients with marked primary anxiety.

The benzodiazepines have complex metabolic patterns but can be roughly divided into two groups: 1 chlordiazepoxide, diazepam, medazepan, clorazepate and clobazam which have active metabolites and metabolic pathways of oxidation and demethylation and 2 lorazepam, temazepam and oxazepam which have no active metabolites and are inactivated by conjugation with glucuronic acid (Breimer *et al* 1980). In general, glucuronic acid conjugation capacity is maintained in the elderly whereas the ability to oxidise and demethylate drugs wanes. Thus, the half-life of diazepam is, on average, at least twice as long in the elderly as in younger people, whereas that of lorazepam is unchanged. It follows that, if a benzodiazepine is used, it is preferable to try oxazepam or lorazepam as unduly prolonged half-lives are unlikely. Even so, elderly people are more sensitive to benzodiazepines than younger patients (Reidenberg 1980), even allowing for pharmacokinetic differences; in addition, dosages should be conservative (Greenblatt & Shader 1980). Inco-ordination, tremor, ataxia, and confusion should be sought and the dosage lowered if they ensue. Muscle relaxation may be excessive (Linnoila & Vinkari 1976). Benzodiazepines, even in normal doses, can produce dependence with abstinence symptoms of the barbiturate type on withdrawal.

Alternatives to the benzodiazepines include meprobamate and sedative antihistamines, but they are not as effective. Antipsychotic drugs such as thioridazine in low doses have been widely used as antianxiety agents, especially in the elderly. They are quite effective in this context but produce more side-effects, and the danger of eventual tardive dyskinesia cannot be ruled out.

With all these antianxiety agents, patients should be warned about driving and operating dangerous machinery. Interactions with alcohol are often marked.

With hypnotic drugs similar considerations apply. The continued administration of hypnotic drugs is common in the elderly. Sleep requirements wane with age and further problems can arise if the old person spends some time napping during the day. Some indigent elderly spend a lot of time in bed because it is the only place they feel warm. Older people take longer to fall asleep than younger people, have more frequent awakenings, and have little and sometimes no deep (slow-wave) sleep. Chronic administration of hypnotics to induce sleep can itself lead to insomnia. Whenever attempts are made to discontinue or merely to reduce the dose of hypnotic, rebound insomnia may ensure with disturbing effects on the old person. Thus, the use of hypnotics in the elderly for sleeping disorders should be minimal. If the insomnia is associated with depression or anxiety, treatment should be of the primary affective disorder, with perhaps the bulk of the dose of the antidepressant or anxiolytic at night to induce sedation and sleep.

The main indication for hypnotics is in the short-term management of acute stress- or situational-related insomnia in the absence of a primary affective state. The commonest hypnotics are now the benzodiazepines, although there are still many old people being maintained on barbiturates. The two benzodiazepines most widely used as hypnotics are nitrazepam (in Europe) and flurazepam (in the USA). Nitrazepam is fairly long-acting with a mean half-life of over 24 hours, and longer in the elderly. Although flurazepam itself has a short half-life of a few hours, its main metabolites have long half-lives. Thus, both nitrazepam and flurazepam have cumulative effects in the elderly even when given in modest dosage. Daytime sedation is likely and may be appropriate if the patient is anxious or agitated; however this is a drawback in patients who wish to maintain their alertness during the day. For the latter, the bulk of elderly insomniacs, a shorter-acting compound such as temazepam or triazolam may be more appropriate.

Many other compounds have been used as hypnotics in the elderly. Alcohol is a favourite self-administered nostrum (Black 1969) and may help lessen anxiety and induce sleep (Ching-Piao 1971, Ching-Piao *et al* 1973, Mishara & Kastenbaum 1974). However, sleep later in the night may be more broken after alcohol and its diuretic effect is troublesome in the elderly. The barbiturates depress respiration to some extent and may also lead to confused states. Glutethimide, methyprylon, ethchlorvynol and methaqualone have all been used as hypnotics in the elderly but their merits are not evident. Chlormethiazole, with its short duration of action, has achieved popularity in some countries: results seem quite good and its dependence potential seems low in the modest dosages used.

Apart from morning sedation and forgetfulness, hypnotics carry the danger of producing confusion and unsteadiness of gait in the night if the patient wakes up to go to the toilet. General measures such as subdued lighting and clear signs lessen this problem but even so the use of powerful hypnotics in the elderly is not to be embarked on lightly.

DRUGS AFFECTING MENTAL FUNCTIONING

Central nervous system stimulants

Caffeine is a mild cerebral stimulant and widely used as a 'pick-me-up'. However excessive use of coffee can produce symptoms of anxiety, especially in the elderly. More powerful stimulants include pentylenetetrazol, magnesium pemoline, methylphenidate and amphetamine. Pentylenetetrazol is an analeptic agent which is sometimes used in elderly patients to increase their alertness and thereby enhance motivation and ability to learn. Methylphenidate and amphetamine are sympathomimetic stimulants: the former has been extensively used to treat the elderly, especially in the USA. Uncontrolled studies were mildly encouraging but controlled studies have been few so that the possible value of these drugs remains controversial (Crook 1979). Against the reports of enhancement of new learning must be set the drawbacks — increased sympathomimetic activity with some of the drugs, decreased appetite, increased irritability, and perhaps psychotic manifestations. In most patients the drawbacks outweigh the advantages but occasionally a patient with cognitive deficits does well on a stimulant drug such as methylphenidate or magnesium pemoline.

Vasodilators

Vasodilator drugs have been advocated in the treatment of 'arteriosclerotic' dementia but the rationale is unclear. Arteriosclerotic blood vessels are incapable of dilating and the general bodily vasodilatation results in a lowering of blood pressure and hence a diminution, not an increase, in cerebral perfusion (Regli *et al* 1971).

The rationale for using vasodilators in arteriosclerotic dementia was extended to senile and Alzheimer's dementia because cerebral blood flow is diminished in these conditions (Obrist *et al* 1970, Simard *et al* 1971). However, the diminution is a consequence, not a cause, of the dementia so increase in blood flow is not likely to exercise any useful effect.

The three drugs most widely used as vasodilators in the treatment of dementia are papaverine, isoxsuprine and cyclandelate. The results with papaverine suggest some improvement in mental functioning (Dunlop 1968, Bazo 1973, Smith *et al* 1968) but it is doubtful whether this justifies the side-effects, namely postural hypotension, flushing, dizziness, headaches, and sweating (Stern 1970). Cyclandelate has been available for over 25 years and many studies have examined its effects. Unfortunately, almost all have been uncontrolled or the assessment of change in mental function has been cursory. Of those studies which reach adequate criteria of design, execution and interpretation (Yesavage *et al* 1979), several show some positive effects of the drug on mental functioning, but only a few report practical benefit (Hall 1976, Fine *et al* 1970, Young *et al* 1974, Judge *et al* 1973). This problem bedevils much of the work in the area of dementia. Although bloodflow may alter (Eichhorn 1965), test results may improve (Ball & Taylor 1967, Smith *et al* 1968), or mood may lighten or stabilise, the practical consequences—both in the day-to-day management of the patient and in longer term prognosis—are nugatory. Some trials were negative (e.g. Westreich *et al* 1975). Isoxsuprine has been evaluated in even fewer trials and there is little firm evidence that it has beneficial effects, let alone that these are of practical value (Affleck *et al* 1961). This beta-adrenergic stimulant may actually decrease cerebral blood flow and it has the expected side-effects of hypotension, flushing, and tremor.

Hyperbaric oxygen has been used extensively to improve cerebral oxygenation in patients with multi-infarct dementia. Despite early encouraging uncontrolled studies, controlled evaluations have failed to establish any therapeutic utility (Thompson *et al* 1976, Goldfarb *et al* 1972).

Mixed vasdodilator/cerebral 'activators'

These drugs have complex actions which produce some vasodilatation but in addition alter cerebral metabolism in an ill-understood way. It is believed that they improve the utilisation of glucose and oxygen, thereby improving dementia especially of the vascular type. Naftidrofuryl improves the oxidative capacity of animal brains and alters the metabolism of glucose; it also protects against the metabolic effects of hypoxia. When 300 mg of the drug was given to human volunteers exercising on a bicycle ergometer, blood pyruvate levels were found to be significantly greater and lactate/pyruvates ratios were significantly reduced, suggesting that the drug can enhance cellular oxidative activity (Shaw & Johnson 1975). Parallel results were obtained in patients with arterial occlusive disease. Several controlled trials against placebo have been carried out in a variety of patients, mainly elderly people with mental deterioration and confusion, sometimes associated with cerebral vascular disorders. Overall, naftidrofuryl proved superior to placebo, improving such variables as ability to concentrate, memory, social adaptation, alertness, and intellect (Admani 1978, Branconnier & Cole 1977, Bouvier *et al* 1974, Judge & Urquhart 1972, Gerin 1974, Brodie 1977). However, not all the studies showed the same pattern of improvement and improvement in test function or in general condition was not always paralleled by useful clinical improvement. In some instances, deterioration seemed to slow. Quite evidently, further studies are needed to establish this drug's role in the therapeutics of old age.

Dihydroergotoxine is a mixture of three hydrogenated alkaloids of ergot. It has complex neuronal effects which are perhaps related to its actions on enzyme systems in the brain, together with improved cerebral circulation. Despite its widespread use in several countries, it is not well-documented and controlled trials are few (Hughes *et al* 1976, McDonald 1979, Jennings 1972, Rao & Norris 1972). A wide variety of functions have been assessed and, in general, drug effects are scanty and rather inconsistent from trial to trial (Gaitz *et al* 1977, McConnachie 1973, Rehman 1973). Overall, some improvement occurs in social skills and general activity (Thibault 1974), but cognitive function is not generally augmented (Roubicek *et al* 1972). As the most beneficial outcomes have been reported in patients with depression and retardation, it may be acting primarily as an antidepressant (Rosen 1975). Indeed, although these compounds are alpha-adrenergic antagonists, they also inhibit the re-uptake of catecholamines — an action of standard antidepressants. Side-effects include hypotension and sinus bradycardia and prolonged use may lead to vascular insufficiency and even gangrene of the extremities, particularly in patients with pre-existing vascular insufficiency.

Cerebral 'activators'

Meclofenoxate is a drug which modifies cerebral neuronal metabolism without producing vasodilatation. It reduces the need of the brain for oxygen and is claimed to improve memory function. Evidence for its efficacy in improving tests functions is not compelling and its clinical effectiveness is unestablished (Oliver & Restell 1967); further studies are needed (Gedye *et al* 1972).

Piracetam, deanol, propranolol, procaineamide (Gerovital) (Jarvik & Milne 1975), and various vitamins have all been advocated in the treatment of cerebral deterioration in the elderly. No adequate evidence supports their use although some encouraging results have been reported (e.g. Gustafson *et al* 1978, Cohen & Ditman 1974, Zung *et al* 1974, Mindus *et al* 1976).

FUTURE DEVELOPMENTS

The area of intellectual deterioration in old age was relatively poorly researched until quite recently. However, interest has focussed recently on Alzheimer's disease (Bowen *et al* 1977). Neurochemical studies have shown that the typical neuropathological changes are associated with a deficit in choline acetyltransferase, the enzyme which synthesises acetycholine (Davies & Maloney 1976, Perry *et al* 1977). The postsynaptic muscarinic receptors remain intact, suggesting a presynaptic neuronal degeneration (Davies & Verth 1978). It is not clear whether other neurotransmitters are also involved (Adolfsson *et al* 1979). The aetiology of the degeneration is similarly unclear but may be related to abnormalities in microtubular protein.

Acetylcholine is important in memory functions — anticholinergic drugs such as atropine and scopolamine impairing memory (Drachman 1977, Drachmann & Levit 1974), cholinomimetic drugs enhancing it. Thus, compounds increasing brain acetylcholine levels have been suggested in the treatment of Alzheimer's dementia, as L-dopa is used in parkinsonism. Choline availability governs the synthesis of acetylcholine and the neuronal uptake of choline may be impaired in Alzheimer's disease. However, increasing choline concentrations in the body does seem to result in increased acetylcholine turnover in the brain. Another way of increasing acetylcholine concentrations is to administer lecithin.

It is too early to evaluate the effect of lecithin administration. Results in studies where choline or lecithin has been given over a very short time to patients with Alzheimer's disease have not been encouraging (Glen 1980). In patients with well established disease, little change has been noted. In earlier, mild cases, some improvement in test functioning and in some behavioural measures was noted. Thus, the utilisation of the increased choline supplies may be deficient, either because uptake is a limiting factor or because the neurones are unable to synthesise acetylcholine in any significantly increased amounts (Glen & Whalley 1979).

An alternative approach is to block the breakdown of acetylcholine with a cholinesterase inhibitor. Unfortunately, there is no long-acting compound capable of crossing the blood–brain barrier. Physostigmine (eserine) is short-acting and has to be injected. Some improvements in memory have been reported in patients with Alzheimer's disease given physostigmine or the direct muscarinic agonist, arecoline. The latter approach is potentially the most rewarding as it does not depend on acetylcholine synthesis for its therapeutic mode of action. Further developments of cholinomimetic drugs will be awaited with interest.

REFERENCES

ADMANI A.K. (1978) New approach to treatment of recent stroke. *British Medical Journal* ii, 1678–9.

ADOLFSSON R., GOTTFRIES C.G., ROOS B.E. *et al* (1979) Changes in the brain catecholamines in patients with dementia of Alzheimer type. *British Journal of Psychiatry* **135**, 216.

AFFLECK D.C., TREPTOW K.R. & HERRICK H.D. (1961) The effects of isoxsuprine hydrochloride (Vasodilan) on chronic cerebral arteriosclerosis. *Journal of Nervous and Mental Diseases* **132**, 335–8.

ALTMAN H., METHA D., EVENSON R.C. *et al* (1973) Behavioral effects of drug therapy on psychogeriatric in patients. I. Chlorpromazine and thioridazine. *Journal of the American Geriatrics Society* **21**, 241–8.

ANDERSON W.F. (1974) Administration, labelling and general principles of drug prescription in the elderly. *Gerontologia Clinica* **16**, 4–9.

AYD F.J. (1974) Single daily dose of antidepressants. *Journal of the American Medical Association* **230**, 263–4.

AYD F.J. (1975) The depot fluphenazines: a reappraisal after 10 years clinical experience. *American Journal of Psychiatry* **132**, 491–500.

BALL J.A.C. & TAYLOR A.R. (1967) Effect of cyclandelate on mental function and cerebral blood flow in elderly patients. *British Medical Journal* iii, 525–8.

BAZO A.J. (1973) An ergot alkaloid preparation (Hydergine) versus papaverine in treating common complaints of the aged: double-blind study. *Journal of the American Geriatrics Society* **21**, 63–71.

BENDER A.D. (1964) Pharmacological aspects of aging: A survey of the effect of increasing age on drug activity in adults. *Journal of the American Geriatrics Society* **12**, 144–34.

BENDER A.D. (1965) A pharmacodynamic basis for changes in drug activity associated with aging in the adult. *Experimental Gerontology* **1**, 237–47.

BENDER A.D. (1967) Pharmacologic aspects of aging: additional literature. *Journal of the American Geriatrics Society* **15**. 68–74.

BENDER A.D. (1968) Effect of age on intestinal absorption. Implications for drug absorption in the elderly. *Journal of the American Geriatrics Society* **16**, 1331–9.

BENDER A.D. (1974) Pharmacodynamic principles of drug therapy in the aged. *Journal of the American Geriatrics Society* **22**, 296–303.

BIRKETT D.P. & BOLTUCH B. (1972) Chlorpromazine in geriatric psychiatry. *Journal of the American Geriatrics Society* **20**, 403–6.

BLACK A.L. (1969) Altering behavior of geriatric patients with beer. *Northwest Medicine* **68**, 453–6.

BLAZER D. (1980) The diagnosis of depression in the elderly. *Journal of the American Geriatrics Society* **28**, 52–8.

BOUVIER J.B., PASSERON O. & CHUPIN M.P. (1974) Psychometric study of Praxitene. *Journal of International Medical Research* **2**, 59–65.

BOWEN D.M., SMITH C.B., WHITE P. *et al* (1977) Chemical pathology of biochemical measurements on human post-mortem brain specimens. *Brain* **100**, 397–426.

BRANCONNIER R.J. & COLE J.O. (1977) A memory assessment technique for use in geriatric psychopharmacology: drug efficacy trial with naftidrofuryl. *Journal of the American Geriatrics Society* **25**, 186–8.

BREIMER D.D., JOCHEMSEN R., VON ALBERT H.H. (1980) Pharmacokinetics of benzodiazepines; short-acting versus long acting. *Arzneimittelforschung* **30**, 875–81.

BRODIE N.H. (1977) A double-blind trial of naftidrofuryl in treating confused elderly patients in general practice. *Practitioner* **218**, 274–8.

CHING-PIAO C. (1971) Psychiatric treatment of geriatric patients: 'pub' or drug? *American Journal of Psychiatry* **127**, 1070–5.

CHING-PIAO C., STOTSKY B.A. & COLE J.O. (1973) Psychiatric treatment for nursing home patients: Drug, alcohol and milieu. *American Journal of Psychiatry* **130**, 543–8.

COHEN S. & DITMAN K.S. (1974) Gerovital H3 in the treatment of the depressed aging patient. *Psychosomatics* **15**, 15–19.

COLE J.O. & STOTSKY B.A. (1974) Improving psychiatric drug therapy. A matter of dosage and choice. *Geriatrics* **29**, (6) 74–8.

CROOK T. (1979) Central-nervous-system stimulants: appraisal of use in geropsychiatric patients. *Journal of the American Geriatrics Society* **27**, 476–7.

CROOKS J., O'MALLEY K. & STEVENSON I.H. (1976) Pharmacokinetics in the elderly. *Clinical Pharmacokinetics* **1**, 280–96.

DAVIES P. & MALONEY A.J.F. (1976) Selective loss of central cholinergic neurons in Alzheimer's disease. *Lancet* ii, 1403.

DAVIES P. & VERTH A.H. (1978) Regional distribution of muscarinic acetylcholine receptor in normal and Alzheimer's type dementia brains. *Brain Research* **138**, 385–92.

DAVIS J.M., FANN W.E., EL-YOUSEF M.K. *et al* (1973) Clinical problems in treating the aged with psychotropic drugs. *Advances in Behavioral Biology* **6**, 111–25.

DAWSON-BUTTERWORTH K. (1970) The chemopsychotherapeutics of geriatric sedation. *Journal of the American Geriatric Society* **18**, 97–116.

DRACHMAN D.A. (1977) Memory and cognitive function in man: does the cholinergic system have a specific role? *Neurology* **27**, 783–90.

DRACHMAN D.A. & LEVITT J. (1974) Human memory and the cholinergic system. *Archives of Neurology* **30**, 113–21.

DUNLOP E. (1968) Chronic cerebrovascular insufficiency treated with papaverine. *Journal of the American Geriatric Society* **16**, 343–9.

DUNN C.G. & GROSS D. (1977) Treatment of depression in the medically ill geriatric patient: a case report. *American Journal of Psychiatry* **134**, 448–50.

EICHHORN O. (1965) The effect of cyclandelate on cerebral circulation: a double-blind trial with clinical and radio-circulographic investigations. *Vascular Diseases* **2**, 305–15.

EISDORFER C. (1975) Observations on the psychopharmacology of the aged. *Journal of the American Geriatric Society* **23**, 53–7.

EISDORFER C. & FANN W.E. (1973) *Psychopharmacology and Aging*. Plenum Press, New York.

FINE E.W., LEWIS D., VILLA-LANDA I. *et al* (1970) The effect of cyclandelate on mental function in patients with arteriosclerotic brain disease. *British Journal of Psychiatry* **117**, 157–61.

FRIEDEL R.O. (1978) Pharmacokinetics in the geropsychiatric patient. In *Psychopharmacology: A Generation of Progress*, ed M.A. Lipton, A. DiMascio, and K.F. Killam, 1149–505. Raven Press, New York.

GAITZ C.M., VARNER R.V. & OVERALL J.F. (1977) Pharmacotherapy for organic brain syndrome in late life. Evaluation of an ergot derivative vs placebo. *Archives of General Psychiatry* **34**, 839–45.

GEDYE J.L., EXTON-SMITH A.N. & WEDGWOOD J. (1972) A method for measuring mental performance in the elderly and its use in a pilot clinical trial of meclofenoxate in organic dementia. *Age and Aging* **1**, 74–80.

GERIN J. (1974) Double-blind trial of naftidrofuryl in the treatment of cerebral arteriosclerosis. *British Journal of Clinical Practice* **28**, 177–78.

GERSHON S. (1973) Antianxiety agents. *Advances in Behavioral Biology* **6**, 183–7.

GLEN A.I.M. (1980) The pharmacology of dementia. *Hospital Update* **10**, 977–88.

GLEN A.I.M. & WHALLEY J. eds (1979) *Alzheimer's Disease: Early Recognition of Potentially Reversible Deficits*. Churchill Livingstone, Edinburgh.

GOLDFARB A.I., HOCHSTADT N.J., JACOBSON J.H. *et al* (1972) Hyperbaric oxygen treatment of organic mental syndrome in aged persons. *Journal of Gerontology* **27**, 212–17.

GREENBLATT D.J. & SHADER R.I. (1980) Effects of age and other drugs on benzodiazepine kinetics. *Artzneimittelforschung* **30**, 886–90.

GREENBLATT D.L., DOMINICK J.R., STOTSKY B.A. *et al* (1968) Phenothiazine-induced dyskinesia in nursing-home patients. *Journal of the American Geriatric Society* **16**, 27–34.

GUSTAFON L., RISBERG J., JOHANSON M. *et al* (1978) Effects of piracetam on regional cerebral blood flow and mental functions in patients with organic dementia. *Psychopharmacology* **56**, 115–17.

HALL M.R.P. (1973) Drug therapy in the elderly. *British Medical Journal* iii, 582–4.

HALL P. (1976) Cyclandelate in the treatment of cerebral arteriosclerosis. *Journal of the American Geriatrics Society* **24**, 41–5.

HANSEN J.M., KAMPMANN J. & LAURSEN H. (1970) Renal excretion of drugs in the elderly. *Lancet* i, 1170.

HOLLISTER L.O. (1975) Drugs for mental disorders of old age. *Journal of the American Medical Association* **234**, 195–8.

HUGHES J.R., WILLIAMS J.G. & CURRIER R.D. (1976) An ergot alkaloid preparation (Hydergine) in the treatment of dementia: critical review of the clinical literature. *Journal of the American Geriatrics Society* **24**, 490–7.

IRVINE R.E., GROVE J., TOSELAND P.A. *et al* (1974) The effect of age on the hydroxylation of amylobarbitone sodium in man. *British Journal of Clinical Pharmacology* **1**, 41–3.

JARVIK L.F. & MILNE J.F. (1975) Gerovital-H3: A review of the literature. In *Aging* eds S. Gershon and A. Raskin, 203–27. Raven Press, New York.

JENNINGS W.G. (1972) An ergot alkaloid preparation (Hydergine) versus placebo for treatment of symptoms of cerebrovascular insufficiency: double-blind study. *Journal of the American Geriatrics Society* **20**, 407–12.

JUDGE T.G. & URQUHART A. (1972) Naftidrofuryl — A double-blind cross-over study in the elderly. *Current Medical Research Opinion* **1**, 166–72.

JUDGE T.G., URQUHART A. & BLAKEMORE C.B. (1973) Cyclandelate and mental functions: a double-blind cross-over trial in normal elderly subjects. *Age and Aging* **2**, 121–24.

KANTOR S.J. & GLASSMAN A.H. (1980) The use of tricyclic antidepressant drugs in geriatric patients. In *Psychopharmacology of Aging,* ed C. Eisdorfer, and W.E. Fann, 99–118. MTP Press, Lancaster.

KLOTZ U., AVANT G.R., HOYUMPA A. *et al* (1975) The effects of age and liver disease on the disposition and elimination of diazepam in adult men. *Journal of Clinical Investigation* **55**, 347–59.

LEAROYD B.M. (1972) Psychotropic drugs and the elderly patient. *Medical Journal of Australia* **1**, 1131–3.

LINNOILA M. & VINKARI M. (1976) Efficacy and side effects of nitrazepam and thioridazine as sleeping aids in psychogeriatric in-patients. *British Journal of Psychiatry* **128**, 566–9.

LIPPINCOTT R.C. (1968) Depressive illness: identification and treatment in the elderly. *Geriatrics* **23**, (11), 149–52.

MCCONNACHIE R.W. (1973) A clinical trial comparing 'Hydergine' with placebo in the treatment of cerebrovascular insufficiency in elderly patients. *Current Medical Research and Opinion* **1**, 463–8.

MCDONALD R.J. (1979) Hydergine: a review of 26 clinical studies. *Pharmakopsychiatrie* **12**, 407–22.

MINDUS P., CRONHOLD B., LEWANDER S.E. *et al* (1976) Piracetam-induced improvement of mental performance. *Acta Psychiatrica Scandinavica* **54**, 150–60.

MISHARA B.L. & KASTENBAUM R. (1974) Wine in the treatment of long-term geriatric patients in mental institutions. *Journal of the American Geriatrics Society* **22**, 88–94.

NOVAK L.P. (1972) Aging, total body potassium, fat-free mass, and cell mass in males and females between ages 18 and 85 years. *Journal of Gerontology* **27**, 438–43.

OBRIST W.D., CHIVIAN E., CRONQVIST S. *et al* (1970) Regional cerebral blood flow in senile and presenile dementia. *Neurology* **20**, 315–22.

OLIVER J.E. & RESTELL M. (1967) Serial testing in assessing the effect of mec-lofenoxate on patients with memory defects. *British Journal of Psychiatry* **113,** 219–21.

PERRY E.K., PERRY R.H., BLESSED G. *et al* (1977) Necropsy evidence of central cholinergic deficits in senile dementia. *Lancet* i, 189.

RAMSAY L.E. & TUCKER G.T. (1981) Drugs and the elderly. *British Medical Journal* **282,** 125–7.

RAO D.B. & NORRIS J.R. (1972) A double-blind investigation of hydergine in the treatment of cerebrovascular insufficiency in the elderly. *Johns Hopkins Medical Journal* **130,** 317–24.

REGLI F., YAMAGUCHI T. & WALTZ A.G. (1971) Cerebral circulation. Effects of vasodilating drugs on blood flow and the microvasculature of ischemic and nonischemic cerebral cortex. *Archives of Neurology* **24,** 467–74.

REHMAN S.A. (1973) Two trials comparing 'Hydergine' with placebo in the treatment of patients suffering from cerebrovascular insufficiency. *Current Medical Research and Opinion* **1,** 456–62.

REIDENBERG M.M. (1980) Drugs in the elderly. *Bulletin of the New York Academy of Medicine* **56,** 703–14.

RITSCHEL W.A. (1976) Pharmacokinetic approach to drug dosing in the aged. *Journal of the American Geriatrics Society* **24,** 344–54.

ROBINSON R.A. (1967) Some problems of clinical trials in elderly people. *Gerontologia Clinica* **3,** 247–57.

ROSEN H.J. (1975) Mental decline in the elderly: pharmacotherapy (ergot alkaloids versus papaverine). *Journal of the American Geriatrics Society* **23,** 169–74.

ROUBICEK J., GEIGER C. & ABT K. (1972) An ergot alkalloid preparation (Hydergine) in geriatric therapy. *Journal of the American Geriatric Society* **20,** 222–9.

SALZMAN C., KOCHNASKY G.E. & SHADER R.I. (1972) Rating scales for geriatric psychopharmacology — a review. *Psychopharmacology Bulletins.* **8,** no 3, 3–50.

SALZMAM C., SHADER R.I. & HARMATZ J.S. (1975) Response of the elderly to psychotropic drugs: predictable or idiosyncratic? *Psychopharmacology Bulletin* **II,** no 4, 48–50.

SATHANANTHAN G.L., FERRIS S. & GERSHON S. (1977) Psychopharmacology of Aging: Current Trends. *Current Developments in Psychopharmacology* **4,** 250–64.

SHAW S.W.J. & JOHNSON R.H. (1975) The effect of naftidrofuryl on the metabolic response to exercise in man. *Acta Neurologica Scandinavica* **52,** 231–7.

SIMARD D., OLESEN J., PAULSON O.B. *et al* (1971) Regional cerebral blood flow and its regulation in dementia. *Brain* **94,** 273–88.

SMITH W.L., LOWREY J.B. & DAVIS J.A. (1968) The effects of cyclandelate on psychological test performance in patients with cerebral vascular insuficiency. *Current Therapeutic Research* **10,** 613–18.

SMITH W.L., PHILIPPUS M.J. & LOWREY J.B. (1968) A comparison of psychological and psychophysical test patterns before and after receiving papaverine HCL. *Current Therapeutic Research* **10,** 428–31.

STERN F.H. (1970) Management of chronic brain syndrome secondary to cerebral arteriosclerosis, with special reference to papaverine hydrochloride. *Journal of the American Geriatric Society* **18,** 507–12.

THIBAULT A. (1974) A double-blind evaluation of 'Hydergine' and placebo in the treatment of patients with organic brain syndrome and cerebral arteriosclerosis in a nursing home. *Current Medical Research and Opinion* **2,** 482–87.

THOMPSON L.W., DAVIES G.C., OBRIST W.D. *et al* (1976) Effects of hyperbaric oxygen on behavioral and physiological measures in elderly demented patients. *Journal of Gerontology* **31,** 23–8.

TOBIN J.M., BROUSSEAU E.R. & LORENZ A.A. (1970) Clinical evaluation of haloperidol in geriatric patients. *Geriatrics* **25**, (6), 119–122.

TRIGGS E.J., NATION R.L., LONG A. *et al* (1975) Pharmacokinetics in the elderly. *European Journal of Clinical Pharmacology* **8**, 55–62.

TSUANG M.M., LU L.M., STOTSKY B.A. *et al* (1971) Haloperidol vs thioridazine for hospitalized psychogeriatric patients: double-blind study. *Journal of the American Geriatric Society* **19**, 593–600.

WALLACE S., WHITING B. & RUNCIE J. (1976) Factors affecting drug building in plasma of elderly patients. *British Journal of Clinical Pharmacology* **3**, 327–30.

WESTREICH G., ALTER M. & LUNDGREN S. (1975) Effects of cyclandelate on dementia. *Stroke* **6**, 535–8.

YESAVAGE J.A., TINKLENBERG J.R., HOLLISTER L.E. *et al* (1979) Vasodilators in senile dementias. A review of the literature. *Archives of General Psychiatry* **36**, 220–4.

YOUNG J., HALL P. & BLAKEMORE C.B. (1974) Treatment of the cerebral manifestations of arteriosclerosis with cyclandelate. *British Journal of Psychiatry* **124**, 177–80.

ZUNG W.W.K., GIANTURCO D., PFEIFFER E. *et al* (1974) Pharmacology of depression in the aged: evaluation of Gerovital H-3 as an antidepressant drug. *Psychosomatics* **15**, 127–31.

CHAPTER 5

The Dementias of Old Age

Raymond Levy & Felix Post

The diagnosis and management of demented patients are the bread and butter of the psychiatry of old age and almost all the chapters in this volume deal with various aspects of the dementias of late life. Also, in accordance with the importance of the subject, there have been several recent publications which have dealt with it most expertly and exhaustively, among them one from the Office of Health Economics (1979) dealing mainly with British experience and a review chapter by Jarvik (in press) from the North American angle. Biological aspects are particularly well discussed in Lishman's (1978) textbook of organic psychiatry.

The present chapter does not attempt to deal exhaustively with the subject which pervades the whole book. Instead, an attempt will be made to furnish the reader with points of reference concerning terminology, epidemiology, clinical features, management and outlook for the future.

DEFINITIONS

Dementia should be narrowly and precisely defined. Especially in later life, many persons suffer impairment of memory, of learning ability, abstract thinking, problem solving, as well as decline of affectivity and social awareness. These defects may be associated with brain disorders, with somatic illnesses impairing cerebral functioning (Chapter 3), with toxic effects (Chapter 3), or with emotional disturbances (Chapter 6). Since no lasting damage to neurones or brain structure has occurred, this kind of impairment is usually fully reversible, occasionally spontaneously, but more usually with appropriate treatment. When the onset is sudden and the duration short, the conditions have been defined as *acute confusional states*. Slower development or longer duration is often indicated by using the term *subacute confusion*. Under unfavourable circumstances, arising from delayed treatment or from the occurrence of cerebral damage, there may be only incomplete mental recovery. The patient is left with various cognitive and personality defects which may, however, remain stationary over many years. The patient is not progressively *dementing,* but is certainly *demented.* Examples of these end-states are the sequelae of severe head injury and of tardily treated myxoedema or subdural haematomata.

In this chapter, the term 'dementia' will be reserved for progressive conditions with a gradual decline of cognitive and other cerebral functions leading ultimately to death. Dementias thus defined are always associated with detectable neuronal or other structural brain pathology associated with a disease process.

The psychiatrist working with old people will obviously encounter patients with dementias which have started before the age of 65 — the various kinds of presenile dementias. With the exception of Alzheimer's disease which will be discussed under senile dementia, these will not be described here but have been described briefly in Chapter 1. The main concern will be with the recognition and management of two groups of disorders: the *senile dementias* and the *multi-infarct dementias*. The International Classification of Diseases — ICD9 (WHO 1978) — includes these under Senile and Pre-Senile Organic Psychotic Conditions (290) but, unfortunately, perpetuates an outmoded subdivision and terminology. For example, separate subcategories are given for senile dementia: simple type (290.0), senile dementia, depressed or paranoid type (290.2), and senile dementia with acute confusional state (290.2). It is difficult to see any justification for maintaining such subcategories since any dementing patient may, at times, show depressive or paranoid symptoms. Where a confusional state is superimposed, it would be preferable to include a second diagnosis since the system allows for one under 293.0 Acute Confusional State. The ICD9 also uses the term 'arteriosclerotic dementia' (290.4) for what is now more commonly referred to as multi-infarct dementia.

EPIDEMIOLOGY

Like other major mental illnesses, the dementias of old age occur with roughly equal frequencies in all human populations which have been studied, regardless of culture and race. Clearly, their number has become a problem only in civilisations with a high adult survival rate. In the United Kingdom, it is estimated (Central Statistical Office 1979) that the population over the age of 74 will increase between 1977 and 1991 from 2.9 to 3.6 million. In the USA, a similar increase has been forecast (Redick & Taube 1980). As will be shown below, some 20% of these very old people will develop clear-cut dementia.

The preponderance of old women over old men in the population will increase further and disproportionately, also, as will also be shown, old women are especially prone to senile dementia. Even in industrialised Western countries, incidence is far lower than prevalence. Only a small proportion of dementing old people come to the notice of medical services on account of behaviour disturbance or psychological impairment and one in five dements is at present cared for in public institutions rather than in the community.

These and other methodological considerations have been exhaustively discussed by Kay & Bergmann (1980), who have also compared prevalence figures yielded by a number of competently carried out surveys. In summary, the following emerged: prevalence figures for dementia in old age vary between 3% and 14% overall and between 20% and 30% in those over the age of 80. Although there are, of course, more women than men at risk, women are only significantly more often demented over the age of 80. Below that age, dementing disorders are somewhat more common in men. Multi-infarct dementias predominate in men below the age of 75. Above 75, senile dementia is as frequent as multi-infarct dementia but senile dementia is much more frequent in females. The above observations apply to well established dementia, but in view of the difficulties of early diagnosis, figures for the prevalence of early or mild dementia differ considerably between studies.

SENILE DEMENTIA

General considerations and aetiology

There has been considerable dispute over the years about whether this condition really exists as a disease. Several issues can be isolated from this continuing debate: 1 the distinction from normal ageing, 2 the relationship to Alzheimer's disease, 3 the attempt to attribute the condition to extracerebral causes, and 4 the largely cosmetic attempts to invent new names to avoid the use of what is felt to be a derogatory term. It is now generally agreed that, although age-related, the condition is quantitatively and probably qualitatively different from normal ageing. This is evidenced by the high proportion of elderly people who remain cognitively intact. The distinction from Alzheimer's disease is more problematical. Alzheimer himself considered his eponymous disease as a variant of senile dementia but opinions have been divided ever since. There is little doubt that, from the neuropathological point of view, there is little to distinguish the two conditions (see Chapter 1) and the same neurochemical abnormalities have been observed in both. On the other hand, there have been suggestions that there might be genetic differences. In particular, Larsson *et al* (1963) have implicated a major dominant gene in the transmission of senile dementia and Sjogren *et al* (1952) have favoured polygenic inheritance for Alzheimer's disease. The current view held by the majority of workers in the field is that Alzheimer's disease and senile dementia are one and the same and this is reflected by the increasing use of the term senile dementia of Alzheimer type

(SDAT). Nevertheless, the age of onset may have a bearing both on the progress of the disease and on the clinical picture, younger patients being more likely to show focal parietal or temporal lobe dysfunction and tending to be more severely affected and dying more rapidly (Constantinides *et al* 1978, Jacoby & Levy 1980a, Naguib & Levy 1982). The attempt to implicate largely extracerebral causes was particularly popular among British geriatricians in the seventies and led to the use of the term 'chronic brain failure' (Caird & Judge 1974). It is to be hoped that it will now be given a quiet burial. Other attempts to use alternative terminology include the North American 'chronic brain syndrome' which now appears to be on the decline (DSM III 1980) and the largely administrative British neologism 'elderly mentally infirm'. The latter is now enshrined in a number of official government publications concerning the allocation of resources and is mentioned here for the benefit of perplexed readers who may not be familiar with its use.

As far as causative factors are concerned, no firm evidence has yet been advanced to support any apart from hereditary predisposition. Larsson *et al* (1963) suggested that the aggregate mortality risk in the most closely observed group of relatives was of the order of 4.3 times that for the general population. A useful, more recent summary of the genetic evidence is given by Zerbin-Rüdin (1975).

Clinical features and recognition

Senile dementia has a slow and gradual onset and may be very difficult to recognise at an early stage. Indeed, there are suggestions that subjects who develop the condition may show poor cognitive performance as much as 20 years previously (Jarvik & Blum 1971). Although neurotic and depressive symptoms are rarely seen as precursors of dementia, restlessness, irritability, increasing egocentricity, suspiciousness, and dysphoric states, as well as atypical obsessive compulsive disorders may occasionally occur before any intellectual impairment has become obvious. It is therefore good practice to subject every ageing patient to a brief memory and orientation questionnaire such as that devised by Quershi & Hodgkinson (1974). However, clinical and psychological tests are of limited value in the recognition of incipient dementia unless they are administered at spaced intervals.

The problem of *benign senescent forgetfulness* has been well summarised by one of the originators of the concept (Kral 1978). Slowing and decline of learning and of mnestic abilities are general phenomena of ageing (Chapter 2) and older people are often well aware of their difficulties with recall, particularly of names. Such difficulties may be exacerbrated by anxiety which is sometimes provoked by psychological testing. There are some useful distinctions between benign and pathological memory defects. For instance, subjects with benign forgetfulness may forget part of an experience or a task, but never the whole of it. They tend to retain insight into their disability and usually respond well to cues; this is in contrast to dementing patients who fill in memory gaps with various kinds of confabulation and tend to mix up recent and past events. Normal age changes tend to be patchy whereas those in dementia more often develop as an orderly march of events. The differences between the memory dysfunction of dementia and that due to ageing have been fully documented by Miller (1974).

Related to the concept of benign senile forgetfulness is that of *doubtful dementia*. A community survey (Bergmann *et al* 1971) has shown that, when followed-up, only few subjects originally described as doubtfully demented, developed overt dementia. Most of the subjects so described turned out to have been underprivileged, unintelligent old people, often with neurotic–depressive complaints. There is an urgent need to develop reliable ways of diagnosing senile dementia in the early stages so that any methods which are developed to arrest or slow down the progress of the disease may be applied before incapacitating and irreversible damage has occurred.

At the moment, patients are likely to be brought to our knowledge only after disabilities have become obvious to families and family doctors. In that situation, the main task is to differentiate senile dementia from other disabling conditions. It is obviously essential to assess and record the patient's mental state with special emphasis on cognitive performance. In this regard, a brief screening test is essential. An example of such a questionnaire covering orientation, memory for past personal events, for general events, and for recent personal events is that which has been used in our unit for many years (Institute of Psychiatry 1973). There are a number of equally useful questionnaires, some of which have been subjected to detailed validation (Chapter 2). It is important to record the patient's answers verbatim so that they can be reviewed as a whole. In this way, a particular pattern of defects may emerge and one may assess whether these are patchy or global; also, mild perseveration may be spotted. Where previous intelligence is in doubt, a brief vocabulary test (e.g. the Mill Hill) should be administered as poor performance in the recall of general events may be merely a reflection of low verbal intelligence rather than a sign of dementia. A simple and easily administered performance test (the coloured version of Raven's Progressive Matrices) may be acceptable to the patient. Comparison with the verbal score may highlight the discrepancy between verbal and non-verbal performance — often thought to be characteristic of organic deterioration — although it should be pointed out that, recently, increasing doubts have been cast on the significance of such discrepancies (Jarvis 1978). These simple tests have the advantage that they can be administered in a less anxiety-producing setting by nursing staff familiar to the patient. For more subtle changes or where legal problems such as those of testamentary capacity arise, a clinical psychologist will be required to administer standardised and fully validated measures (Chapter 2). A brief examination of linguistic and spatiotemporal ability and right–left orientation should never be omitted, e.g. the meaning of simple objects as well as more complex ones, a demonstration of the use of such things as a key, a telephone dial, etc., the copying of simple designs and the drawing of a clock face. Finally, physical examination should be recorded in detail. It is only through carefully recorded assessments of all such patients that we will be able to accumulate the clinical data which are so essential to a greater understanding of senile dementia and perhaps isolate prognostically and therapeutically different subtypes.

However, for the differential diagnosis of the condition, the history of its development is far more important. It is essential to discover why a particular patient is referred for consultation. This is rarely due to the presence of mild memory failure which is usually passed off as being due to old age. There may have been a sudden recent deterioration, particularly in behaviour, but more often changes in social or psychological situation in a family may have made the burden of care too severe. In order to date the onset, it is necessary to enquire specifically about the earliest signs of failure, which may not have been considered as important by relatives at the time. The picture which emerges tends to be relatively uniform. Disorientation is usually the first defect and this is often first noted in unfamiliar circumstances, e.g. during a holiday. Urinary incontinence as such is rare as an early defect in dementia, but occasionally micturition may have occurred in an inappropriate place. Restriction of interests and anecdotal, repetitive talk may have been noticed. In some, but by no means all, patients a character change will have begun to occur: egocentricity, irritability, emotional lability, suspiciousness and accusatory behaviour. Concurrently, there may have been accumulating evidence of memory decline, e.g. missing or muddling of appointments, failure to recall the events of the previous day, loss of possessions and, occasionally, misidentification of persons. Domestic skills and home as well as bodily care are likely to have begun to deteriorate, but it is well known that superficial social skills may be preserved for a long time, masking marked cognitive and psychomotor defects. These include failure to recall not only the previous day but discussions and tasks occurring in the course of clinical examination. The patient is usually unaware of these defects (preservation of insight is only seen in early and mild cases) and answers besides the point, e.g. by rendering the doctor's name in a changed form or by filling in memory gaps by simple confabulations. Although it is generally believed that memory for past events is preserved, this is often not the case.

Some patients may become troublesome on account of *delusions and hallucinations*. Classically, these occur in restless, wandering patients who collect and hide objects, accusing others of theft when they cannot find them. Men may develop rather ludicrous but potentially dangerous delusions of jealousy. The appearance of illusions and hallucinations, especially of a visual nature with varying levels of awareness and increased restlessness which increases at night, almost always suggest a complicating acute confusional state due to physical illness.

The recommended careful search for the earliest symptoms of dementia and their dating is not only of academic interest. It allows us to gauge the speed with which the condition is progressing and to arrive at an estimate of prognosis. Where mild defects have been present over many years without marked worsening, any precise differentiation between benign forgetfulness and senile dementia becomes irrelevant, especially in very old people.

A complete and well documented history is also essential for the differential diagnosis of senile dementia at the clinical level (special investigations will be outlined below and are referred to in Chapter 3).

Functional conditions of recent onset which need to be excluded are affective illnesses, especially depressive pseudodementia, and late paraphrenia; details are discussed in Chapter 6. What needs to be stressed here is that where depression, elation, overactivity, or paranoid delusions and hallucinations complicate dementia, there is always some evidence indicating the earlier presence of cerebral deterioration though it may not have been regarded as important by relatives or friends. Where there is no such preceding evidence of cognitive decline, the presence of intellectual defects may be ignored for the purposes of treatment which should be directed primarily at the basic anxiety, depression, or paranoid state.

The earlier differences between multi-infarct and senile dementia tend to disappear in the later stages. In the absence of localised paresis, it may be difficult to differentiate focal neurological defects from the rigidities, Parkinson-like states and occasional fits suffered by some senile dements. In any case, postmortem studies have repeatedly demonstrated that some 25% of elderly dements had infarcts as well as typical Alzheimer changes. Recent CT studies (Jacoby & Levy 1980a) have shown that infarcts may remain 'silent' during the patient's life. Preservation of insight in multi-infarct as against senile dementia is not a reliable differentiating feature. Even the classical step-wise progression associated with infarcts may occasionally be seen in 'pure' senile dementia.

In the past, certain clinical sub-divisions of senile dementia were described. Comment has already been made on the doubtful validity of separating depressive and paranoid forms from so-called 'simple' senile dementia as is done in ICD9. Another doubtful entity which was made much of in the past is 'presbiophrenia'. This condition was said to occur in physically healthy old people with severe defects in memory and orientation associated with marked euphoria, restlessness and overactivity, and with a special propensity towards collecting and hoarding rubbish. It seems likely that in the future it may become possible to isolate subtypes which have greater validity. It is already becoming clear that patients with difficulties pointing to parietotemporal damage have a much worse prognosis in terms of progress of the condition and life expectancy (McDonald 1969, Naguib & Levy 1982).

MULTI-INFARCT DEMENTIA

General considerations and aetiology

The term multi-infarct dementia has now displaced that of arteriosclerotic dementia as increasing evidence has accumulated to demonstrate the presence of infarcts of various sizes and situations in postmortems of patients diagnosed as having arteriosclerotic dementia. Indeed, it is extremely doubtful whether, in the absence of such infarcts, cerebral arteriosclerosis produces any detectable psychiatric disability. The relationship between this type of dementia and raised systemic blood pressure is well known. There is new evidence that hypertension may also be associated with a dementia in which the predominant damage is seen in the deep white matter of the brain (Janota 1981). This has often been referred to under the name of Binswanger's disease but it is not yet clear whether this condition can be considered as nosologically separate. The aetiology of these conditions is discussed in textbooks of general medicine which deal with the causes of arterial disease and hypertension in general.

Clinical features and recognition

Except in the cases of 'silent' infarcts mentioned above, this form of dementia is seen more frequently by geriatric physicians than by psychiatrists. It should only be diagnosed in the presence of evidence of clear focal deterioration of the brain substance due to cerebral infarcts. Hachinsky *et al* (1975) have devised a scale which provides an 'ischaemic score' indicating the relative importance of such damage as a contributor in any particular case of dementia.

 Occasionally, there may be prodromal changes in general health or personality, such as loss of weight, declining physical fitness, and increasing irritability. The onset, however, is sharply indicated by the occurrence of a cerebral infarct. Where this causes a paresis or dysphasia or other focal defect, there is no difficulty with recognition. A greater problem arises where the patient or informants report falls or faints without any neurological sequelae. Apart from the results of special investigations, the occurrence of 'strokelets' is indicated by a history of such falls or faints followed by brief episodes of bewilderment, drowsiness, repetitive stereotyped actions or emotional lability. Some strokes are not associated with any changes in the level of awareness and, even where unconsciousness has occurred, there may not always be any cognitive and personality changes detectable on clinical examination. This state of affairs may continue for many years until the patient's death, perhaps from extracerebral causes. There may be an increased propensity to the development of affective symptoms but otherwise the psychiatrist is likely to encounter only patients who are exhibiting the well known stepwise progression of a multi-infarct dementia. Following each cerebral insult, the patient passes through a period of confusion, sometimes with illusions or fleeting delusional ideas, usually of a paranoid nature. Recovery occurs in a few days but after each stroke it is followed by residual mental impairment which becomes increasingly disabling. Dysphasias, dysgnosias, and dyspraxias may be superimposed on the memory defect. After the first or subsequent strokes, mono- or hemiplegia may furnish the physical factors which lead to referral to geriatric physicians (see Chapter 3).

In the absence of obvious neurological signs, occasional post-infarct patients may appear to present with functional psychiatric illnesses. Affective disorder may be wrongly diagnosed by the inexperienced clinician who is struck by the sometimes well-marked emotional lability. It is sometimes possible to demonstrate this by making a joke while the patient is in the middle of a bout of crying when one can make them laugh heartily and occasionally uncontrollably — something which is almost never exhibited by patients suffering from true depression. The emotional state of some patients is silly and facile and there is no manic or depressive thought content. Paradoxical laughter or crying occur as a rule only in the presence of pseudobulbar palsy. More difficult to differentiate from the flow of talk of psychotic patients is receptive aphasia presenting with incoherent overproduction of speech, i.e. jargon aphasia with logorrhoea. This illustrates the need in the examination of all elderly patients for the inclusion of some simple and preliminary tests of temporal and parietal lobe functions as described in many texts (e.g. Institute of Psychiatry 1973).

SPECIAL INVESTIGATIONS

These are discussed at some length by Marsden (1978) who lists the following set of investigations as being appropriate to exclude treatable conditions: blood count and film, ESR, WR, and serology; thyroid function tests, electrolytes and liver functions tests, plasma creatinine, vitamin B_{12}, chest and skull X-ray, EEG, radioisotope brain scan, CT scan, and CSF examination.

It should, however, be stressed that Marsden refers mainly to patients under 70 and does so from the viewpoint of a neurologist. In patients presenting to a psychiatrist, the yield of such detailed investigation is likely to be extremely low and discretion should be exercised in selecting what is appropriate in the light of a full history and physical examination.

In view of current interest about the place of *CT scanning* in the investig-ation of dementia, this will be singled out for greater attention. There is little doubt that CT scanning has made an important contribution to our basic knowledge about the relationship between structural alterations in the brain and clinical symptomatology (Jacoby *et al* 1980, Jacoby & Levy 1980a, 1980b). It would also seem that where special programmes which record local brain density are available (Naeser *et al* 1980, Bondareff *et al* 1981) predictive use can be made of the density of the parietal lobes. Thus, Naguib & Levy (1982) have shown that, in a follow-up study of 40 carefully examined subjects, those who survived had significantly higher parietal lobe densities than those who did not. However, the value to individual patients is rather more doubtful. In our experience, unsuspected intracerebral pathology is occasionally detected but this is seldom correctable and, even when it is, this rarely leads to improvement in the mental state. These comments apply particularly to the existence of *communicating hydrocephalus* which requires further investigation by ventricular cisterography. We have never seen this condition presenting in a psychiatric context in spite of a diligent search since reading the first description by Hakim & Adams (1965). To return to CT scan results, these do allow for correct categorisation into demented or non-demented groups in some 80% of cases but the overlap is great and misclassification does occur in a sizeable minority of cases. In general, it would appear that enlarged sulci are often seen in benign forget-fulness whereas enlarged ventricles are more often associated with senile dementia. The introduction of methods which make use of the numerical output of the scanner rather than its visual representation may alter things in the future.

MANAGEMENT

Different aspects of the management of dementia have been dealt with in other chapters. In particular, Mr Woods (Chapter 2) discusses psychological management, Dr Hemsi (Chapter 9) social management, Professor Grimley Evans (Chapter 3) the treatment of associated physical disease, and Profes-sor Lader (Chapter 4) the place of drugs in the management of dementia. This section will therefore deal only with a few matters which have not been covered.

As was mentioned above, it is always worth treating associated psychiatric symptoms. In restless and agitated patients we have found prom-azine or thioridazine to be of value since these are well tolerated and seldom produce dystonic reactions or other extrapyramidal effects. If the response is not adequate, it may occasionally be necessary to use haloperidol and some writers have commented on the high tolerance of demented elderly subjects to this drug. Paranoid symptoms may sometimes be alleviated by the use of major tranquillisers and associated depression very frequently responds to small doses of tricyclic antidepressants (e.g. imipramine) — often resulting in a remarkable improvement in general behaviour. When such drugs are used, the blood pressure should be carefully monitored.

Many patients with dementia suffer from sleep disturbance or may show an inverted sleep rhythm. In these circumstances, chlormethiazole is as useful a drug as any, and short-acting benzodiazepines such as lorazepam or oxazepam may also be used. Although some psychiatrists working with old people recommend the avoidance of nitrazepam because of its long half-life, if it is used with caution this may well help to produce mild tranquillisation during the day. A careful watch should be made for the occurrence of ataxia or general unsteadiness and a drop in blood pressure.

Finally, it should be stressed that, although the use of drugs in the treatment of the basic dementing process has been disappointing, this may largely be due to the fact that it has hitherto been based on faulty premises and, furthermore, has been administered to very advanced cases. Advances in our knowledge of the neurochemistry of dementia offer great hope for the future. However, if these are to be applied effectively, it will be necessary to detect the disorder long before patients have presented to the psychiatrist or, indeed, to their own general practitioner. It is important that such putative remedies as are employed should be rigorously tested over a long period and given in adequate doses. We should learn from the experience of L-dopa which was originally abandoned for use in parkinsonism because it was used in what are now considered to be far too small doses. It is also possible that since different neurochemical disturbances are gradually being uncovered (e.g. deficiencies in adrenergic as well as cholinergic transmitters), it may eventually be possible to isolate subgroups which require different pharmacological treatment or possibly even sometimes treatment with a combination of substances.

The general impression of most workers in this field is that research in dementia has reached the 'take-off' phase and that one can confidently expect that great strides will be made in the next few years which may well transform our understanding of the condition and of its management.

REFERENCES

ALZHEIMER A. (1907) Uberine Eigeuartige Erhrankgung der Hirurinder. *Allgemeine Zeitschrift für Psychiatrie* **64**, 146–8.

ALZHEIMER A. (1911) Uber Eigenartige Krankheitsfalle des Spataren Aeters. *Zeitschrift für die Gesamte Neuroligie und Psychiatrie* **4**, 356–85.

BERGMANN K., KAY D.W.K., FOSTER E.M. *et al* (1971) A follow-up study of randomly selected community residents to assess the effects of chronic brain syndrome and cerebrovascular disease. *Proceedings of the V World Congress of Psychiatry*. Excerpta Medica, Amsterdam.

BONDAREFF W., BALDY R. & LEVY R. (1981) Quantitive Computed Tomography in Senile Dementia. *Archives of General Psychiatry* **38,** 1365–8.

CAIRD F.I. & JUDGE T.G. (1974) *Assessment of the Elderly Patient.* Pitman Medical, Tunbridge Wells.

CENTRAL STATISTICAL OFFICE (1979) *Social Trends,* no. 9. HMSO, London.

CONSTANTINIDES J. (1978) Is Alzheimer's Disease a Major Form of Senile Dementia? Clinical, Anatomical and Genetic Data. In *Alzheimer's Disease: Senile Dementia and Related Disorders,* eds R. Katzman, R.D. Terry and K.L. Bick, Raven Press, New York.

DSM III (1980) *American Psychiatric Association, Diagnostic and Statistical Manual for Mental Disorders,* 3rd edn, American Psychiatric Association.

HACHINSKY V.C., ILIFF L.D., ZILKHA E. (1975) Cerebral Blood Flow in Dementia. *Archives of Neurology* **32,** 632–7.

HAKIM S. & ADAMS R.D. (1965) The Special Problem of Symptomatic Hydrocephalus with Normal Cerebrospinal Fluid Pressure: Observations on Cerebrospinal Fluid Dynamics. *Journal of Neurological Sciences* **2,** 307–27.

INSTITUTE OF PSYCHIATRY (1973) *Notes on Eliciting and Recording Clinical Information.* Oxford University Press.

ISAACS B. & CAIRD F.I. (1976) 'Brain Failure' — A Contribution to the Terminology of Mental Abnormality in Old Age. *Age and Ageing* **5,** 241–4.

JANOTA I. (1981) Dementia, Deep White Matter Damage and Hypertension: 'Binswanger's Disease'. *Psychological Medicine* **II,** 39–48.

JACOBY R.J. & LEVY R. (1980a) Computed Tomography in the Elderly: 2. Senile Dementia: Diagnosis and Functional Impairment. *British Journal of Psychiatry* **136,** 256–9.

JACOBY R.J. & LEVY R. (1980b) Computed Tomography in the Elderly: 3. Affective Disorder. *British Journal of Psychiatry* **136,** 270–5.

JACOBY R.J, LEVY R. & DAWSON (1980) Computed Tomography in the Elderly: 1. The Normal Population. *British Journal of Psychiatry* **136,** 249–5.

JARVIK L.F. (1982) Diagnosis of Dementia in the Elderly. A 1979 Perspective. In *Review of Gerontology and Geriatrics,* ed C. Eisdorfer. Springer, New York.

JARVIK L.F. & BLUM J.E. (1971) *Cognitive Decline as Predictors of Mortality in Twin Pairs: A 20 year Longitudinal Study of Ageing in Prediction of Lifespan,* eds E. Pulmore and F.C. Jeffers. D.C. Heath, Lexington.

JARVIS M. (1978) Verbal and Performance Discrepancy as a Predictor of Brain Damage as Assessed by Computed Tomography. MPhil thesis, London University.

KAY D.W.K. & BERGMANN K. (1980) Epidemiology of Mental Disorders Among the Aged in the Community. In *Handbook of Mental Health and Aging,* eds J.E. Birren and R.B. Sloane. Prentice-Hall, Englewood Cliffs, N.J.

KRAL V.A. (1978) Benign Senescent Forgetfulness. In *Alzheimer's Disease: Senile Dementia and Relating Disorders,* eds R. Katzman, R.D. Terry and K.L. Bick. Raven Press, New York.

LARSSON T., SJOGREN T. & JACOBSON G. (1963) Senile Dementia: A clinical, Socio-Medical and Genetic Study. *Acta Psychiatrica Scandinavica* (suppl.) **167,** 1–259.

LISHMAN W.A. (1978) *Organic Psychiatry.* Blackwell Scientific Publications, Oxford.

MCDONALD C. (1969) Clinical Heterogeneity in Senile Dementia. *British Journal of Psychiatry* **115,** 267–71.

MARSDEN C.D. (1978) The Diagnosis of Dementia. In *Studies in Geriatric Psychiatry,* eds A.D. Isaacs and F. Post. John Wiley, New York.

MILLER E. (1974) Dementia as Accelerated Ageing of the Nervous System. Some Psychological and Methodological Considerations. *Age and Ageing* **3**, 197–202.

NAESER M.A., GEBHARDT C. & LEVINE H.L. (1980) Decreased Computed Tomography Numbers in Patients with Presenile Dementia. *Archives of Neurology* **37**, 401.

NAGUIB M. & LEVY R. (1982) Prediction of Outcome in Senile Dementia. A Computed Tomography Study. *British Journal of Psychiatry* (In Press).

OFFICE OF HEALTH ECONOMICS (1979) *Dementia in Old Age*. White Crescent Press, Luton.

QUERSHI K.N. & HODKINSON H.M. (1974) Evaluation of a Ten Question Mental Test in the Institutionalised Elderly. *Age and Ageing* **3**, 152–7.

REDICK R.L. & TAUBE C.A. (1980) Demography and Mental Health Care of the Aged. In *Handbook of Mental Health and Ageing*, eds J.E. Birren & R.B. Sloane. Prentice-Hall, Englewood Cliffs, N.J.

SJOGREN T., SJOGREN H. & LINDGREN A.G.H. (1952) Morbus Alzheimer and Morbus Pick. A Genetic, Clinical and Patho-Anatomical Study. *Acta Psychiatrica et Neurologica Scandinavica* (suppl.) **82**, 1–52.

WORLD HEALTH ORGANISATION (1978) *Mental Disorders: Glossary and Guide to their Classification in Accordance with the Ninth Revision of the International Classification of Diseases*. Geneva.

ZERBIN-RÜDIN (1975) Genetics in Modern Perspectives. In *The Psychiatry of Old Age*, ed J.G. Howells. Brunner Mazel, New York.

CHAPTER 6

Functional Disorders
I. Description, incidence and recognition

Felix Post

For practical purposes it remains appropriate to set functional conditions apart from disorders related to deterioration or disease of the brain. Clinically, in the vast majority of patients clear cut differences exist between these two types of disorder, and in the few instances where the immediate distinction is not possible this is often due to both conditions being co-existent. In such cases further progress will reveal the extent to which coarse brain changes had been, and continue to be, responsible for the psychopathology.

For a deeper understanding, especially of psychiatric conditions affecting persons with ageing nervous systems, it is helpful to recognise that organic and functional disorders are not as different in kind as is dreamt of in mind–body dichotomy. It is suggested that mind should be conceptualised as nothing more than self-awareness made possible in humans far more than in other species by many evolutionary developments, mainly that of language (for a fuller discussion see Leach 1970). Mind should no longer be regarded as an entity apart from biological and especially from cerebral functioning. At the present, it is probably not possible to reduce the mechanisms of language production and of awareness to physics and chemistry, but this may well become feasible in future ' . . . in terms that are not within the range of physical processes as presently understood' (Chomsky 1972).

This and the next chapter are based on this kind of materialistic and mechanistic theory. Perceptual input in the widest sense, of everything that is experienced, results in molecular changes in the neurones of the receptive areas of the brain and, secondarily, in those registering and elaborating this input. In particular, signals interpreted as threats will activate molecular neurone changes in brain areas concerned with arousal, mood, and its cognitive elaborations. In some genetically predisposed persons, and in those sensitised by previous experiences, these alterations of arousal and of mood may become persistent rather than only short-lasting, and some of the associated microbiological changes affecting neurotransmitter molecules have been demonstrated in patients with the more severe affective illnesses.

176

It is quite likely that similar findings will also be made in relation to less severe deviations of mood states, especially those occurring in the anxiety which is thought to fuel many minor psychiatric — so-called neurotic — conditions. By contrast, microbiological changes of transient and structural brain alterations of persistent or progressive organic psychosyndromes are not localised to areas subserving mood and arousal, but are in most instances widely spread through the brain. On the other hand, in severe functional psychoses, neuronal dysfunctioning may also spread more widely into brain areas concerned with level of awareness, with vegetative functions, and with memory and other intellectual functioning: hence the bewilderment and confusion, parkinson-like facies, and pseudodementia of some severely depressed patients, to give just one example.

This lack of sharp lines of demarcation will be reflected in discussing the functional disorders of late life as a series of conditions representing increasing disruptions of the personality. As the occasion arises, the additional role of the ageing or the deteriorating brain will be introduced, and incidence together with some aspects of aetiology will be discussed. Management, treatment, prognosis, and speculative aetiological considerations will be dealt with separately in the following chapter, at the end of which references for both chapters will be listed together. This unconventional presentation may at first seem confusing. It has been chosen to avoid repetition, because along with the continuum of the functional disorders and illnesses many aspects of their management, of the results of treatment, and of aetiology have much in common.

PERSONALITY DEVIATIONS AND DISORDERS

The equipment with which a person enters upon the last stages of life will go a long way towards determining his level of psychic adjustment. Physical ill health will be a potent factor in psychological malfunctioning and breakdown, as well as in the response to treatment. Personality structure does not break down on account of ageing alone or without physical deterioration, especially of the brain. However, the personality with which a person enters late life will not only make him more or less vulnerable to functional psychiatric disorders, but will also determine their form and content.

Severe, life-long personality deviations may develop into late paraphrenia, and this will concern us later. Apart from this rare development one has to admit to almost complete ignorance when asked the question, 'What happens to psychopaths as they grow older?' There is a general impression that deviating personalities normalise as they grow older, but for obvious reasons there are no prospective studies to support this. The antisocial actions of those with abnormal personalities certainly diminish markedly once adolescence and early adult life are left behind: criminality declines significantly with rising age; many explosive and aggressive persons are reported in retrospect as having 'settled down'. On the other hand, one suspects that inadequate people deteriorate steadily as they grow older, and that many of them find their way to and remain in doss-house types of environment. If, as has been suggested, some aspects of personality ageing are associated with a shift from extraversion to introversion, improvement of aggressive personalities and further decline of inadequate people could be explained by diminished reactivity towards the environment. Unfortunately, psychological research has not confirmed earlier findings pointing in this direction—and that includes the related 'disengagement hypothesis' (Thomae 1980).

We know a little more about personality disorders in the survivor group aged 65 and over. In relation to some less severe personality deviations, there have been occasional serendipitous long-term findings: it was possible to re-assess the parents originally rated during a study concerning their children at a time when the parents' ages ranged from 60 to 82 (Maas & Kuypers 1974). Most of these, by then, elderly persons were functioning well psychologically and were healthy; those who were not had shown indications of personality and health problems as young adults. It was the more pathological or maladaptive personality traits and life-styles that persisted from early adulthood onwards. Poor health was an important factor in the living pattern of the elderly, and influenced this even more adversely when 'poor health' had been a concern to the subjects (who grew old in spite of this!) 40 years earlier. A similar pattern was observed in persons followed over 12 years during the 8th and 9th decades of life (Thomae & Schmitz-Scherzer 1979). Those who had been more competent in terms of activity, cognitive functioning, health, and independence tended to make a better adjustment and were more intelligent and less rigid during the subsequent years of their old age.

In a community sample of persons aged 65–80 Bergmann (1971, 1978) found that some 6% exhibited longstanding personality deviations without super-added psychoneurotic symptomatology. In broad terms, he encountered two types of personality deviation. For the first of these he was unable to find a better term than 'inadequate': they were persons who since early life had 'failed to live up to the standards of society' in terms of work record, marital history, interests, and socio-economic independence. Some had also been anxiety prone or had exhibited tendencies towards hysterical conversion phenomena or rigid obsessionality. They continued to present a focus of care and attention for families or other persons, and perhaps preserved their self-esteem by accepting their dependence with gratitude. More clearly defined was the second group of persons with deviant personalities, who might best be called 'paranoid': they had been refusing to conform to social expectations, always rejecting friendship and help, and denying their own obligations. Their attitudes were extra-punitive and hostile. However, they continued to adopt a strategy, a 'fighting stance', by means of which they were often successful in withstanding the vicissitudes of old age. Possibly, this kind of personality deviation is commoner in old men, and may include the 'independent old people' living alone found as a small group in earlier surveys conducted by geriatricians.

Sexual difficulties and deviations

A detailed review of the recent literature on sexual interests and activity in the aged has been prepared by Elias & Elias (1977). Contrary to what one might expect, age decline of sexual functions in mammalians including man has not been found to be due to any age-related decline in the production of sex hormones. Before this occurs, age-related changes in the nervous system have begun to affect sexual behaviour. This is in keeping with an increasing realisation in human sexology that, in contrast to sexual development, later sexual behaviour depends on psychological (i.e. CNS) and social factors rather than on hormone levels. Thus, after the age of 50, psychologically evoked penile erections become increasingly unusual. Morning erections are maintained, but REM sleep erections decrease in frequency. By the time the 60s have been reached, penile erection has become entirely linked to physical contact, and all other libidinal and coital functioning has become increasingly slowed. According to Comfort (1980) this is as far as physiological age changes in the sexual functions of males go. All other decline in male sexuality and especially, of course, the occurrence of impotence are never due to age changes alone: they are related to physical disease and physical noxa (prescribed drugs, alcohol, etc.). Even more important, conflicts relating to sexual activity are aggravated by psychosocial age factors of an obvious, traditional kind, as well as by depression in the widest sense of the word.

Much less is known about sexual functioning in old women but probably, apart from lack of opportunity, sexual activity is impeded in them to an even larger extent by physical general illness, as well as by conditions affecting the internal and external genitalia: some of the latter, may in fact, be the result of disuse atrophy. Under favourable circumstances female orgasmic capacity may be retained into the highest age.

All this having been said, only between 15–25% of persons over 75 claim continued successful sexual intercourse (Comfort 1980). The large majority fall by the wayside on account of lack of opportunity, physical illness (and its treatment), and psychogenic inhibition which, in most instances, has also been interfering with sexual functioning throughout earlier life. Possibly for this reason, I have always been struck by the great rarity of complaints concerning impotence or other sexual difficulties in clinic patients over 60, much in contrast with younger attenders and their spouses. Perhaps within the setting of the 'permissive society' old people may soon bring sexual problems more frequently, and the psychiatrist's understanding of sexual functioning in the elderly may prove useful for therapy.

This stage may have been reached for older men with problems related to *homosexuality*. The sparse literature on homosexuality in late life, which is entirely limited to 'gay' men, has been summarised by Kimmel (1977). More recently, a slightly fuller summary has been given by Corby & Solnick (1980). Kimmel reported on his contact with 14 clients aged 55–81, mostly in their early sixties. A retrospective review confirmed that homosexuals generally showed as many different life-styles as heterosexuals. Some had been ambisexual, but only about half of Kimmel's subjects had had long lasting homosexual relationships, and only one ever set up a permanent shared home. Most of them had been living alone for many years, and many reported traumatic relationships. They had suffered due to social pressures — especially the five ever-married subjects. Elderly male homosexuals are, therefore, a vulnerable group, and the circumstances which may lead them to seek perhaps not so much treatment as counselling are well described by this author.

Since the subject of *sexual misdemeanours* by elderly men was last summarised (Post 1967), few further experiences have accumulated. In spite of the stereotype of the 'dirty old man', it has been confirmed that exhibitionism and other indecent actions especially towards children are far less often perpetrated by old than by younger men. In San Francisco (Epstein *et al* 1970) out of a total of 256 sexual offences only five were by individuals over 60: two were for indecent exposure, two for sexual advances to children, and one woman of 65 was arrested for an act of indecent behaviour in the street (no information about her mental condition seemed to have been recorded). Old men with behaviour disorders of this kind occurring for the first time in late life are said to have had overtly normal sexual past histories. It is thought that lessening coital capacity had made them unacceptable to women, but that friendly children with their immature sexuality did more easily respond to the old mens' advances. In a recently treated case, however, exhibitionism was triggered off by female children's legs in the street, as well as those of small grand-daughters in the home. Against expectation, in this (as in similar cases) there was no evidence for cerebral impairment leading to diminished control, nor did such impairment appear during lengthy follow-up; the disordered behaviour failed to recur after a sufficiently high regular dose of anti-androgen had been prescribed and taken.

Senile recluses

These are rarely discussed in the literature (Macmillan & Shaw 1966, Clark *et al* 1975). Their annual incidence has been estimated to amount to only 0.5 per 1000 persons over 60 living in their own homes. They come to notice because neighbours become concerned with the nuisance caused or because a final illness is suspected. In fact, nearly half of them die soon after admission, usually to a geriatric facility. Where psychiatric or psychological assessment had been possible, a characteristic picture tended to emerge. Men and women have been found to be equally affected. Most lived alone, but a few shared their seclusion with a sibling, more rarely a spouse. Senile recluses as a group are of average or above average intelligence, and possibly persons belonging to the middle and upper classes predominate. Poverty is conspicuous by its absence: considerable sums of money are often found hidden among the filth and shambles of the home. Recluses have always been independent, quarrelsome, and secretive people, who come increasingly to reject contact with others except perhaps an occasionally visiting relative: they may literally barricade themselves in their homes and only venture out occasionally. Unlike Diogenes they certainly never go out with a lamp into the marketplace in broad daylight ' . . . to seek men' so the term 'Diogenes' syndrome', which has begun to gain currency, seems to be inappropriate; in addition, senile seclusion is no syndrome, it marks the end stage of a personality disorder. At the time of assessment about half the patients were regarded as otherwise normal; the rest seemed to have become paraphrenic psychotics or senile dements by the time they were assessed. It has been claimed that the survivors can be rehabilitated, even in day hospital settings, and that, when there were two recluses living together, removal of the dominant partner would result in normalisation of the remaining one, as in cases of *folie à deux.*

Addictive disorders

Apart from dependence on day and night sedatives with their deleterious after-effects (Chapter 4) and the more harmless abuse of laxatives, alcoholism is the only serious dependency problem in late life. Its medical aspects are discussed in Chapter 4 and the alleged beneficial effects of alcohol together with the management of aged alcoholics will be briefly dealt with in the next chapter.

A number of investigations (summarised by Mishara & Kastenbaum 1980) have led to the following conclusions concerning the use and abuse of alcohol in late life. As a group, older people drink less than younger ones and, in particular, there are fewer elderly heavy drinkers. In general, lifelong drinkers seem to reduce their intake after the age of 50 for a variety of reasons, of which increasing financial stringency is the most obvious. In addition, ageing people may become aware that alcohol tends to diminish further their decreasing capabilities, and may begin to fear its effects also on account of their growing health consciousness. In fact, at least one study (Barnes 1979) has shown that mortality risks in old people who drink moderately are decreased as compared with those of total abstainers!

Not all characteristics marking problem drinkers at an earlier age apply in later life. Problems arising at work, with neighbours, and with members of the family (except perhaps with a spouse) are less prominent; but, as for younger persons, older problem drinkers are recognised as such by the occurrence of shakes, debilitating hangovers, blackouts, and memory loss, as well as of an inability to conduct everyday tasks without drinking or without planning daily activities around a drinking routine. Finally a problem drinker is a person with alcohol-related diseases, and an alcohol problem is frequently missed in persons presenting with physical disease (and also with psychiatric conditions, especially masked depressions).

Alcoholism among the elderly has begun to cause serious concern in the USA (for a summary see Simon 1980). A household survey in New York State revealed the peak ages of incidence at 45–54 and again at 65–75 — by which age the male : female predominance had decreased to 3 : 2. In a San Francisco psychiatric screening unit there were some 23% with the diagnosis of alcoholism among those over 60, and a further 5% were regarded as heavy social drinkers. In the same city, four of every five arrests of persons over 60 were for drunkenness as against one out of two of all age groups, even though probably no more than 11% of alcoholics over 60 had started to drink heavily only late in life.

There are no studies following younger problem drinkers into old age but alcoholism is, of course, known to shorten life; probably only the physically and mentally toughest alcohol abusers reach their 70s or 80s. The study of alcoholics seen in old age by Rosin & Glatt (1971) has been confirmed in its conclusions by other workers (Mishara & Kastenbaum 1980) and a predictable picture emerges. Surviving early-onset alcoholics exhibit the same personality problems and defects with which one has long been familiar, while late-onset alcoholics are usually reported as having had stable personalities and life records. Alcohol was only resorted to in response to the stresses of late life, often in a setting of depression. On the other hand, alcoholic addiction, may also be induced by assiduous relatives in an attempt to still the anxieties of old persons in their care, and to cope with hypochondriacal behaviour, e.g. faint feelings. Also depression may be a symptom rather than a cause of chronic intoxication, and so may, of course, be confusion. Like iatrogenic drug effects, alcohol abuse will have to be increasingly considered in the diagnosis and management of disturbed old people.

NEUROSES

So far we have dealt with deviations of personality, and with habit and conduct disorders of a kind which only occasionally cause discomfort or suffering to the individual himself, and which do not immediately arouse the concern of doctors and other health workers. If one feels the need for precise definitions, one may hold that the conditions discussed so far are not 'diseases', though they may lead on both to functional and organic psychiatric illnesses.

We move more closely towards 'illness' when we consider the neuroses: they almost always cause suffering to the individual and often to those close to him. Neuroses arise in vulnerable personalities which are under pressure and stress, and they are usually only episodically disabling. Even chronic neuroses tend eventually to be self-limited and they lose many of their disabling aspects in later life (Müller 1969).

Neurotic symptoms of a mild and sporadic kind affect many 'normal' people. It is therefore not surprising that these forms of personality malfunction show similar changes with age as do personalities. On account of psychomotor slowing and of the impairment of learning new material of all kinds, older people become less outgoing and more restricted to their families and to their inner selves. For this reason disorders which forcefully impinge on others are commonest in younger persons: impulsive acting out in terms of aggression and delinquency, as well as dramatic hysterical-conversion symptoms or self-injuring actions. These disorders diminish as people grow older. Inward directed neurotic symptoms become more often a source of discomfort or suffering, and some may arise for the first time only late in life. Hysterical symptoms become more somatised as in Briquet's syndrome and anxiety tends to crystallise into phobic and obsessional symptoms. As we shall see, hypochondriacal and depressive symptoms finally become the commonest neurotic phenomena in old age, related to increasing concern with the interior of the body and, more speculatively, inward turning of aggression.

All these clinician's impressions are highly conjectural and are at best based on what have been called proto-theories of personality ageing by Neugarten (1977) in an important summary paper.

A French clinician (Goda 1979) has recently remarked on the lack of flamboyant and hysterical symptomatology in the aged. In addition to speaking of neurotisation of personality through ageing, he pointed out that the neurotic disorders of late life approached Freud's 'actual neuroses', with much exhaustion and depression as well as somatic complaints. From a different angle, Jarvik & Russell (1979) have pointed out how very rare acute anxiety states with sympathetic discharges were in the elderly. Probably this was because stresses which provoke fight or flight were less likely to be experienced in the settings of later life. The stresses were much more often long-term and not suitable to be reacted to with fight or flight. A more appropriate reaction was 'freeze' — not an adaptive response to an outer danger, but as a period of inactivity, of 'playing possum' for a while, until adjustment to the stress occurred after a favourable issue of the situation.

Kraepelin called the mental disorders of old age the darkest area of psychiatry. This is no longer the case, but the neuroses of old age certainly continue to be the most invisible part of our specialty! It is well known that family doctors rarely refer elderly neurotics. Our experiences with them have remained very limited, and the only hard facts are those culled by Klaus Bergmann as part of the Newcastle studies of elderly community residents. His work (Bergmann 1971, 1978) may be summarised to the following effect. From a total research population a random sample of some 300 subjects aged 64–80 was drawn. All subjects in whom the research team had earlier diagnosed either an organic or a functional psychosis had been excluded. The remainder were studied by means of a semi-structured psychiatric interview, a personality questionnaire yielding self-ratings, and a social worker's enquiry.

Only 49% emerged as entirely psychologically stable. In 6% longstanding personality deviations were diagnosed and in 45% neuroticism was registered because at least two of the following were present: episodic tension, somatic anxiety symptoms, phobic propensities, episodes of depersonalisation, obsessional phenomena, and episodic depressive states. In just over half (i.e. in 21% of the whole sample) there was evidence of lifelong neuroticism, while it was noted that in the remaining 24% of the whole sample neuroticism had become manifest only after the age of 60. However, only a small proportion of subjects with operationally defined neuroticism were in any significant way distressed by neurotic symptoms: 18% with a male : female ratio of 1 : 6.5. Clinically significant, late-onset neuroses were found in only 11% of the sample (male : female ratio 1 : 4.5). Longstanding neurotics had exhibited all kinds of symptomatology, such as chronic or episodic anxiety, depression, phobic or obsessional symptoms, as well as past tendencies towards conversion or dissociation. By contrast, the only diagnostic labels at all appropriate for late-onset neurotics were either of depression or of anxiety, with depression greatly predominating. This finding — to the effect that when neurotic symptoms manifested themselves for the first time only in late life they were almost always associated with an affective change — had been noted by an earlier worker. His investigations had, however, been limited to patients seen in a general practice and in a psychiatric hospital unit (McDonald 1967).

It is to be noted that lifelong neurotics were found to differ beyond chance expectations from late-onset neurotics in a number of characteristics. Persons with lifelong propensities to neurotic disabilities had tended to suffer from neurotic symptoms in childhood, were often late children, and had problematic relationships with their parents. They were not differentiated from late life neurotics in terms of genetic factors or earlier life adjustment (including marital record). On the other hand, early-onset neurotics stood out with a high frequency of hypochondriacal preoccupations and complaints in spite of generally enjoying better physical health than either late-onset neurotics or normals. By contrast, late-onset neurotics (though also hypochondriacal in attitude) were more often afflicted with real physical disabilities, and in particular with cardiovascular defects, and thus had a higher mortality risk. They also tended to be disadvantaged by lower incomes, felt more lonely, and restricted themselves to domestic overactivity, which was ineffectual in that it was associated objectively with diminished self-care.

DEPRESSIONS

In sharp contrast with the neuroses of late life, illnesses with depression as their main feature have been well studied during the last twenty years. Here the difficulty lies in achieving a judicious selection. An extended discussion of the subject was completed recently (Post 1982).

Historical perspective

Willmuth (1979) sketched out the ideas which have been held in the past. The term 'melancholia' had, of course, different meanings at different periods, but Willmuth thought there was strong evidence that the physicians of antiquity were well aware of senile depression as a condition apart from dotage. In the Middle Ages many of the persecuted and executed witches were possibly senile depressives. (Some, infact, were the victims of pseudologic children.) By the nineteenth century, humoral pathology had given way to brain pathology, and depression in the elderly was increasingly regarded as a stage of dementia of old age. However, Kraepelin and others began to abandon this view around the beginning of the present century. The earlier finding of Griesinger that full return of cognitive powers and memory quite often accompanied recovery from senile depression was increasingly often confirmed. It should be stated that depressive illnesses in old age have been much more generally and effectively recognised in the last 30 years or so, not on account of improved knowledge, but on account of better teaching of matters of which knowledgable psychiatrists had been aware for a long time.

Incidence and prevalence

Data are difficult to interpret because investigators have different ideas about what constitutes depression. It has been pointed out (Gurland 1976) that — where cases are defined by psychiatrists — milder, so-called neurotic, depressions have their greatest incidence between the ages of 35 and 45, while psychotic depressions manifest themselves for the first time most frequently between 55 and 65. After that age first depressions become increasingly rare, especially after the age of 75. However, when a label of depression is attached on the basis of complaints in surveys not necessarily conducted by psychiatrists, the highest prevalence has been found in persons over 65. Thus 34% of the elderly voluntary subjects of an American study (for a summary see Gianturco & Busse 1978) complained of episodes of depression initially, and 70% of the survivors had experienced 'depressions' after a 15 year follow-through. However, in spite of this there appeared to have been no suicide attempts and no hospital admission for depression in this cohort. Possibly more clinically relevant were findings of community surveys of the elderly in Edinburgh (Williamson 1978) and Newcastle (Kay *et al* 1964) reporting a prevalence of depressive illness in 5.4 and 2.4% respectively. Depression was more frequently diagnosed where subjects attended a geriatric clinic (14%) or had applied for local authority help (32%) (Goldberg 1970). An interesting investigation was reported by a Finnish team led by a psychiatrist with special interest and expertise in late life depression (Stenback *et al* 1979). Their subjects were men and women born in Helsinki in 1903 who were studied when they had just reached their 70th birthday. It was possible to interview 93% in a semi-structured fashion and just over half also agreed to complete the Beck Depression Inventory. On this 48.3% scored as depressed, but it has often been pointed out that the somatic components of the Beck scale tend to lead to unduly high scores in the elderly (Zemore & Eames 1979; for a useful discussion of depression scales see Gilleard *et al* 1981). On clinical interview, only 23.3% were classified as mildly or moderately depressed, and not a single member of this survivor cohort was severely depressed or had ever suffered from a bipolar affective psychosis. The same author (Stenbeck 1980) has recently summarised the world literature of geriatric depression and, in the section on epidemiology, he stressed the difficulties which arise on account of gradations between three conditions 1. mild mood disorders not affecting behaviour 2. depressions of a neurotic kind and severity, and 3. those of a severely disruptive, psychotic type. The severest melancholic illnesses were probably encountered not in real old age, but between the ages of 45 and 60, with later recurrences showing lessening severity of symtomatology. It has even been suggested that depressions in old age are no more frequent than in younger ages. Be that as it may, my own earlier and recent (Post 1972) follow-through studies of hospital-treated depressives over 60, have shown that only 25% of patients failed to have further depressive breakdowns within the next three years, and lengthy intervals between recurrent attacks seem more rarely encountered than in clinical practice with younger patients. Up to the age of 75, depression is the most frequent condition seen in psychogeriatric practice.

Symptomatology

It has been generally thought (and most recently confirmed in Japan by Kawashima 1979) that, as depressives become older, their symptomatology was more often characterised by less retardation but more agitation, hypochondriacal contents, anxiety, self-reproach and suicidal proclivities. However, employing standardised and validated measures of the present mental state, Gurland (1976) reported that the only feature found significantly more often in older depressives was hypochondriacal symptomatology.

My own research (Post 1972) was unfortunately limited to depressives over 60 who had required admission to a psychiatric unit; it was planned to allow comparison with an earlier series of inpatients at a time when there was little ambulant treatment of elderly depressives. On the basis of symptomatology alone, three types of depressive picture could be clearly differentiated. However, what stood out was that only few patients complied with clinical pictures which have been regarded as characteristic of 'senile melancholia': either empty, apathetic states or agitated conditions with stereotyped utterances of abysmal guilt, self-reproach, and self-belittlement, often with nihilistic delusions. Such conditions are still seen occasionally, but modern psychiatric practice is far more concerned with patients exhibiting a less dramatic psychopathology.

To return to my (1972) research sample of nearly 100 consecutive admissions three main points may be made.

1.   Some 37% had severe and psychotic depressions. Many conformed to the 'classical' picture: at different times they were both severely retarded and agitated; their general bearing, their psychomotor activity (especially facial expression and lack of mobility), and their talk clearly communicated a mood of great sadness and despair, and usually also of overwhelming dread or fear. With most patients there were considerable feeding problems, loss of weight and sleeplessness. Sudden, but often not very effective, attempts at self-injury might have occurred before, but also after admission. Usually, the patients voiced numerous depressive delusions of a kind with which the reader will be familiar from textbooks and clinical practice. On exploration, it would usually emerge that the patient regarded himself as thoroughly bad and worthless — exaggeratedly blaming himself for past failures or transgressions. He believed himself impoverished, shabbily and dirtily clothed and was convinced that others noticed that he was filthy and smelly. On further exploration it emerged that he often thought that this was due to retention of rotting food inside his body due to obstruction of his bowels or other portions of his alimentary or perhaps his urinary tract. Occasionally, these delusions were nihilistic in a subtle form: a shrinking of organs or of their muscles. More rarely, and grossly, there were beliefs that abdomen, chest, or skull were literally empty. At the opposite pole, one can encounter

delusions of enormity, of bowels not having been opened for months and of the inundating damage that their opening is certain to cause — such are rarely encountered nowadays. Religious guilt delusions have also become less common. In one-fifth of this severely psychotic group (which made up 37% of the research series) no delusional content could be discovered. These patients were usually very apathetic and practically mute, verging on stupor, and had perhaps been lying in bed at home for weeks or months before admission; occasionally they were severely restless in an apparently empty fashion. In either case, these patients betrayed the depth of their psychosis through severe feeding and sleep disturbances. Possibly, delusional thought content was present but inaccessible.

2. Some 24% of consecutive depressives were labelled as intermediate psychotics. Only two-thirds of them clearly communicated some depression and/or anxiety with their somatic concomitants; the remainder were in no way obviously depressed. All of them, however, were suffering from some delusional ideas, often of similar type and severity as the severely psychotic depressives. Frequently, the mildness or absence of communicated disorders of mood could be explained in terms of a 'burnt out' quality of these often more longstanding cases. Certainly perplexity, which was a frequent feature of the severely psychotic patients, was rarely obvious. These intermediate psychotics seemed more resigned, though sometimes they were hostile, exhibiting an 'aversion depression'. Quite often, they felt shunned or even persecuted from the background of their guilt, poverty, or pollution delusions. These paranoid features may pose difficulties of diagnosis, especially in relation to so-called schizo-affective illnesses. Rarely, the patient may utter only one stereotyped nihilistic statement like, 'I am nothing, I am not Mrs . . . ., I am nothing.'

3. Lastly, 39% of patients were labelled as neurotic depressives simply because their preoccupations could not be regarded as delusional. They were given vent in reiterative and importuning complaints about unpleasant somatic sensations, especially in the lower abdomen. The patients would seek repeated assurance confirming the absence of physical disease, of whose presence they were by no means firmly convinced. In more than half of these cases, even mild depression was hardly noticeable, but some underlying feelings of lowered self-esteem and of self-reproach could usually be uncovered on exploration, even though patients often seemed to blame others. After unsuccessful family doctor or outpatient treatment, these 'neurotic' and often histrionic patients had come to require inpatient care on account of their importuning behaviour, restlessness, and nocturnal disturbance. Patients of this kind are beginning to be well recognised by geriatricians as persons who exhaust and exasperate their families and friends, and who make themselves disliked in hospitals and homes. Williamson (1978) advised that the 'unlikeable' patient should always be suspected of depression. He also pointed out that intractable pain may be a symptom of

'masked' depression, and that depression may render much more unbearable post-herpetic and other physically caused pains. I would add that tinnitus in an agitated old person is often rendered no longer noticeable after antidepressant treatment.

Suicide

At younger ages the ratio of suicide to para-suicide is 1 : 10, but this is reversed above the age of 65. Between 25 and 30% of all suicides occur after that age, while in countries for which suicide statistics are available only 10–15% of the population is over 65 years old. Attempted suicides among the elderly amount to only 5% of those counted at all ages, and many of them are probably not just calls for help but indeed, 'botched' suicides of old people with impaired mental abilities (see Shulman 1978). Moreover, in the follow-up of attempted suicides, ultimately fatal suicidal acts were found to have occurred twenty times more often in older as against in younger men. In the USA it was found that suicide rates rose consistently with age only in white males, especially when they were no longer or never married. Three-quarters of them had visited their doctors within a month of the suicide, and a retrospective review showed that in 60% there had been cues pointing to suicidal preoccupations, mainly in relation to depression (Miller 1978). It is generally accepted now that, in contrast to younger people, suicidal ideas and behaviour are almost always related to clinical depression.

Diagnosis

Recognition and differential diagnosis need be discussed only in relation to transient and personality-related mood disorders, to senile mental impairment, and to schizo-affective conditions.

The strain imposed by neurotically complaining old people in family or institutional settings may, usually only as a last resort, lead to psychiatric consultation. By then the patient will have become thoroughly unpopular and a list of longstanding problems will be offered by the informants. The presence of potentially treatable depression is indicated when carefully aimed enquiry elicits that a worsening or a change in the longstanding maladjustment had recently occurred. The fresh appearance of circumscribed psychoneurotic symptoms, especially phobias and obsessions but also of alcohol abuse or hypochondriasis, are usually associated with depression in the group with which we are concerned. Equally important, but more difficult to elicit, are loss of previous interests, activities, appetite, and sleep. Though sleep in the elderly may be briefer and more interrupted than in younger persons, elderly depressives like younger patients, report both early waking and sleep onset difficulties. In contrast to normal elderly, those with depression have been found to exhibit sleep EEGs with considerable shortening in REM latency, reduced sleep efficiency, and an increased number of shifts and arousals throughout the night (Kupfer *et al* 1978). It has been claimed that a depression scale introduced at the Duke Medical Center is useful for differentiating clinical depression from dysphoric disorders of persons over 65 (Blazer 1980).

In more severely depressed patients, accounts of declines in memory and self-care, as well as the clinical discovery of cognitive defects, may raise strong suspicions of the presence of an organic mental syndrome with depressive overlay. Depressive symptomatology during the early stages of the dementias of late life does occur, of course, but by no means as frequently as was assumed by earlier clinicians.

Depressive pseudodementia

In depression, cognitive impairment is sometimes noted at the height of the illness, but this is no longer noticeable following remission. The term 'depressive pseudodementia' was probably first used in relation to the functional psychoses of late life by Madden *et al* (1952), but the seminal publication on this condition was that of Kiloh (1961), who contrasted it both with the kind of pseudodementia and the Ganser syndrome seen in younger patients — conditions which he regarded as on the borderline between hysteria and schizophrenia. I summarised the aspects and significance of depressive pseudodementia in the elderly more recently (Post 1975) and there has also been a useful contribution by Wells (1980).

In summary, pseudodementia is a feature frequently encountered in elderly patients with the more severe kinds of affective illness. In a Japanese sample (Kawashima 1979), 18% exhibited the condition, and transient confusional states were also noted in 17% in relation to drug effects and to physical illness. This Japanese figure may be too high: many agitated or severely retarded depressives only appear confused or demented because they are barely able to co-operate in attempts to assess their cognitive functioning. The term 'pseudodementia' should be reserved for patients who *can* be assessed and who show only a few but striking failures in orientation and memory. In my experience, this is the case in only about 10% of cases, though in one series 16.5% would have been classified as 'organic' if their faulty performance on a new word learning test had been the sole criterion of diagnosis. In fact, small but statistically significant failures on a number of psychological tests were discovered in a high proportion of psychotically ill depressives before treatment (Cawley *et al* 1973).

In differentiating organic brain syndromes from affective illnesses with prominent cognitive defects, the following observations have been found useful: in the case of pseudodements, informants are always aware of the presence of memory and orientation defects. Moreover, they can usually date their onset, and describe rapid worsening from then on up to the time of referral. In one series, eight out of ten patients were reported to have shown losses in social and domestic skills apparently related to loss of mental ability. By contrast, the frequency with which relatives are unaware of patient's cognitive defects during the development of the confirmed dementias of late life is notorious. Even when cognitive decline had been noted, the date of the onset is usually difficult to fix, and social skills remain well preserved until dementia is well advanced. The pseudodements themselves forcibly complain of their memory and other cognitive difficulties — they may almost parade them — in contrast to the frequent anosognosia of true dements. On open-ended questioning, pseudodements tend to give clear chronological accounts of their illness and past life. In the main, 'don't know' answers are given only to direct questions. Pseudodements tend to get distressed and make little effort on simple tasks, while dements do their best and only finally exhibit a catastrophy-reaction. Clearly defined defects of temporoparietal functions like dysphasia, dyslexia, and failure of left–right discrimination are unusual in pseudodements. Near-miss and past-the-point answering, as well as patchiness and variability occur both in true and in pseudodementia. On more detailed examination, the memory defects of pseudodements have been shown to have a different structure from those defined in true dements by Whitehead (1974), Kahn *et al* (1975), and by others. In socially and intellectually deprived old people dementia may be wrongly suspected (Bergmann *et al* 1971). At the other end of the scale, highly intelligent and educated depressives with patchy cognitive defects may have to be observed over a longish period before incontrovertible evidence of cerebral defects emerges: possibly the delay is due to their unusual compensatory abilities.

Perhaps the main point to be made about pseudodementia is that it should not be considered too seriously. The treatment of an affective condition is strongly indicated even in the presence of lasting or progressive cerebral pathology. The same should be said in relation to paraphrenic and schizo-affective disorders, whose differentiation from brain syndromes will be discussed briefly later.

MANIC ILLNESSES

In the Western world these are much rarer than depressions, and it used to be thought that manics were even less frequently encountered among the elderly. They certainly were not specifically studied before one of my colleagues took up the subject (see Shulman & Post 1980 for a more detailed account). Shulman discovered that over a ten year period, 67 patients aged 60 or over had been admitted (to the Bethlem–Maudsley Hospitals) with a diagnosis of mania, retrospectively confirmed on the basis of strict criteria. At other centres, the proportion of manics among elderly affectively ill patients has been reported as between 6.5 and 19%. The female : male ratio was 2.7 : 1, an even higher female preponderance than that found in depressives but not as high as in late life paraphrenics. Only six of the 67 patients had experienced a manic illness for the first time before the age of 40. That had also been their first mental breakdown, and none of them subsequently experienced purely depressive illnesses, but only manic or mixed manic-depressive conditions. All patients beyond that age of first onset had suffered depressions as well as mixed illnesses and pure manias. In 42 of 61, the first attack had been purely depressive and, on average, ten years had elapsed before the appearance of manic symptoms, always after 45 and mostly around 60; a quarter had a latency for manic symptoms of between 25 and 47 years. Eighteen out of 42 patients with first depression would have sailed under the false flag of a unipolar psychosis before (after more than the three 'statutory' depressive attacks) the bipolar nature of their illness declared itself by the appearance of manic symptoms.

Obviously, this case note study did not lend itself to a descriptive analysis. From a personal impression, purely euphoric clinical pictures with an infectious affect are unusual in the elderly. Depression is never far removed, and this may be the reason for the predominance of surly, hostile affects in elderly manics. Coupled with this, flight of ideas is often slow and fragmented, and may become recognizable only on studying a recorded sample of spontaneous speech. It may be missed if the flow is broken by impatient interruptions on the psychiatrist's part! Grandiose delusions tend to be of a banal sort and mainly limited to financial matters or (in men) sexual prowess. The differential diagnosis is from an acute brain syndrome, and from the euphoric and overactive type of senile dementia, presbiophrenia, to use an old fashioned term. This is made more difficult by the patient's inability or unwillingness to submit himself to a cognitive assessment; however, not only severe mania but also hypomania is always of recent onset in a setting of previous intellectual preservation. The main reason why a manic disorder may be missed in the elderly is failure to consider it when confronted with an overactive, troublesome and seemingly confused old person.

PARAPHRENIC ILLNESSES

When schizophrenia-like symptoms first occur late in life, disintegration of personality functions tends to be limited: catatonic symptoms are most unusual and so are stereotyped psychomotor disorders. Incongruity and flattening of affect are, in the aged, perhaps more difficult to recognize and seem to be either absent or unobtrusive; so are dilapidation of speech and the underlying formal thought disorder. Prominent are delusional ideas (much more rarely true autochthonous delusions) and the associated hallucinosis. The delusional ideas are always of a persecutory kind, and the banality of their content has often been noted: they are not grandiose, religiose or relating to personal identity, but mainly concern domestic issues and possessions, including personal dignity and sexual virtue. Paranoid psychoses in old age, therefore, approximate to what has been singled out in a purely descriptive sense as the paraphrenic type of schizophrenia. Paranoid, schizophrenia-like, and schizophrenia states as seen in the aged have been comprehensively dealt with recently (Post 1980) and only the essential features will be discussed here. Those which relate to causation and management will be discussed in the following chapter.

Incidence

Persistent persecutory states are relatively rarely encountered in psychogeriatric practice: the Newcastle survey discovered not a single paraphrenic still living in the community studied, and among a sample of 300 persons coming to the notice of a local authority, there were only eight paranoid cases (Goldberg 1970). Kay & Roth (1961) calculated that only about 10% of elderly persons admitted to mental hospitals were paraphrenic. Paraphrenia of late life is so uncommon that it has come to be studied in the United States only quite recently (Bergen & Zarith 1978, Bridge & Wyatt 1980). About four in every five late paraphrenics are women.

Clinical aspects

Persecutory delusions and hallucinations are encountered in a number of different settings. They are fleetingly present in some acute confusional states, and somewhat more lastingly in subacute brain syndromes. Some patients suffering from dementing illnesses of late life exhibit well structured and persistent paranoid pictures, which are only later erased by the increasing dementia. Elderly depressives, and occasionally manics, may exhibit paranoid and schizophrenia-like symptoms. Finally, these phenomena may occur without lasting affective admixtures and without increasing cognitive impairment; patients of this kind have been termed (in the strict sense) late or senile paraphrenics. Regardless of the clinical setting, I have gained a strong clinical impression that persecutory delusions and hallucinations are encountered in patients in the form of three well differentiated syndromes, which remain stable in terms of history and on follow-up.

Persecutory states are least disruptive when they are limited in content to only one or two themes. Patients suffering from such a simple paranoid psychosis believe themselves to be subjected to annoyance by their neighbours or, much more rarely, by their relatives. Out of envy or on account of their own past attitude of aloofness, others want them out of their homes and instigate various nuisances: thefts are committed against them, and they may have to put up with nasty odours, knockings or specially installed noisy machinery. Occasionally, they are insulted by neighbours or in the street. Jealous delusions of old men about their wives are particularly troublesome and potentially quite dangerous. In many cases, patients suffering from these simple paranoid psychoses seem to harbour delusional ideas only, but usually there are also some, mainly auditory, hallucinations and these are occasionally shared by a spouse or a daughter. Delusional perceptions may include the disappearance of objects, their mysterious removal from one place to the other, or the imagined presence of stains or of infestations (delusional parasitosis). Probably, the majority of old people with such simple paranoid psychoses never come to the notice of doctors, let alone psychiatrists. Their families tend to humour them, as do the police. Hospital admission is rarely required, except perhaps in the case of patients living alone or becoming more than verbally aggressive. In my own series (Post 1980) less than a third of patients hospitalised for persistent persecutory states suffered from this limited kind of condition.

In over two-thirds of patients, the overt mental disturbance was so great that continued survival outside a psychiatric facility would have seemed unlikely. About half suffered from schizophrenia-like symptoms, not just isolated paranoid delusions and hallucinations, but states of severe panic or aggressiveness in response to widespread psychotic experiences: accusing or denigrating voices; cars circling the building with headlights shining into their rooms; gases being pumped into their homes; children crying underneath the floorboards; telescopes or rays being directed at them; enemies about to break into their house, etc. Finally, the remaining half of patients with severely disruptive paranoid psychoses (over one-third of all patients in my inpatient series) were indistinguishable from younger paranoid schizophrenics. In addition to symptoms of the kind enumerated above, they exhibited some of the features which Schneider suggested as of first rank importance when making the diagnosis of schizophrenia. In the age group with which we are concerned they are limited to true delusions of passivity, thought withdrawal, and thought broadcasting — all experiences suggestive of dissolution of ego boundaries. Most frequently and most easily ascertained is a third person auditory hallucinosis, when the patient believes that he overhears remarks about him or a running commentary on his actions by one or more persons, referring to the patient by name or more usually as 'he' or 'she'. As with younger patients, it is important to register these symptoms as 'first rank' only where the patient describes their experiences without or with only slight leading.

As we pointed out earlier, these three syndromes are not limited to patients that might be labelled as late paraphrenics, but can also occur as prominent features of organic mental illnesses and occasionally of affective psychoses. The presence of 'true' paranoid schizophrenia symptomatology would seem to betoken a greater personality disruption than that of either simple paranoid or schizophrenia-like psychoses. Patients suffering from either of these two last conditions quite frequently lose their current symptoms (without insight) when transferred to hospital or other sheltered surroundings, at any rate for a time. By contrast, 'Schneider-positive' patients in my experience always continue to hold their delusional beliefs and to experience their hallucinations without interruption after admission to hospital. Even in the elderly, the content of their psychoses may be less commonplace and domesticated than is the case with simple paranoid and schizophrenia-like psychotics, and in every aspect these patients with first rank symptoms closely resemble paranoid schizophrenics of earlier onset.

SCHIZO-AFFECTIVE ILLNESSES

Among my series of inpatients with paranoid illnesses of late onset (which included also a few cases with confirmed chronic brain syndromes of various kinds), 57% displayed some depressive features, which were well marked in 23% (Post 1980). In differentiating depressive or manic from schizophrenic-paranoid symptoms we are taught to look for the underlying affect. The paranoid delusions of manics are either related to ideas of grandeur or present a reaction to attempts at restraining the patient's overactivity. In depression, the persecutions are felt to be deserved (police prosecution for imagined misdeeds, shunning of and critical remarks about the patient, who is deluded about being poverty stricken or dirty and smelly, etc.). In paraphrenia the patient is not elated with pressure of thought and overactivity; he is sometimes euphoric but more often dysphoric. He feels himself persecuted in a position of delusional superiority, which causes envy and enemity. In terms of response to the treatment and of further course these criteria have not been found reliable in the elderly. Patients who turn out to be paraphrenics may have depressive types of paranoid beliefs and experiences, and vice versa.

I submitted to long-term review (Post 1971) all those patients over 60 who had been admitted during the course of three years in whom difficulties had been encountered at some stage in differentiating between a depressive and a paraphrenic psychosis. In most instances the diagnostic problem had been settled by the time either the antidepressive or antischizophrenic treatment had been initiated, and the research sample came to consist of only 4% of all patients consecutively admitted in the course of three years. Thus, a mere 29 patients came under close investigation and were operationally called schizo-affectives. This thorny concept will not be discussed here. Attempts to define or to deny the existence of a schizo-affective entity in younger patients have been made by Procci (1976) and quite recently by Kendall & Brockington (1980). Half of my schizo-affectives proved to run a course in which the mixture of depressive and paraphrenic symptoms remained a constant feature; in the other half, schizo-affective episodes alternated with purely depressive and purely paraphrenic ones. There was a strong impression that a schizophrenia-like symptomatology predominated, with only a few patients exhibiting simple paranoid or paranoid schizophrenic first rank symptoms. Possibly rather more schizo-affectives than late paraphrenics were also suffering from various forms of mild or slowly developing changes in cerebral pathology.

CHAPTER 7

Functional Disorders
II. Treatment and its relationship to causation and outcome

Felix Post

It was shown in the preceding chapter that the functional psychiatric conditions of late life can be most fittingly regarded as a continuum of overlapping symptom clusters and not as disease entities, each with its distinct and separate aetiology, course and response to treatment. These overlap just as much as the syndromes themselves. Most aspects of management apply to all functional disorders, and there are only a few specific therapies which need be described only in relation to the relatively uncommon severe and psychotic illnesses.

Of over-riding importance is a skilled approach to the patient and his family to promote a therapeutic relationship between them and the doctor, as well as with his non-medical colleagues. In the following, this general approach, which applies to all elderly psychiatric subjects, will be described first in relation to the minor disorders whose treatment is based on heuristic assumptions concerning their aetiology, but uncertain as to its effectiveness. However, all that has been learnt about the management of less ill patients is fully applicable to that of psychotic patients, and in their case often highly effective specific therapies will be discussed, the actions of which will be related to theoretical considerations of aetiology and long-term outcome. It is hoped that this presentation will do greater justice to the complex clinical reality than traditionally structured accounts.

NEUROTIC AND ALLIED CONDITIONS

Probably too much as been made in the past of alleged differences in the psychology of older and younger people (see Chapter 2). Differences that do exist tend to be generational rather than biological. These, however, need to be known and allowed for in the psychiatrist's approach to the older patient. In accordance with Lawton's (1976) advice, the following points should serve as a guidelines.

For well-known reasons, members of the older generation tend to be even more resistant to the ideas of psychological medicine than younger people. However, good therapeutic rapport can be achieved with older people, provided one is aware of the stronger taboos they feel especially with regard to ease of self-revelation and of discussion of sexual matters. In this area, too, less permissiveness in older persons has been shown by Willesey *et al* 1977 to be due to social rather than ageing factors. Where a psychotherapeutic approach is attempted, it has to be kept in mind that old people do have greater difficulties with problem solving and with abstraction. Patients may thus have to be guided by repetition, and too much abstraction in formulating their problems should be avoided. Anxiety further impairs cognitive ability in the elderly and should only be sparingly evoked in therapy. Allowance should thus be made not only for obvious and for concealed hearing difficulties, but also for slowness in comprehension. Life review should probably be encouraged only cautiously, as it is likely to bring up preponderantly negative past experiences. Denial is often the preferred style of the elderly and should be respected. It is one of the reasons why old people are often unaware of social facilities available to them, especially of non-official ones, and so they may need active help and intervention. Psychiatrists working with elderly people should only rarely avoid contact with a patient's significant others, and should never be reluctant to seek help from social workers.

More specifically in relation to psychotherapy, the prescription given by Davis & Klopfer (1977) seems to be sensible: relatives, while they may sometimes scapegoat the patient, are more often very distressed and have to cope with their own problems. Apart from practical matters, they should only be involved when there is an acute situational crisis. At that stage, '. . . the therapist may serve as a kind of referee and avoid blaming anyone but looking for cause and effect and offering various options for solution.' This recommendation of sparing contact with the families of elderly neurotics is not in conflict with individual and group support of family members caring for dementing and other patients beyond the reach of psychotherapeutic endeavours. Sometimes therapy with a relative may be helpful in the management of the elderly patient.

Social work

Where the role of social work is concerned, it is worth remembering that the effectiveness of the trained social worker in comparison with that of untrained personnel has been conclusively demonstrated (Goldberg 1970); voluntary workers need trained supervision. Obvious family and practical problems apart, doctors are most likely to seek a social worker's help under the impression that the elderly patient's greatest problem is loneliness, and that this should be relieved. A tremendous amount has been written about loneliness in the elderly to the effect that people may live alone and be lonely, that they may live alone and not be lonely, and that they may not live alone, and yet be lonely. The complaint of loneliness has many meanings, and these have been elucidated by Bergmann (1978) on the basis of his community study. First of all, mentally and physically healthy old people may be lonely because they have outlived friends and relatives. Secondly, there are lonely persons, who with or without loss of intimate contacts, are suffering from immobilising physical or mental disorders (or frequently from both). Finally, there is a small group of persons who are not isolated from others, who have no physical or mental infirmities, and who yet complain about loneliness; their problem has not as yet been understood. When confronted with the complaint of loneliness it is therefore necessary to discover which of these features are relevant, and to devise therapeutic strategies accordingly: medical treatment to increase mobility, psychiatric management to combat depression and anxiety, and attempts at re-socialising only those for whom physical or psychic factors seem to be relatively unimportant. In fact, Bergmann found that functional psychiatric patients attracted more and inappropriate social services than seemed rational, sometimes more than the far more seriously disabled persons in the community with organic mental conditions. Moreover, social workers' support given to anxious-depressive clients was frequently especially inappropriate: domiciliary services rather than social work attempting to render these clients more sociable.

Personality disorders

Turning to personality disorders of old people coming to psychiatric notice, management will probably have to limit itself to the provision of an environment which will reduce the problems caused. However it is especially important to assess and treat first of all any neurotic symptomatology, especially depression which may have led to recent and more disruptive 'decompensation' in longstanding maladjusted persons.

Sexual disorders

I cannot recall a single patient over 60, who came for help with impotence or frigidity. Patients were referred only because they had aroused concern on account of exhibitionism and/or sexual transgressions towards children. Regular contact with such patients in an atmosphere of sympathetic understanding and managment by spouses (where existant) or families frequently reduces or even abolishes the behaviour. Where it does not, I found the use of an anti-androgenic preparation, such as cyproterone acetate (Androcur) 100–200 mg daily, very successful and without side-effects over several years' observation on the minimal effective maintenance dose.

Alcohol

Before discussing the treatment of alcoholism, attention should be drawn to the allegedly beneficial effects of alcohol in old people. It has been called 'balm of autumn' and 'milk of old age' while, even under Islamic Law, Arab physicians like Avicenna have recommended wine (Mishara & Kastenbaum 1980). In our time, there have been investigations which demonstrated that 3–6 ounces of wine, when given as a regular daily medication, improved sociability, sleep, and concomittantly some cognitive functions (Mishara & Kastenbaum 1980). These authors point out in their comprehensive book that, in the case of elderly problem drinkers, we do not yet possess the basic data needed before introducing therapeutic programmes. There seems to be a consensus to the effect that aversive (including disulphram) therapies were too risky in the elderly. Where there is good evidence for alcohol having become a problem only in relation to a circumscribed and a fairly recent anxious depressive change, treatment of this depression does often lead to a satisfactory reduction of drinkng; however, it should be remembered that 'depression' is frequently simulated by hangover effects and that antidepressants will cause further trouble under these circumstances. The management of causative psychosocial background problems will always be difficult, but should be attempted. From personal experience I would say that complete withdrawal and continued abstinence from alcohol are always indicated in patients of the age group with which we are concerned. Alcoholics will be seen by us largely because they themselves or their families have come to a point where they want help, and under these circumstances withdrawal and supervision are usually successful without admission. Whatever their claims of motivation, elderly alcoholics living on their own always need admission and usually subsequent discharge into some form of sheltered or institutional surroundings. Regardless of social settings, aged problem drinkers of long or recent standing tend, as members of a survivor group, to have relatively well structured personalities, and are more likely to respond to a psychotherapeutically orientated approach than most younger alcoholics: I have again and again been impressed with the favourable response, both short-term and long-term, of aged alcoholics. Where an acute confusional state seems related to alcoholism, gradual withdrawal of alcohol is perhaps a safer procedure than immediate withdrawal covered by drugs like chlormethiazole (BMJ Editorial 1981).

Neuroses

In considering the treatment of the neuroses, it should be remembered that only few elderly neurotics are referred for treatment, either because (in the case of longstanding disorders) their social support has recently broken down or because neurotic symptoms have appeared only recently, when they almost always do so in an anxious-depressive setting. Where antidepressant or anxiolytic therapies, as well as attempts to deal with psychosocial problems, have failed, specifically aimed psychotherapy should be considered. By its nature, psychotherapy is directed towards assumed causes, either in psychodynamic terms (hang-ups) or as faulty learning. The literature on psychotherapy with the elderly has grown considerably, mainly in the USA. Much of it is discursive and exhortatory: Freud's advice against treating older persons with his method is unfavourably commented upon, and hopes for success of psychotherapy in the elderly are held out. Only few writers have based their work on their personal experience with old patients; nevertheless a good deal can be discovered in their publications, which will be of use to psychiatrists with psychotherapeutic experience in treating younger patients.

In planning strategies of psychotherapy, Kahana (1979) has found it useful to divide older patients with neurotic symptoms into three groups: first, essentially healthy ageing persons, in whom therapy aimed at effecting changes in their psychic structure can be successful. Second, there are the larger number of debilitated aged including not only persons with chronic brain syndromes, but also those with debilitating general conditions, as well as chronically unhappy and socially deprived old people. Finally, there is a much smaller intermediate group, mainly with more recent situational problems.

In the case of severely debilitated aged an approach described by the late Alvin Goldfarb may be useful in the hands of some therapists: in a brief series of short sessions the illusion is created in the patient that he has vanquished the therapist, who figures as on omnipotent parent. Thus self-esteem is enhanced and the patient's aggravatingly complaining behaviour reduced. In some of these apparently hopeless situtions, I have certainly found it useful to tell the patient that his problems are far too difficult for me, and to continue supportively in this submissive spirit over long periods, with the patient usually keeping his appointments and becoming a smaller burden to his family. In a report on the effect of sets of therapeutic interviews conducted by voluntary workers under the weekly supervision of a psychotherapist, the point is made that even dementing patients sense whether the encounter with the therapist is mechanical or genuinely human. It is claimed that the psychotherapeutic conversations with patients diminished their resentment and promoted their acceptance of their situation (Bircher *et al* 1978).

Valuable advice on the conduct of psychotherapy in essentially well preserved old people is given by several authors. Among many other important technical matters, Ingebretsen (1977) points out that obtaining insight and giving support have to be carefully balanced, varying from individual to individual. Past life should be supportively evaluated, but forgiveness should be granted only up to a point. At the same time acceptance of a patient's past life by the therapist will increase the patient's self-esteem and enable him better to deal with his anxieties. A recurrent theme concerns the fact that almost invariably the therapist is younger than the patient, who may look upon him not as a protective, let alone omnipotent, parent but as a child. Counter-transferences thus obviously have to be guarded against. These may also be created through the strain on the therapist of sessions filled with ' . . . the trials and tribulations encountered in most ordinary events of every day living' (Wilensky & Weiner 1977). To guard against one's counter-transferences it is necessary to recognise the intensity of affect which accompanies such experiences in old people. Dream therapy with the aged is proposed by Brink (1977), who points out that along with a reduction of REM sleep, there is lower dream recall in the old. Their dream contents reveal preoccupations with diminished resources and loss, and Brink's suggestion is that in old patients dreams should not be used in Freudian or Jungian fashion, but that associations should be encouraged towards recent events, and the patient should also be led to discover the motivations involved in the dream content. He gives two examples where, over time, dream content was altered by suggestions and autosuggestion, and concurrently the patients' waking attitudes, feelings, and behaviour were changed for the better.

Regular therapeutic sessions of largely open groups are a feature of many psychogeriatric units on both sides of the Atlantic. Very little has been published about results, and that which has is found in relatively inaccessible journals. I have gained the impression that these ward groups certainly give the psychiatrist an additional dimension for understanding his patients: in one report, patients attending a therapeutic group were given more medication than their matched controls! Group therapy with the elderly in the community tends to have attendance problems. Those that did attend regularly tended to improve in their anxious-depressive complaints and attitudes, but this was not related to form of therapy, e.g. relaxation versus life review (Ingersoll & Silverman 1978), or focussed as against more diffuse therapy. On the whole, the more directive approaches are favoured, and a useful discussion is offered by Krasner (1977) who recommends that patients should first be treated individually, and that this can be tailed off in favourable cases as group treatment progresses. In this way, excessive disturbance of the group can (if thought wise) be avoided, and transference and resistance phenomena occurring in the patient can be dealt with individually.

Behaviour therapy of phobic and obsessional disorders, which are not infrequently encountered in older patients, seems decidedly under-reported, but personal experience suggests that it may well be as effective as in younger patients. Behavioural modification is recommended for patients whose rigidity blocks effective coping through obsessive and phobic thinking (Brink 1978). An interesting case report is offered by Garfunkel (1979) of a patient with longstanding situational phobias. What amounted to a practically complete and lasting cure was produced by five months of treatment, with biweekly sessions only at first. Imaginal desensitisation was used, and the difficulties arising from this are described. In my experience, graded in-vivo desensitisation to phobic situations has proved the method of choice, with few patients failing to benefit from efforts directed by a trained worker (usually a clinical psychologist) aided by nursing staff, voluntary workers, and members of the patient's family.

The third group of patients distinguished by Kahana (1979) were well retained old people breaking down in a crisis. Almost always, depressive symptomatology predominated and, to avoid repetition, discussion of crisis intervention will be postponed to when we shall be dealing with the psycho-therapeutic approach to depressive illnesses in the next section.

MAJOR PSYCHIATRIC ILLNESSES

Depressive illnesses

The relationship between aetiology, symptomatology, therapeutic modalities and outcome has been fully discussed on many occasions (Post 1972, 1975, 1982). A full repetition would be out of place in a general text, and an attempt will be made to give a more concise account.

Causation

There seems to be overwhelmingly strong evidence in the case of younger depressives that their breakdowns tend to follow closely upon disruptive life events and stresses (Paykel 1982). Our investigations into these aetiological factors were carried out at a time when a sophisticated methodology had not yet been worked out. The following common sense assumption was made: where a person over 60, who had been at risk of developing a depressive illness (conservatively speaking) for the preceding 30 years of his life, had become for the first time (or in repetition of widely spaced previous occasions) clinically depressed within a few weeks or months of an incisive event, the probability that this event had been causal rather than coincidental seemed very high. Guarding carefully against the possibility that life events may be engineered by patients during the nascent phases of their depressions, and not relying on psychodynamic pointers, our various investigations yielded precipitating events in anything between 65 and 80% of patients.

In a third of patients these events, as emerging from the accounts of informants, were what have been termed exit events: bereavements (especially widowing), the moving away of children and close friends, and occasionally, only the threat of bereavement, such as a spouse's sudden severe illness even if followed by recovery. In about a quarter of cases the impact made on the patient by his own sudden illness — an intimation of mortality —. was the triggering event, while in contrast to some other writers we did not find that longstanding ill-health and invalidism could be clearly implicated as a cause of clinical depression. Other precipitating events were loss of status (especially retirement, which as we know is weathered by most people), moving away from the old home, and some other less clearly definable psychological stresses not previously experienced by the patient.

The association of physical illness with depression has been well recognised, and is for obvious reasons particularly strong in late life. Suicide had been found very significantly associated with terminal illness (Barraclough 1971), and possibly cancer may be a factor in depression even before the patient has become aware of its presence. Heart disease is also likely to evoke depression, and the number of physical disorders including drug effects which may be accompanied or masked by depression is legion. (For a full account and discussion of possible mechanisms see Salzman & Shader 1979.)

In many instances, the impact of physical illness as a precipitant of depression is not directly at the level of brain chemistry but via its psychological effects. Turning to speculations on the psychological 'causes' of depression in our age group, it has been suggested (Fassler & Gaviria 1978) that there is a normal depression which is part of the ageing process, and that this amounts to a sense of dejection which arises from the elderly person engaging in a survey of his past life (areas of failure and frustration rather than of achievement and gratification), as well as through his recognising and appraising his own physical image. Most people make an adjustment as age advances and this normal depression is overcome. On the other hand, it may be fostered by an undue slowing down of mental processes, which makes people withdraw from social activities, and renders them more introspective and prone to boredom. This may well be the background on which clinical depressions arise in response to disruptive live events. However, bereavement may cause lasting depression even in socially involved and financially secure elderly persons: 25% of such widows interviewed 21 months after their husband's death still seemed depressed (Heyman & Gianturco 1973). A measure of loss of control (attempting to objectify Seligman's concept of learned helplessness) was found to be associated with depression only in elderly men, but not in women (Hanes & Wild 1977). Psychodynamic mechanisms operating in late life depressions through failure in coping have been summarised and inconclusively ventilated by Salzman & Shader (1979).

Psychotherapeutic management of depression

The recent literature on this topic was found to yield only very few accounts describing what was actually done in psychotherapy with elderly depressives and with what success. Depression was the usual disorder encountered in crisis situations — the third group of cases whose discussion we had postponed (p. 203). Kahana (1979) describes how, in the course of a few sessions and in a setting of positive transference, insight into various intrapsychic problems and improvement in the patient's ability to deal with them were achieved. A case is also quoted where, through patient listening and also through obtaining information from the family, a recent interpersonal problem was unearthed, and where the therapist did not shy away from giving positive advice and instructions. Kovacs (1977) found that distress reactions sometimes occurred when old people were subjected to unreasonable demands from relatives. The patient may originally only complain of insomnia. Two cases are used to describe Kovacs' methods of discovering the underlying upset and his direct method of therapy is outlined: this involved peremptory instructions and advice to the patient. He warns that one has to feel very sure of one's ground before employing such methods. In managing more firmly established depressive illnesses, Goldstein (1979) also advocated a strong-arm approach: the doctor should be perceived as caring, loving, but powerful, and he should expect the patient to function at his optimum level. Capabilities should be assessed, and the patient should not be allowed to function below them. While not pushing patients beyond their capacities, regression should be countered by pressure to perform. Feelings of helplessness and moanings about losses should be combatted. Goldstein warns that often staff are more upset by harsh measures than patients; these have included removal of mattresses, also threats of starvation, e.g. for refusal to go to the dining room. Relatives must be made aware of the patient's capabilities and taught to say 'no', to ignore frantic pleadings and 'urgent' telephone calls. A more gentle approach is advocated by Karpf (1977) who regards depression as a danger signal, which allows psychological preparation for age decline and death, or coping with loss of a loved object in the psychoanalytic sense. He does not give explicit advice on how ' . . . first to help the patient to achieve ego-integrity, and second, to uncover the existential sadness inherent in the aged who are near death'. An investigation of two types of group therapy in comparison with an untreated matched sample was reported by Michaels (1977). Recently bereaved and depressed outpatients were treated either by a catharctic method, in which grief, loss, death and dying were worked through, or only social and topical discussion was encouraged. Both groups improved in terms of depression scale scores more than untreated controls, and the author claims that the catharctic approach was more successful than the placebo group treatment.

The work quoted concerning psychotherapy of both neurotic and of depressive conditions seems to indicate that there is plenty of scope for psychotherapists willing to work with elderly people. I would, however, like to cite Kahana (1979) who stresses that there is no place for a psychotherapist with the elderly who shies away from directive intervention, drug therapy, or even electroconvulsive therapy. A psychotherapeutic approach improves compliance with these measures.

Somatic therapy

Somatic therapies of depressive states do not differ in any important way from those with which the reader will be familiar from his experience with younger patients. Only a few additional matters need be discussed here (see also Chapter 4).

Antidepressant drugs have powerful actions on cerebral functions and toxic effects are easily produced in the ageing brain by average or even small dosages: delirious or schizophrenia-like states, and, in the elderly, even more dangerous unsteadiness of gait and falling attacks. It is, therefore, of interest that the depressive states of debilitated old people in a geriatric ward were reported to have responded well to thioridazine 25–200 mg daily and that 30% did not relapse after the treatment was discontinued (Maurer 1973). Also reported has been an investigation in which no drugs were used at all in a similar group of physically debilitated depressives: 15 sessions involving the promotion of physical contact and measures to increase communication were found to improve depression-scale rating significantly in comparison with an untreated control group (Power & McCarron 1975). When antidepressant preparations are employed in elderly patients, it is advisable for the doctors to use one preparation only over a long time in order to get to know its therapeutic and side-effects thoroughly. Moreover, it should be a preparation whose plasma concentration can be measured in a laboratory to whose services one has easy access. Ideally, plasma concentration should be measured if after two weeks of treatment there are no signs of response. (I am aware that this matter may still be controversial, and for further details, including choice of preparation, cardiotoxic effects, etc. see Chapter 4, also Jacoby 1981.) In the treatment of elderly depressives my first choice has recently been a tricyclic preparation, amitriptyline, but there may well be more suitable antidepressants (Chapter 4). If, after 4–5 weeks on the recommended therapeutic plasma level there has been no worthwhile improvement, I have prescribed electroconvulsive therapy. Where this was resisted, a monoamine oxidase inhibitor has been tried and there have been a few patients who responded, and even some (and this was confirmed on long-term follow-up) who have been successfully maintained only on a combination of tricyclic and MAOI drugs.

As a treatment of first choice, electroconvulsive therapy has been used only in the most severe and life-endangering psychoses. The treatments were administered no more frequently than twice a week, gradually more widely spaced but continued until remission had been obtained. The average number of treatments has been eight, but up to 18–20 have very occasionally been given with ultimate success. Unilateral (non-dominant hemisphere) applications of electrodes produce fewer cognitive and especially memory defects immediately after conclusion of therapy (Strömgren 1973), but in a sample of patients recently reported by Weeks *et al* (1980) of whom few were between 60 and 70, there were no longer any signs of impairment several weeks after treatment regardless of whether its application had been unilateral or bilateral. All the same, the use of unilateral electroconvulsive therapy is strongly recommended in elderly patients because the period of confusion immediately after each individual treatment, during which most accidents and injuries occur, is so much shorter (Fraser & Glass 1978). On the other hand, where unilateral electroconvulsive therapy seems to fail, further bilaterally induced convulsions may lead to success, possibly because a failure of producing fits by the unilateral method had not been spotted.

Psychosurgical procedures are now only rarely recommended, partly on account of the present climate of opinion, but largely because elderly depressives 'resistent' to drugs and electroconvulsive therapy are usually physically (and not only cerebrally) much impaired and not fit for brain operations. However, even now there is the occasional 'hopeless case' who responds gratifyingly and psychosurgery should not be banished from the thoughts of psychogeriatricians!

Outcome and prognosis

These have been little studied. This is surprising when one recalls that, up to the age of 75, the majority of elderly people seen in the psychiatric clinic suffer from some kind of depression. Apart from my own (1972) publication, which also summarises an earlier investigation, I have only been able to trace one paper by Cole & Hickie (1976), which will be discussed later, and one by Angst & Frey (1977). This Swiss study had been preceded by another one of patients diagnosed as depressives at the Lausanne clinic in earlier adult life. It was shown that depressions tended later in life to become less severe and less frequently recurring. Angst & Frey followed severely ill depressives for 13–17 years after their admission to the Burghölzli Clinic. There were 59 with onsets before 40, and 100 with first depressions after that age, mostly between 50 and 69. Comparing these two groups it was found that their course was very similar, with a practically equal number of phases. But, in contrast with the earlier work just mentioned, late-onset depressions became more often chronic and 12–13% ended in suicide. They calculated, however, that the risk of suicide was lower than in early-onset cases.

It was unfortunate (for reasons which will become clear presently) that my own studies were also confined to elderly depressives who had come to require inpatient treatment. In the earlier study, at a time when electroconvulsive therapy and leucotomy were the only specific remedies available, only 6 of 81 depressives without cerebral pathology failed to become fit for discharge. Nowadays, there is only the very rare patient who fails to remit to some extent during his first treatment episode. We know nothing precise, quantitatively or qualititatively, about outcome for the vast majority of ageing depressives who are treated by their family doctors or in psychiatric outpatient clinics and day hospitals. One may, however, assume that most do well as only few need admission. Nevertheless for them the future is far from rosy, and has not been strikingly improved in any way since the introduction of thymoleptic preparations; however, these have probably reduced the number of patients needing admission (for details see Post 1972). A cohort of nearly 100 depressed hospital patients over 60 years of age were followed for three years after discharge. They had required admission, occasionally immediately, but usually only after unsuccessful drug treatment. All could be discharged but only 26% remained completely well throughout the subsequent three years. Further attacks with good recoveries were suffered by 37%, but 25% were found not to have made complete recoveries on follow-up: they remained anxious, worrying, unhappy in their adjustment, often sleeping and eating poorly, hypochondriacally complaining, and in many instances going through further attacks of more circumscribed depressive illness. Finally, 12% remained depressively ill throughout, though not necessarily with long periods in hospital. Three of the 92 patients ended by suicide, and four made suicide attempts.

These disappointing results were achieved in spite of carefully devised and energetically pursued treatment and after-care. At first one at a time, and later in combination if required, tricyclics, monoamine oxidase inhibitors, as well as electroconvulsive therapy were all employed during the index admission and often also during the follow-through period. One patient had psychosurgery, and a few had lithium maintenance treatment, which was just beginning to be introduced. Regular social work supervision was shown not to prevent recurrences, but did lead to an earlier institution of further treatment. Surveying it all, only 24% of patients required no further treatment after discharge or after antidepressant drugs had been discontinued soon after discharge. The remainder required treatment episodically or continuously. There is an inescapable conclusion: severely ill, aged depressives almost always require long-term supervision, which may become even more demanding if it becomes confirmed that carefully monitored lithium maintenance will prevent frequent and serious recurrences. In consolation, it might be pointed out that recent and more careful work has shown that (pace textbooks!) younger depressives also face an uncertain future.

Conclusions

To round off of the subject a few theoretical speculations on the classification of and the predisposition to depressive illnesses of late life may not be out of place. It would be of considerable practical value if these illnesses could be classified on the basis of aetiology and symptomatology to yield indications for the most appropriate kind of therapy as well as useful predictions of long-term course. As we saw (Chapter 6) it was relatively easy and straightforward to distribute on the basis of the mental state alone over a few subgroups a cohort of elderly depressive inpatients. Some of these groupings were characterised by the presence of delusions as well as of depression of varying severity, and others by an absence of delusions and the presence of only minimal depression or of more prominent anxiety. The first groups of patients exhibited clinical characteristics traditionally associated with psychotic and 'endogenous' depressions, while patients belonging to the other groupings fitted well (as far as symptomatology was concerned) into the stereotype of neurotic depressives. It is of interest that far more sophisticated analyses of younger depressives employing cluster techniques have similarly yielded a well defined group of patients with the characteristics of endogenous depression, and in addition other more diffuse clusters without these features. Andreason *et al* (1979) summarised these findings and reported their own, largely confirmatory results; however, they also indicated that their groupings did not correlate with differing family histories, therapies, or short-term outcomes. They concluded that more thorough family studies and long-term follow-up should be carried out to discover whether the clusters obtained by them did in fact represent true subtypes.

I had earlier attempted this (Post 1972) with disappointing results. In the case of patients over the age of 60, the long-term course pursued by patients with psychotic symptomatology did not differ from that followed by neurotic depressives. Regardless of clinical picture, certain variables have been shown and have been confirmed (Jacoby 1981) to be of adverse prognostic import: age over 70, physical senility, and — related to both — the presence of serious and progressive physical diseases, by no means necessarily affecting the brain. These adverse prognostic indicators, while holding for group comparisons, have been found to be of no use in predicting the further course taken by individual patients.

With regard to therapy, as expected the initial modality had more often been electroconvulsive therapy in the case of the more severely ill psychotic depressives, though some had eventually responded only after tricyclic or other drugs had been used (Post 1972). Neurotic depressives always received drug therapy as a first choice of treatment, but many required electroconvulsive therapy later. This, rather than drug therapy, had been successful in rendering many of the neurotic depressives fit for discharge, and only insignificantly less often than had been the case with psychotic patients. (In this series we had been careful not to give electroconvulsive therapy and drugs concurrently during the index illness, not only for reasons of research, but because it always seems important with an eye on future recurrences to establish whether a patient is more likely to respond to electroconvulsive therapy or to antidepressants.) Family histories of affective disorders were also only insignificantly more often registered in psychotic as against in neurotic depressives. Early loss of a parent and other childhood deprivations were not more characteristic of neurotic depressives. No type of precipitating life-event was found to have been more common in them as compared with the psychotics, whose illnesses are traditionally regarded as more 'endogenous'. In fact, precipitating events, especially bereavements, had been registered more often (albeit insignificantly so) in patients with positive family histories! There was only one set of background variables on which the neurotics differed significantly from the psychotics: in the last mentioned, previous neurotic and other personality difficulties and deviations were by no means uncommon, but they were found very significantly more often in neurotic depressives.

Thus, it has not proved possible to subdivide elderly depressives into clinical subtypes with differing aetiology, therapeutic needs or outcome. Attempts in samples of elderly depressives to obtain a bimodal distribution of patients indicating a dichotomy between psychotic-endogenous and neurotic-reactive illnesses have consistently failed (Jacoby & Levy 1980).

My conclusion is that all elderly depressives sufficiently ill to require hospital admission have some endogenous predispositions; if that were not so, practically all old people would come to suffer depressive illnesses sooner or later! Possibly the illness takes its clinical features from the personality it strikes. Furthermore, in the case of elderly neurotic depressives studied in the community, Bergmann (1971) commented on the frequency with which they often exhibited 'endogenous features' such as early waking, feeling worse in the morning, sudden onset, short duration, and weight loss. There is an important caveat, however, arising from one of the (1972) observations to the effect that in my material manic developments had occurred in 14 of 56 psychotic depressives as against in only 3 of 36 neurotics. There thus remains a lingering suspicion that, in spite of its lack of practical significance, there may after all be some theoretically important factors which differentiate endogenous depressions from the rest. In this connection, Martin Roth in a recent review (1979) made the percipient forecast that biochemical indices may come to make more important contributions to the classification and rational treatment of late life depressions than clinical analyses.

Finally, another area of ignorance should be briefly defined. It surrounds the questions as to why so many people fall ill with depressions only in late life (for details see Cawley *et al* 1973). An answer to this question has been sought by comparing depressives over the age of 60 who had suffered attacks earlier in life with patients whose depressions had occurred for the first time only as they grew old. Against expectation, late-onset depressions are no more often precipitated by life-events related to the vulnerable position of the aged than depressive attacks recurring since an earlier age. Also, late-onset depressives tend to have had more stable and more firmly structured personalities than early-onset patients. At the same time, most studies have shown that a family history of affective disorders is more rarely elicited in late- as compared with early-onset cases, and there is little evidence for late life depression having a specific heredity. (For a summary seen Mendelwicz 1976.) Therefore, the first emergence of depression in late life could not be explained either in terms of especially severe environmental stresses encountered during old age or of constitutional defects, and so another possibility had to be reconsidered: that increasing predisposition to late-onset depressive illnesses and to more frequent and prolonged depressive recurrences with advancing years may be due to age changes in the brain.

We saw in the preceding chapter that in the recent past the association between affective disorders and the dementias of old age was over-valued. Possibly, there is a special link between multi-infarct dementia and depression via a common diathesis, but several follow-up studies of aged depressives have shown that dementias of any kind occur in them at a later stage no more frequently than in the general run of the elderly (see Post 1974). This was confirmed more recently by Cole & Hickie (1976), but they also discovered that minor disorientation and memory defects in depressives over 70 when observed in late- rather than in early-onset cases tended to be associated with a lower discharge rate (and in the case of those who remitted) with 'significant declines of living arrangements'. They wondered, therefore, whether these late-onset depressives might not be afflicted with some ' . . . more subtle cerebral changes'. This possibility was both earlier and more recently investigated in co-operation with and by my colleagues (Cawley *et al* 1973, Davies *et al* 1978, Hendrickson *et al* 1979, Jacoby & Levy 1980) with the following results: It was only weakly confirmed that cognitive defects discovered at the height of late life depressions improved less on remission in late as against in early-onset patients. However, elderly depressives as a group scored lower even after remission than normal controls on a vocabulary test of intelligence. Elderly depressives during the illness and also on remission had delayed auditorily evoked cortical potentials similar to, but to a smaller extent than senile dements. All but one of nine depressives with enlarged cerebral ventricles demonstrated by computed tomography had had their first attack of affective illness after the age of 60: they were also older and symptomatically more of an endogenous type. These patients had a higher death rate than the rest, but not from primarily cerebral causes (Jacoby 1981). Finally, there are many age-related changes in the hormonal and cerebral amine systems, as well as in cholinergic and monoaminergic transmitters and in monoamine oxidase activity, which reflect predisposing factors to depression (summarised by Ordy & Brizzee 1975). Thus there is mounting evidence to support a hypothesis according to which increased propensity to depression is related not to coarse brain deterioration, but to age changes in the central nervous system and its neuroendocrine associations.

Manic illnesses

The treatment, outome and aetiology of manic illnesses during late life have not been specifically studied so far. Probably treatment and its immediate results do not differ from those of younger manics, except that unpleasant side-effects to drugs are more easily produced. At the time of writing, haloperidol seems to be the drug of immediate choice for more severely disturbed and overactive patients, although neurological complications tend to be produced when the daily dose exceeds 9 mg over any length of time. In most patients there is no over-riding urgency in suppressing psychotic behaviour, but at the same time, and in contrast to the majority of depressives, hospital admission is always indicated, if necessary under initial compulsion. Provided there are none of the usual physical contraindications, lithium therapy should be commenced, and will usually induce amelioration in the great majority of patients within a few days. In our retrospective sample of 67 cases (Shulman & Post 1980), 27 had received adequate lithium therapy, and all but three benefitted considerably. (For the special risks of lithium administrations in elderly patients see Chapter 4.) Patients surviving any length of time almost invariably suffer further attacks of mania, depression, or mixed manic depressive psychosis. Provided an adequate lithium plasma level can be maintained (as a rule at the lower end of the range recommended for younger patients), further attacks can be prevented or at least ameliorated to an extent which makes re-admissions unnecessary. The same impression has been obtained for the efficacy of maintenance therapy with lithium salts in frequently recurring depressions. In both bipolar and unipolar affective patients, attempts at discontinuing maintenance therapy have in my experience always led to serious and prolonged recurrences within a few weeks.

Regarding aetiology, the only available findings concern the relationship between mania and neuropathology. Only three of the 67 patients followed were found to have demented: all were women. By contrast eleven men had at one time (but only rarely immediately preceding a manic attack) suffered from a variety of cerebral insults, ranging from cerebral trauma, infection and anoxia, to cerebrovascular accidents. The existence of secondary or symptomatic mania in relation to cerebral pathology has recently been postulated by a number of writers mainly in relation to younger patients (for references see Shulman & Post 1980).

Paranoid, schizophrenia-like, schizophrenic and schizo-affective illnesses

The treatment, outcome and aetiology of these illnesses have been fully set out recently (Post 1980). A more streamlined account will be attempted here and only important and easily accessible references will be given.

Findings relating to the course taken in late life by longstanding schizophrenic patients will not be summarised again. All that need be repeated is that their symptoms tend to become far less disruptive with increasing age but that, at the same time, the life adjustment of two-thirds of schizophrenics remains severely impaired: only few achieve stable marriages or other good relationships, and only two-fifths continue to live outside institutions of one kind or another (Post 1980).

Management

The main obstacle encountered in the management of paranoid patients arises, of course, from their lack of insight. Referral to a psychiatrist is unlikely before a social crisis, sometimes of a severe kind, has occurred. Actual violence in such a situation is much rarer than in the case of younger paranoids and, as a rule, a parley of some sort is possible in the setting of a domiciliary visit. Only a small proportion of patients are persuaded by their friends to accompany them to the outpatient clinic. Regardless of the setting of the first encounter, the same guidelines apply as with younger paranoid psychotics: one's profession should not be concealed and the patient usually needs little encouragement to display his disorder. However, some patients deny all symptoms and disturbances when interviewed on their own, but they will give free rein to their paranoid ideations when seen together with prompting relatives. Other than encouragement, interjections should be avoided by the doctor, and patients should be allowed to finish their story. It is imperative not to contradict or even to argue any points. I have found a useful gambit to admit my puzzlement about what the patient has just told me, and to concede that it is beyond my powers to deal with the persecutions: however, since the patient is obviously nervously disturbed by his experience, the use of a calming medication and attendance for further discussions are recommended to him. This non-critical approach, which the patient will be unlikely to have encountered before, frequently fosters sufficient rapport for the patient to accept medication. However, this is very unlikely to be taken with adequate regularity by patients living on their own or not closely supervised by their families. A temporary stay with them may be possible and, in any case, as we saw earlier some simple paranoid and schizophrenia-like illnesses remit with purely environmental re-location or, at any rate, these patients become more manageable when away from the source of imagined persecution. In the case of patients living alone, whose medication cannot be supervised, it is often possible with the help of their social workers to get them to accept informal admission. On the other hand, there are very many instances where all attempts at achieving co-operation will fail completely. Compulsory admission (a 28 day order will usually suffice) should be most firmly recommended. Reluctant relatives and social workers should be assured of the likelihood of early, and mostly excellent, results of treatment.

When outpatient treatment can be instituted with sufficient supervision, it is particularly advisable to avoid any adverse drug reactions, even though improvement will in this way often be delayed. Depending on the size and general fitness of the elderly patient, I would start with a twice daily dose of thioridazine, 25 or 50 mg. Once every fortnight, I would increase the total daily dose by 25 or 50 mg until (before further stepping up has become due) the patient's active symptoms have disappeared on both his own and his friends' report. At this stage the patient is likely to continue to hold on to his delusional beliefs, but he will cease to act on them. In the enfeebled and especially in those patients where the paraphrenic symptomatology has emerged in a setting of a relatively early dementia, suppression of disturbing symptoms may occur after a few days on as little as 50 mg of thioridazine daily. It is unsafe to exceed 500 mg of this preparation and, if relatively high dosages fail to produce a useful remission, more potent preparations should be tried even though they are, of course, much more likely to precipitate unpleasant neurological complications. Again it would be ill advised to exceed, e.g. trifluoperazine 25–30 mg daily. Failure at this stage should indicate admission, as combined oral and depot treatment should not be attempted in the older age groups in patients who cannot be observed at least once a day. At this stage the patient, whose co-operation has been maintained by means of a gentle and psychologically sophisticated approach, is unlikely to refuse a short admission to hospital. As soon as the patient no longer experiences any hallucinations or produces either fresh delusions or enlarges upon old ones, dosages should be reduced gradually until 'active' symptoms begin to appear once again. Maintenance doses will lie somewhat above this level, in most cases between 25 and 100 mg of thioridazine or 1–5 mg of trifluoperazine.

Where treatment is only feasible after admission to hospital, it may not infrequently be discovered that the patient obtains immediate and lasting relief from all his psychotic experiences, though this is most unlikely to occur where these had been of a Schneider-positive type. In any event, any treatment should be started but, in order to assess response, nights away from hospital back into the patient's usual, unsheltered environment will have to be risked. Obviously, in hospital, dosages can be increased more quickly and depot injections alone or combined with oral therapy can be instituted. The reader should use any method and type of preparation with which he is familiar in younger patients, and no specific advice will be given here. The patient is discharged on his tailor-made maintenance regime.

Neurological complications cannot always be avoided but few patients seem to be aware or distressed by them. All the same, annual drug 'holidays' should be attempted (see Mehta *et al* 1977). It was found that two-thirds of patients who had been successfully maintained, relapsed within an average of 20 months following cessation of treatment, but that most of them recovered after its resumption (see Post 1980).

Outcome

It can be categorically stated that before the introduction of major tranquillising drugs, paranoid illnesses in elderly patients, which were not related to the development of organic-cerebral deterioration or secondary to an affective phase, invariably persisted for the remainder of the patient's life. I can only recall a single patient who remitted spontaneously, only to relapse after a year or so. With modern treatment, one can expect long-term freedom from all symptoms in one-third of cases, half of whom may even gain and preserve full retrospective recognition of the pathological nature of their ideas and experiences. In over one-third there will be fluctuating returns of paranoid symptoms, but in one-quarter it will turn out that, in spite of initial response, the psychotic disturbance is not relieved in the long run. These results (Post 1966) were obtained before depot injections were used and they may well be better now. The later development of one of the dementias of old age may well be higher than in the general elderly population but, as we shall see, many of these patients are odd people and often deaf; their cognitive state may be difficult to differentiate from the intellectual changes which were responsible for the concept of dementia praecox. Apart from organic cerebral disorders and severe deafness, poor past interpersonal adjustment is an unfavourable prognostic. Full response to initial treatment with even only a modicum of insight is a favourable sign. Over-riding all this, success depends mainly on continued adequate drug maintenance and a variety of personal and social factors favouring this. The effects of major tranquillisers seem to be purely symptomatic and equally good in simple paranoid, schizophrenia-like, and 'true' paranoid-schizophrenic psychoses. At best, the patients become symptom free, but most of them remain handicapped by their previous personalities. In spite of flexibly used therapies, schizo-affectives have a much poorer prognosis (Post 1971).

The aetiology of late paraphrenic illnesses

There is little but speculation concerning the aetiology of late paraphrenic illnesses. The outstanding fact is an overwhelming predominance of women with persistent paranoid illnesses, and this would seem to indicate the presence of sex-linked hereditary-genetic factors. Dementing patients with persistent paranoid symptomatology — like younger 'organic' paranoids — lack schizophrenic heredity and so probably do paranoid affectives. A specific hereditary loading in schizo-affective illnesses has not been found with any undue frequency in the age group with which we are concerned, but elderly schizo-affectives stand out in terms of frequent family histories of many kinds of psychiatric conditions (Post 1971). Late paraphrenics, regardless of type of clinical picture, significantly more often have schizophrenics among their parents, siblings, and children than do members of control populations, but less frequently than early-onset schizophrenics (summarised in Post 1980). The predominance of previously 'schizoid' personalities and the relatively weak (but significant) hereditary loading with schizophrenia suggests that the late paraphrenic illnesses are delayed forms of disorders somewhere along the schizophrenic spectrum.

Other aetiological factors have been fully discussed recently by Cooper *et al* (1976), Cooper (1976), and in summary by Post (1980). Briefly, the great majority of late paraphrenics have been found to have suffered from life-long personality defects and deviations. In contrast to late life depressives, they tend to have shown few circumscribed neurotic symptoms or traits; some have had earlier episodes of psychological disturbance, which may have been mild and unrecognised schizophrenic 'thrusts'. Objectively, the chief indicator of the earlier personality dysfunctioning of late paraphrenics is their low marriage rate, the frequency of delayed marriages, and the small number of surviving children. Equally impressive, though more problematic to define, is the rarity of evidence for satisfactory sexual adjustment having ever been attained. Unlike early-onset schizophrenics, late paraphrenics have usually had average work histories and few conflicts with the law. Their personality defects show themselves mainly in failure of building up and maintaining close relationships of any kind. In many of them group membership is limited to confraternities practicing sectarian religions including spiritualism. Most patients are described by their relatives as quarrelsome–aggressive, egocentric–obstinate–domineering, suspicious–jealous–easily feeling persecuted, or shy–sensitive–withdrawn. The illness tends to develop imperceptibly and gradually with increasing age.

Unlike depression, one can rarely convince oneself that the illness has been precipitated by life-events independent of the patient's own behaviour and actions. Where a paranoid psychosis seems to be the sequel of bereavement, one usually finds on closer study that the deceased spouse or relative had either concealed the patient's psychotic state or had shared his delusions. Physically, late paraphrenics are usually healthy old people without reduced life expectation. The only (but important) defects are social deafness and, debatably, visual impairment which are far more common than in healthy or depressive elderly persons. Deafness does not produce the paranoid symptomatology of, for example, auditory hallucinosis via sensory deprivation, and the visual illusions associated with deteriorating eyesight are always recognised as such by the sufferers. Deafness in paraphrenics is almost always of longstanding — the result not of age-linked deterioration of auditory functioning (nerve deafness), but of middle ear disease or degeneration dating from childhood or early adult life. There is good evidence to show that this longstanding deafness may be an important factor in deforming the pre-psychotic personality. Why in such an abnormal personality paranoid, schizophrenia-like, or paranoid-schizophrenic symptoms should arise in old age is, of course, unknown. Plausibly, the development may be related to the increasing age-linked social isolation suffered by schizoid persons far more severely than by old people who had been socially integrated in the past. As in the case of late-onset depressives, subtle cerebral age changes may conceivably lead to a mild degree of mental disintegration. This may allow unconscious psychodynamics, which had previously determined the deviant personality traits, finally to emerge as frankly psychotic phenomena. The mechanisms of dynamic psychopathology in late paraphrenics are usually patently obvious. Such individuals have always been basically hostile towards and shut off from other people and, in the psychosis, they believe themselves to be persecuted and threatened in their privacy and their possessions. In an equal banal fashion, it is especially those patients without or with little in the way of past sex lives whose delusions and hallucinations are of a sexual nature. There is usually no evidence for any earlier overt or latent homosexuality, and the psychotic experiences are of an undisguisedly genital kind. Schizophrenic ways of thinking and experiencing have taken over only late in life and therefore they tend to be less disruptive of personality functioning and more easily subdued by pharmacological means than is the case in younger patients: both continue to suffer from deformed personalities even when their psychotic symptoms have been suppressed or controlled by drugs.

Conclusions

Continuity stands out in all the functional disorders and illnesses discussed in these two chapters. There is continuity in the symptomatology of these conditions and of the sufferers' earlier personalities with them. The pressures and stresses precipitating them tend to be similarly related to continuous biological and social ageing. The need for continuity in their management cannot be overstressed.

REFERENCES

ANDREASON N.C., GROVE W.M. & MAURER R. (1980) Cluster analysis and the classification of depression. *British Journal of Psychiatry* **137**, 256–65.

ANGST J. & FREY R. (1977) Die Prognose endogener Depressionen jenseits des 40. Lebensjahres. *Nervenarzt* **84**, 571–4.

BARNES G.M. (1979) Alcohol use among older persons: Findings from a Western New York State general population survey. *Journal of the American Geriatrics Society* **27**, 244–50.

BARRACLOUGH B.M. (1971) Suicide in the elderly. In *Recent Developments in Psychogeriatrics*, eds D.W.K. Kay & A. Walk. British Journal of Psychiatry special publication no. 6.

BERGER K.S. & ZARIT S.H. (1978) Late life paranoid states: Assessment and treatment. *American Journal of Orthopsychiatry* **48**, 528–37.

BERGMANN K. (1971) The neuroses in old age. In *Recent Developments in Psychogeriatrics* eds D.W.K. Kay & A. Walk. British Journal of Psychiatry special publication no. 6.

BERGMANN K. (1978) Neurosis and personality disorder in old age. In *Studies in Geriatric Psychiatry,* eds A.D. Isaacs & F. Post. John Wiley, New York.

BERGMANN K., KAY D.W.K., FOSTER E. *et al* (1971) A follow-up study of randomly selected community residents to assess the effects of chronic brain syndrome and cerebrovascular disease. *Proceedings of the V World Congress of Psychiatry, Mexico.* Excerpta Medica, Amsterdam.

BIRCHER M., SIX W. & KELLER W. (1978) Experiences in clinical psychotherapy with geriatric patients. *Praxis* **67,** 990–5.

BLAZER D. (1980) The diagnosis of depression in the elderly. *Journal of the American Geriatrics Society* **28,** 52–8.

BRIDGE T.P. & WYATT R.J. (1980) Paraphrenia: Paranoid states of late life. *Journal of the American Geriatrics Society* **28,** 193–205.

BRINK T.L. (1977) Dream therapy with the aged. *Psychotherapy* **14,** 354–60.

BRINK T.L. (1978) Geriatric rigidity and its psychotherapeutic implications. *Journal of the American Geriatrics Society* **26,** 274–7.

BRITISH MEDICAL JOURNAL, editorial (1981) Management of alcohol withdrawal symptoms. *British Medical Journal* **282,** 502.

CAWLEY R.H., POST F. & WHITEHEAD A. (1973) Barbiturate tolerance and psychological functioning in elderly depressed patients. *Psychological Medicine* **1,** 39–52.

CHOMSKY N, (1972) *Language and Mind.* Harcourt Brace Jovanovich, New York.

CLARK A.N.G., MANKIKAR G.D. & GRAY I. (1975) Diogenes syndrome. A clinical study of gross neglect in old age. *Lancet* i, 366–73.

COMFORT A. (1980) Sexuality in later life. In *Handbook of Mental Health and Aging,* eds E.J. Birren & R.B. Sloane. Prentice-Hall, Englewood Cliffs, N.J.

COLE M. & HICKIE R.N. (1976) Frequency and significance of minor organic signs in elderly depressives. *Canadian Psychiatric Association Journal* **21,** 7–12.

COOPER A.F. (1976) Deafness and psychiatric illness. *British Journal of Psychiatry* **129,** 216–26.

COOPER A.F., GARSIDE R.F. & KAY D.W.K. (1976) A comparison of deaf and non-deaf patients with paranoid and affective psychoses. *British Journal of Psychiatry* **129,** 532–8.

CORBY N. & SOLNICK R.S. (1980) Psychosocial and physiological influences on sexuality in the older adult. In *Handbook of Mental Health and Aging,* eds J.E. Birren and R.B. Sloane. Prentice-Hall, Englewood Cliffs, N.J.

DAVIES G., HAMILTON S., HENDRICKSON D.E. *et al* (1978) Psychological test performance and sedation thresholds of elderly dements, depressives and depressives with incipient brain change. *Psychological Medicine* **8,** 103–9.

DAVIS R.W. & KLOPFER W.G. (1977) Issues in psychotherapy with the aged. *Psychotherapy* **14,** 343–8.

ELIAS M.F. & ELIAS P.K. (1977) Motivation and activity. In *Handbook of the Psychology of Aging,* eds J.E. Birren & K.W. Schaie. Van Nostrand Reinhold, New York.

EPSTEIN L.J., MILLS C. & SIMON A. (1970) Antisocial behaviour of the elderly. *Comprehensive Psychiatry* **11,** 36–42.

FASSLER L.B. & GAVIRIA M. (1978) Depression in old age. *Journal of American Geriatrics Society* **26,** 471–5.

FRASER R.M. & GLASS I.B. (1978) Recovery from E.C.T. in elderly patients. *British Journal of Psychiatry* **133,** 524–8.

GARFINKEL R. (1979) Brief behaviour therapy with an elderly patient. *Journal of*

Geriatric Psychiatry **12**, 101–9.

GIANTURCO D.T. & BUSSE E.W. (1978) Psychiatric problems encountered during a long-term study of normal ageing volunteers. In *Studies in Geriatric Psychiatry,* eds A.D. Isaacs & F. Post. John Wiley, New York.

GILLEARD C.J., WILLMOTT M. & VADDADI K.S. (1981) Self-report measures of mood and morale in elderly depressives. *British Journal of Psychiatry* **138**, 230–5.

GODA G. (1979) De la notion névrose en gériatrie. *Revue de la gériatrie* **4**, 71–4.

GOLDBERG E.M. (1970) *Helping the Aged: A Field Experiment in Social Work.* Allen & Unwin, London.

GOLDSTEIN S.F. (1979) Depression in the elderly. *Journal of the American Geriatrics Society* **27**, 38–42.

GURLAND B.J. (1976) The comparative frequency of depression in various adult age groups. *Journal of Gerontology* **31**, 283–392.

HANES C.R. & WILD B.S. (1977) Locus of control and depression among non-institutionalized elderly persons. *Psychological Reports* **41**, 581–2.

HENDRICKSON E., LEVY R. & POST F. (1979) Averaged evoked responses in relation to cognitive and affective state of elderly psychiatric patients. *British Journal of Psychiatry* **134**, 494–501.

HEYMAN D.K. & GIANTURCO D.T. (1973) Long-term adaptation by the elderly to bereavement. *Journal of Gerontology* **28**, 259–62.

INGEBRETSEN R. (1977) Psychotherapy with the elderly. *Psychotherapy* **14**, 319–32.

INGERSOLL B. & SILVERMAN A. (1978) Comparative group psychotherapy for the aged. *Gerontologist* **18**, 201–6.

JACOBY R.J. (1981) Depression in the elderly. *British Journal of Hospital Medicine* **25**, 40–7.

JACOBY R.J. & LEVY R. (1980) Computed tomography in the elderly: 3. Affective Disorder. *British Journal of Psychiatry* **136**, 270–5.

JARVIK L.F. & RUSSELL D. (1979) Anxiety, aging and the third emergency reaction. *Journal of Gerontology* **34**, 197–200.

KAHANA R.J. (1979) Strategies of dynamic psychotherapy with the wider range of older individuals. *Journal of Geriatric Psychiatry* **12**, 71–100.

KAHN R.L., ZARIT S.H., HILBERT N.M. *et al* (1975) Memory complaint and impairment in the aged. *Archives of General Psychiatry* **32**, 1559–73.

KARPF R.J. (1977) The psychotherapy of depression. *Psychotherapy* **14**, 349–53.

KAWASHIMA K. (1979) Clinical study of depressive illness in old age. In *Recent Advances in Gerontology,* ed H. Orimo. International Congress Series no. 469. Excerpta Medica, Amsterdam.

KAY D.W.K., BEAMISH P. & ROTH M. (1964) Old age mental disorders in Newcastle upon Tyne. Part I: A study of prevalence. *British Journal of Psychiatry* **110**, 146–58.

KAY D.W.K. & ROTH M. (1961) Environmental and hereditary factors in the schizophrenias of old age ('late paraphrenia') and their bearing on the general problem of causation in schizophrenia. *Journal of Mental Science* **107**, 649–86.

KENDALL R.E. & BROCKINGTON I.F. (1980) The identification of disease entities and the relationship between schizophrenic and affective psychoses. *British Journal of Psychiatry* **137**, 324–31.

KIMMEL D.C. (1977) Psychotherapy and the older gay man. *Psychotherapy* **14**, 386–93.

KILOH L.G. (1961) Pseudo-dementia. *Acta Psychiatrica Scandinavica* **37**, 336–51.

KOVACS A.L. (1977) Rapid intervention strategies in work with the aged. *Psychotherapy* **14**, 368–72.

KRASNER J.D. (1977) Loss of dignity — Courtesy of modern science. *Psychotherapy* **14**, 309–18.

KUPFER D.J., SPIKER D.G., COBLE P.A. *et al* (1978) Electroencephalographic sleep recordings and depression in the elderly. *Journal of the American Geriatrics Society* **26,** 53–7.

LAWTON M.P. (1976) Geropsychological knowledge as a background for psychotherapy with older people. *Journal of Geriatric Psychiatry* **9,** 221–3.

LEACH E. (1970) *Lévi-Strauss.* Fontana/Collins, London.

MASS H.S. & KUYPERS J.A. (1974) *From Thirty to Seventy. A forty year longitudinal study of adult life styles and personality.* Jossey-Bass, San Francisco.

MCDONALD C. (1967) The pattern of neurotic illness in the elderly. *Australian and New Zealand Journal of Psychiatry* **1,** 203–10.

MACMILLAN D. & SHAW P. (1966) Senile breakdown in standards of personal and environmental cleanliness. *British Medical Journal* ii, 1032–7.

MADDEN J.J., LUHAN J.A., KAPLAN L.A. *et al* (1952) Nondementing psychoses in older persons. *Journal of American Medical Association* **150,** 1567–70.

MAURER A.S. (1973) Management of emotional disturbances in geriatric patients. *Journal of the American Geriatrics Society* **21,** 226–8.

MEHTA D., MEHTA S. & MATTHEW D. (1977) Tardive dyskinesia in psychogeriatric patients. A five year follow-up. *Journal of the American Geriatrics Society* **25,** 545–7.

MENDELWICZ J. (1976) The age factor in depressive illness: Some genetic considerations. *Journal of Gerontology* **31,** 300–3.

MICHAELS F. (1977) The effects of discussing grief, loss, death and dying on depressive levels in a geriatric outpatient therapy group. *Dissertation Abstracts International* **38,** (2–13), 910.

MILLER M. (1978) Geriatric suicide: The Arizona Study. *Gerontologist* **18,** 488–95.

MISHARA B.L. & KASTENBAUM R. (1980) *Alcohol and Old Age.* Grune & Stratton, New York.

MÜLLER Ch. (1969) *Manuel de Geronto-Psychiatrie.* Masson & Cie, Paris.

NEUGARTEN B.L. (1977) Personality and aging. In *Handbook of the Psychology of Aging,* eds J.E. Birren & K.W. Schaie. Van Nostrand Reinhold, New York.

ORDY J.M. & BRIZZEE K.R. (1975) *Neurobiology of Aging. Advances in Behavioural Biology, vol 16,* Plenum Press, New York.

PAYKELL E.S. (1982) Life events and early environment. In *Handbook of Affective Disorders,* ed E.S. Paykell. Churchill Livingstone, Edinburgh.

POST F. (1966) *Persistent Persecutory States of the Elderly.* Pergamon Press, Oxford.

POST F. (1967) Disorders of sex in the elderly. *Practitioner* **199,** 377–82.

POST F. (1971) Schizo-affective symptomatology in late life. *British Journal of Psychiatry* **118,** 437–45.

POST F. (1972) The management and nature of depressive illness in late life: A follow-through study. *British Journal of Psychiatry* **121,** 393–404.

POST F. (1974) Diagnosis of depression in geriatric patients. In *Depression,* eds D.M. Gallant & G.D. Simpson. Spectrum Publications, New York.

POST F. (1975) Dementia, depression and pseudo-dementia. In *Psychiatric Aspects of Neurologic Disease,* eds D.F. Benson & P. Blumer. Grune & Stratton, New York.

POST F. (1980) Paranoid, schizophrenia-like and schizophrenic states in the aged. In *Handbook of Mental Health and Aging,* eds J.E. Birren & R.B. Sloane. Prentice-Hall, Englewood Cliffs, N.J.

POST F. (1982) Affective disorders in old age. In *Handbook of Affective Disorders,* ed E.S. Paykell. Churchill Livingstone, Edinburgh.

POWER C.A. & MCCARRON T. (1975) Treatment of depression in persons residing in homes for the aged. *Gerontologist* **15,** 132–5.

PROCCI W.R. (1976) Schizo-affective psychosis: fact or fiction? *Archives of General Psychiatry* **33,** 1167–78.

ROSIN A. & GLATT M.M. (1971) Alcohol excess in the elderly. *Quarterly Journal of Studies on Alcoholism* **32**, 53–9.

ROTH M. (1979) Some lessons from comparison and contrast of affective disorders in late and earlier life. In *Recent Advances in Gerontology*, ed H. Orima. International Congress Series no. 469. Excerpta Medica, Amsterdam.

SALZMAN C. & SHADER R.I. (1979) Clinical evaluation of depression in the elderly. In *Psychiatric Symptoms and Cognitive Loss in the Elderly*, eds H. Raskin & L.F. Jarvik. John Wiley, New York.

SHULMAN K. (1978) Suicide and parasuicide in old age: A review. *Age and Ageing* **7**, 201–9.

SHULMAN K. & POST F. (1980) Bipolar affective disorder in old age. *British Journal of Psychiatry* **136**, 26–32.

SIMON A. (1980) The neuroses, personality disorders, alcoholism, drug use and misuse, and crime in the aged. In *Handbook of Mental Health and Aging*, eds J.E. Birren & R.B. Sloane. Prentice-Hall, Englewood Cliffs, N.J.

STENBACK A. (1980) Depression and suicide behaviour in old age. In *Handbook of Mental Health and Aging*, eds J.E. Birren & R.B. Sloane. Prentice-Hall, Englewood Cliffs, N.J.

STENBACK A., KUMPULAINEN M. & VAUHKONEN M.L. (1979) A field study of old age depression. In *Recent Advances in Gerontology*, ed H. Orimo. International Congress Series no. 469. Excerpta Medica, Amsterdam.

STRÖMGRON L.Z. (1973) Unilateral versus bilateral electro-convulsive therapy. *Acta Psychiatrica Scandinavica* (suppl. 240).

THOMAE H. (1980) Personality and adjustment to ageing. In *Handbook of Mental Health and Ageing*, eds J.E. Birren & R.B. Sloane. Prentice-Hall, Englewood Cliffs, N.J.

THOMAE H. & SCHMITZ-SCHERZER R. (1979) Constancy and change in personality variables. Findings from a 12 year longitudinal study on ageing. In *Recent Advances in Gerontology*, ed H. Orimo. International Congress Series no. 469. Excerpta Medica, Amsterdam.

WEEKS D., FREEMAN C.P.L. & KENDELL R.E. (1980) ECT: III: Enduring Cognitive Deficits. *British Journal of Psychiatry* **137**, 26–37.

WELLS C.E. (1980) The differential diagnosis of psychiatric disorders in the elderly. In *Psychopathology in the Aged*, eds J.O. Cole & J.E. Bennett. Raven Press, New York.

WHITEHEAD A. (1974) Factors in the learning defect of elderly depressives. *British Journal of Social and Clinical Psychology* **13**, 201–8.

WILENSKY H. & WEINER M.B. (1977) Facing reality in psychotherapy with the aging. *Psychotherapy* **14**, 373–8.

WILLIAMSON J. (1978) Depression in the elderly. *Age and Ageing* **7**, 35–40.

WILLISS F.K., BEALER R.C. & CRIDER D.M. (1977) Changes in individual attitudes towards traditional morality: A 24 year follow-up study. *Journal of Gerontology* **32**, 681–8.

WILLMUTH L.R. (1979) Medical views of depression in the elderly: Historical notes. *Journal of American Geriatrics Society* **27**, 495–9.

ZEMORE R. & EAMES N. (1979) Psychic and somatic symptoms of depression among young adults, institutionalized aged and non-institutionalized aged. *Journal of Gerontology* **34**, 716–22.

CHAPTER 8

Making Services Work: organisation and style of psychogeriatric services

Tom Arie & David Jolley

It is only during the last ten years that there has been widespread acceptance, at least in Britain, of the principle that there should be special psychiatric services for the elderly in each locality. Several factors have contributed, the most important being the 'population explosion' of the elderly, and in particular the very old, in Britain as in all industrial countries. Other factors have been developments in psychiatry which have made available effective biological, psychological, and organisational techniques which are of great relevance for the elderly, but among the beneficiaries of which old people have generally been heavily under-represented. Indeed successive British governments have identified the elderly, the mentally ill, the mentally handicapped, and the chronic sick as among the main priorities of health services development — 'underprivileged' and unfashionable groups are too often neglected both in the deployment of resources and in the interests of professional workers (DHSS 1976a, 1978). Finally, the acceptance in recent decades that health services should generally be planned for defined populations has an obvious relevance to the establishment of district services for elderly people with mental disorders.

Nor has there been much disagreement about the purposes of such services. Prime among these is to help to maintain the mental health of old people where possible, and to contribute to preserving their independence by sustaining, retrieving, and enhancing function. A final responsibility which looms large in Britain (though in many western countries it is commonly the responsibility of nursing homes which function apart from statutory health services) is to provide permanent or intermittent institutional care for those who are so disabled that this is the most practicable and humane way of looking after them. Throughout all these functions 'supporting the supporters' lies as a primary concern alongside the direct welfare of old people themselves.

There is fairly general agreement now about the facilities, and the approximate levels of such facilities, which are necessary for effective services. In this respect, psychogeriatrics owes much to its sister specialty, geriatrics, since the pattern of services which it uses draws on the experience both of geriatrics and of psychiatry. In this chapter, these services will be described in some detail; however, it would be wrong not to say at the outset that what this field needs as much as resources is new ideas. It is difficult to think of any development in the care of the elderly which is as fundamental and fruitful as was the discovery, say, of the day hospital some 40 years ago. It is much to be hoped that more new ideas as basic and far reaching as day hospitalisation will become available before this century is out.

As well as describing the range and development of facilities and experience, this chapter will give much attention to what is perhaps best described as the 'style' of services (Arie 1979, 1980). Style is personal; variety and flexibility are its essence. No-one should lay down the law about style, and yet it is possible to begin to define those characteristics of services which, over and above levels and categories of facilities and personnel, determine whether a service really works.

BACKGROUND

Those who provide psychiatric services for old people need to know the demography of old age in their country and especially in their own locality. The prospective psychogeriatrician must familiarise himself with the local pattern of services, with the agencies — voluntary, private, and statutory — which are involved with the elderly, and with the demography of old age within the population that is to be served and projections of age structure changes during the remainder of this century.

Not even the richest individual can purchase the fulfilment of a dream of eternal youth, but modern-day prosperity has made many years of retirement the reasonable expectation of every citizen, and even extreme old age is now commonplace. The consequences of this unprecedented phenomenon are most apparent in developed societies; for example, during this century alone, the expectation of life at birth for men has increased by over 20 years from just over 48 years to nearly 70, whilst for women the increase has been even greater: from 52 years to over 75. Nearly 15% of the population of Britain is now aged 65 or over, compared with less than 5% at the turn of the century. Large numbers of elderly women are alone, either as spinsters or through having outlived their spouse. In western societies old people often live on as couples in the house that they occupied throughout their married life, and these houses are more likely than those of any other section of the population to lack basic modern amenities; widowhood therefore leaves old women often on their own in cold houses without proper

Table 8.1   Percentage population increase 1970–90 (WHO 1979).

	Industrial world (%)	Developing world (%)
School age	.1.5	28.5
Working age	10.9	28.7
Over 65s	23.7	38.2

indoor sanitation, which are often also too big for their needs (Hunt 1978). In Britain today the elderly are the largest group of the poor (OPCS 1975). The social issues are different in Third World countries, but in those countries the rate of increase of the elderly already exceeds that of other age groups and, as their prosperity grows, the sociomedical problems so familiar in developed countries are already becoming apparent.

Community surveys in many countries have confirmed that not only minor but even major mental disorders are common among old people in their own homes (Parsons 1965, Bremer 1951, Gruenberg 1961). Dementia is present in 5–15% of elderly populations. In Newcastle in the 1960s about 20% of those aged 80 years and over were significantly demented, and whilst the presence of dementia is the main determinant of need for institutional care (Kay *et al* 1964a, 1964b, 1970), there were then seven dements living at home for every one in institutions. Much help for old people is given at home by their immediate family, usually an elderly spouse, a daughter, or daughter-in-law, and the burden carried within such families is often formidable; necessary support from domiciliary services is rarely available in sufficient degree (Grad & Sainsbury 1968. Pasker *et al* 1976).

Whilst dementia, the disabilities of which resemble those of small infants (Arie 1979), produces the most evident need for care, neurotic disorders are even more common, with 10–20% of old people suffering symptoms of a severity sufficient to warrant a formal psychiatric diagnosis (Bergmann 1971). Sharing the social and economic disadvantages of other old people, those suffering from neurotic symptoms arising in old age are more likely to be physically more disabled, and they too have needs for support over and above that which is within the capacity of their immediate circle. Thus they, like those suffering from dementia, are more likely to move into hospital or residential care (Kay *et al* 1970) and need much support to maintain them at home. Their need for domiciliary support was being met in less than one case in four in Newcastle of the 1960s (Foster *et al* 1976).

SERVICES AVAILABLE TO THE ELDERLY IN GENERAL

Much psychiatric morbidity goes unrecognised among old people at home (Williamson *et al* 1964) and even those problems that are identified by family doctors are rarely referred for specialist advice and treatment (Shepherd *et al* 1966). Extramural social services are designed to provide 'welfare', but cannot claim to be sophisticated in the management of psychiatric disorder; even the 'psychiatric social worker' has ceased to exist as such in Britain with the establishment of 'generic' training and, on the whole, generic deployment of social services.

Despite the bias of services towards coping at home, institutions of many kinds admit large numbers of old people. Half the beds in medical and surgical wards of British hospitals are occupied by old people and certain specialties such as orthopaedic surgery, ophthalmology, and genito-urinary surgery, find that more than half their clientele is aged (Slattery & Bourne 1979). In England 'chronic sickness hospitals' have been given over almost entirely to provide the bed base of geriatric medicine, and this is so also in a number of other countries (Brocklehurst 1977). Mental hospitals which were built to provide asylum for the mentally ill before more active treatments were available, are nowadays increasingly occupied by old people whose numbers would grow even further were it not for enforced government rationing and not uncommon reluctance on the part of psychiatrists to admit them (Shulman & Arie 1978). Some 50% of all mental illness beds in England are now occupied by people over 65 years, and the elderly account for between 20 and 40% of psychiatric admissions (DHSS 1976 b).

In Britain, the mental health service is in the process of moving slowly from a base in the mental hospital to a base in the District General Hospital and surrounding community. Economic stringency has slowed down and in some cases arrested this process, leaving a two-tier system of psychiatric care divided between district hospitals and large, often remote, mental hospitals; dangers are already apparent of the latter selectively absorbing the elderly and the demented, with serious potential consequences for quality of care and staff morale. These developments have been reviewed by a government working party of which one of the authors was a member, and which has firmly endorsed the trends towards special psychiatric services for the elderly with facilities in District General Hospitals (DHSS 1980).

Up to the 1950s, residential care for the elderly was provided largely in former workhouses (Townsend 1962). Most of this accommodation has since been replaced by small homes which are much better suited to the needs of the elderly, and the quantity as well as the quality of provision has increased. But the demand far outstrips what is available, and there remain many problems of the quality of life for those who are accepted as residents (Hughes & Wilkin 1980).

Psychiatric disorders are more prevalent among old people in institutions of all sorts than among those at home (Kay *et al* 1962). Symptomatic confusional states are common in acute medical and surgical wards (Bergmann & Eastham 1974, Millar 1981) but dementias and mood disorders loom larger in geriatric wards, among psychiatric admissions, and among the residents of old people's homes. The issues raised by mixing large numbers of mentally abnormal old people with others who are simply physically disabled or ill (geriatric wards) or socially vulnerable (old people's homes) are only now being investigated systematically (Hughes & Wilkin 1980). In England at present there is no significant nursing home sector, either to fill the part of the spectrum between hospital and old people's homes, or as an alternative to one or the other; and the advantages of 'specialist homes' for the mentally confused are not universally accepted (Meacher 1972). Indeed, there is evidence that mixed residential environments can in fact be beneficial to the morale of residents and staff alike, but require flexible arrangements designed to meet the changing needs of residents as they become ill or disabled (Evans *et al* 1981). This flexibility is currently lacking and the residential sector is poorly prepared for the task it is undertaking. For, whilst care staff in London share many characteristics with their counterparts in New York (being women, average age 40 years, married with children at home and frequently born abroad), they are much less likely to have received training in providing for the needs, especially psychological needs, of residents (Godlove *et al* 1980).

Psychiatric services

In Great Britain the psychiatric services have developed from County Asylums which had a history separate from the acute and chronic sick hospitals, largely in isolation from other health facilities (Jones & Sidebottom 1962). Mental hospitals were often deliberately placed at a distance from the large communities, often upwards of half-a-million people, which they served. Some became very big (between 1000 and 2000 beds were not uncommon) and they developed an internal organisation that discouraged intrusion by outsiders and which was apt to foster restricted lives for staff and inmates alike.

Such an arrangement was clearly not well designed to respond to the needs of the elderly when they became mentally ill; yet it was from a mental hospital base that one or two workers such as Duncan Macmillan in Nottingham (1960) and R. A. Robinson in Dumfries (1962) began during the 1960s to develop special psychiatric services for old people. From the late 1960s onwards, the concept of a special old age psychiatry service gained general acceptance, and the innovative services of the late 1960s and early 1970s have been emulated in many parts of the country (Arie 1970, Baker & Byrne 1977, Barton 1965, Blessed 1975, Donovan *et al* 1971, Godber 1975, Langley *et al* 1975, Pitt 1974, Portsmouth 1973, Whitehead 1972). Within the Royal College of Psychiatrists, a Group for the Psychiatry of Old Age (now a Specialist Section) has been an important vehicle in the development and sharing of ideas, and has generated a series of policy statements and guidelines for practice (Royal College of Psychiatrists 1973–80). The

Department of Health and Social Security (DHSS) has, in a series of circulars, issued guidance on facilities of different types, ranging from 'Psycho-Geriatric Assessment Units' (DHSS 1970) to 'Services for Mental Illness Related to Old Age' (DHSS 1972), and has moved progressively towards firm support for these district old age psychiatry services (DHSS 1981). The Health (formerly Hospital) Advisory Service, established in 1969 as an independent body reporting to the Secretary of State (Crossman 1977), sends teams to review psychiatric, geriatric and other services and its Annual Reports (HAS 1970–77) have given further encouragement to these developments, as have its local interventions.

The Department's proposed guidelines (see next section) for the provision of beds and other facilities have not met with universal support, chiefly on the grounds that they were inadequate (Jolley 1977), but have at least served to provide targets for action and debate.

Government guidance on levels of provision and division of responsibility (DHSS 1972)

'Services for Mental Illness Related to Old Age' classified mentally ill old people under three main headings which have been useful in defining responsibility between medical (geriatric), psychiatric, and social services.

1 *Patients who entered hospitals for the mentally ill before modern methods of treatment were available and have grown old in them after many years there.*

Whilst these 'graduates' account for about 20% of our current mental hospital population, their response to rehabilitation is limited and most are likely to live out their lives in hospital. The fate of their successors — middle aged chronic schizophrenics at present supported out of hospital — is uncertain. Many are extremely dependent on older relatives whilst others live in hostels, which demand some degree of independence and, as they themselves become old or their supports fail through infirmity, death, or lack of resources, they will present with new needs for care and supervision. It is hoped that alternatives to a return to the mental hospital will have been created, but there are few or no signs of this alternative provision.

2 *Elderly patients with functional mental illness.*

Old people suffering from neurotic disorders, mood disorders, or paranoid states without serious intellectual decline contribute more than half of elderly referrals to most psychiatric services (Jolley & Arie 1976). They are considered as part of the spectrum of 'general psychiatry' and are provided for from within the ration of facilities that include 0.5 bed per 1000 total population and day hospital places 0.65 per 1000 total population.

3 *Elderly patients with dementia.*

(a) Mild dementia but no significant physical disease or illness.

This is a large category and comprises essentially ambulant demented patients without severe behaviour disorders. Most people within it will be managed in their own homes, unless social circumstances direct that they require residential or day care under the social services department, or an intercurrent physical illness takes them into a medical, surgical, or geriatric ward.

(b) Severe dementia but no other significant physical disease or illness.
The patients are ambulant patients with dementia and gross behaviour disturbances, and they may present problems that require admission to psychiatric care, within a ration of 2.5–3.0 beds per 1000 aged 65 and over in the population.

Psychogeriatric day hospitals (2–3 places per 1000 elderly) may be helpful in the management of patients included in categories (a) and (b).

(c) Dementia, whether mild or severe, with other significant physical disease or illness.
These are essentially non-ambulant demented patients whose care needs are primarily physical, and these are provided by geriatric medical services, using 10 beds and 2 day places per 1000 elderly in the population.

The Royal College of Psychiatrists and British Geriatrics Society produced useful joint comments on these guidelines which continue to provide the framework for services up to the present (Royal College of Psychiatrists 1973b).

Psychogeriatric services

The development of psychogeriatric services during the late 1970s has certainly been facilitated by the reorganisation of the National Health Service in 1974 (Levitt 1976). Health Districts providing comprehensive services for populations of the order of a quarter of a million, co-terminous, where possible, with local authority boundaries or social services areas, have under their Area Authorities administered and planned both hospital and domiciliary services. The recent further reorganisation (in which the Area tier has been abolished) is likely to consolidate still further these population units (DHSS 1979). Such populations containing some 30 000 people over 65, have aimed to become self-sufficient in all but the most specialised services and many have accepted that district psychiatric services for old people are likely to achieve the best use of resources for their mentally ill elderly.

Models of specialised services
(Glasscote *et al* 1977, Arie & Isaacs 1977)

A national survey of psychogeriatric services reports that, at the end of 1980, some 120 consultant psychiatrists had the psychiatry of old age as their main activity, comprising some 10% of all consultant psychiatrists in the National Health Service. Between them they operated 87 defined district services which demonstrate a wide range of style, aspiration, and achievement (Wattis *et al* 1981). Thus some services provide simply a diagnostic clinic with perhaps outpatient, day-patient, or inpatient facility. A few limit their clientele to those suffering from organic mental disorders (Barton 1965, Baker & Byrne 1977), yet the most popular model is one which seeks to tackle all mental disorders presented for specialist attention from a defined population and to provide a comprehensive response to their needs (Arie 1970, Blessed 1975, Godber 1975, Jolley 1981). For such services, domiciliary consultation is usually a lynchpin of their procedure.

By way of example, the service in South Manchester, with a population of some 28 000 aged 65 and over, receives 350 new referrals each year. Three-quarters are women and three-quarters are aged 75 years or more. Two-thirds of new referrals are from general practitioners and these are seen at home within 24–48 hours of a telephone call, or immediately if necessary; referral by letter generally receives a slightly slower response. The remainder of referrals are from other hospital consultants — general physicians or surgeons as well as geriatric physicians. Two-thirds of referrals are of organic psychosyndromes, predominantly dementia, and the remainder have disorders of mood or personality or paranoid states. In addition to new referrals, the Manchester service is involved with 350–400 patients carried over from previous years who are receiving forms of continued support and others (currently 60 per year) re-referred after a period out of contact.

Domiciliary assessment

It is our belief that in a psychogeriatric service all patients referred (and, when possible, all patients re-referred — for things change fast in the clinical condition of mentally disturbed old people) should be initially assessed at home; and that this assessment should be made by a psychiatrist together, when necessary, with other members of the team. Before listing our reasons for this view, which is not always accepted, though it forms the practice of the majority of psychogeriatricians in Britain (Wattis *et al* 1981), it is important to make clear that we believe there is a difference in this respect between *psycho*geriatrics and medical geriatrics. In the case of physically ill old people, there are many occasions when the right course is immediate admission to hospital; it is an unattractive form of 'ageism' to argue that old people even when they have acute medical emergencies should be hospitalised with anything less than the speed and efficiency that we offer to younger people. However, we believe that in psychogeriatrics there are no emergencies which do not benefit from prior assessment on the spot — provided always that such assessment is made available immediately. The worst of both worlds is when admission depends on home assessment, yet such assessment is subject to delays.

We will tabulate our reasons for insisting on the importance of initial home assessment as follows:

1 Psychiatric problems in old people are almost always problems of function — and of function in their normal setting; old people perform quite differently in unfamiliar settings, and what is at issue is not function in an outpatient clinic or hospital ward, but function in that normal setting.

2 Home visiting enables not only the function but the characteristics of that setting to be observed — its amenities or lack of them, whether the place is warm, whether there is food in the larder and signs that it is being eaten, whether the bed is slept in, whether there are accumulations of bottles, etc.

3 It is extremely difficult for general practitioners to communicate all the information necessary to the specialist service. Thus the hospital may feel misled by an inadequate history that has omitted crucial factors, or embarrassed by significant and urgent physical disorders that have been overlooked. It is rarely the case that the general practitioner has failed to see his patient before making a referral, though this does occur occasionally, and many practitioners are very concerned to achieve the best management for their elderly patients but lack confidence and expertise when faced with mental abnormality. It is to be expected that improvements in the time allocated to psychiatry and geriatric medicine in undergraduate curricula and heavy investments in postgraduate courses would rectify this situation. Even so, most specialist psychogeriatricians prefer to gather and check their information at its roots.

4 An on-the-spot visit enables one also to speak to neighbours, local shopkeepers, visiting friends — people who may have been brought on the scene only by the crisis that has generated the referral. The importance of a collateral history in a mentally ill, and especially a confused old person, cannot be overemphasised, and often a home visit proves the best or even the only way of obtaining such a history at the outset.

5 The process of moving an old person, especially an old person who already has a degree of confusion, may exacerbate that confusion and, indeed, threaten life.

6 Hospitalisation of an old person may pre-empt wiser and more appropriate solutions, and may therefore fly in the face of the prime consideration of maintaining an old person as an independent citizen in her own home; the 'hole' in the community left by a person who is removed even temporarily from home has a way of closing rapidly and it may be very difficult to resettle that person however good her recovery.

7 The initial visit may also establish what are the likely resources, material and human, which may assist in eventual resettlement.

Those who do not agree with this policy of universal assessment at home make some significant points, such as that home is not always the best place for a proper and cool physical and mental examination — there are distractions, there may be huge sagging beds which make proper examination difficult or impossible, and investigations are not immediately accessible. To this we would reply that, where it is essential to bring a person up to the hospital for further examination or investigations, this can be arranged subsequently, but in our experience these distractions and inconveniences are rarely insuperable. Blood samples can be taken on the spot or arrangements made for other staff to come and take them later. Hospitalisation for examination and investigation as an outpatient should, we believe, be in addition to the initial home assessment when it is needed rather than in place of it.

Some hold that it is too time-consuming, especially in rural places where distances between home and hospital may be great, to operate such a policy. To this we would reply that our own experiences confirm that such a policy, though certainly demanding, actually saves time as well as being good practice. Time spent in trying to resettle old people who have been inappropriately hospitalised, or of obtaining information which could have been readily obtained at the initial home visit, is often much greater than the time spent on the programme of visiting. As for time, so too for 'costing': for though it may appear expensive for a senior doctor to visit a patient at home and receive payment for his assessment, the resultant efficiency in the most appropriate use of facilities more than counterbalances this expenditure. To this should be added the confidence generated in individuals and in the community by a service for the elderly which can readily be summoned to patients' homes; more will be said about this in our section on 'style'.

There is no doubt that taking a history from relatives is often made difficult by a confused, anxious, and perseverative old person who constantly comes into the room and interrupts. It is our experience that this problem is manageable with tact, and by the expedient of interviewing the relatives before meeting the patient.

In short, both of us in a fairly extensive practice over many years are convinced that such a policy represents both good practice and expediency. Of course, there are countries where administrative or financial considerations make such a policy of home visiting by hospital specialists difficult or even prevent it.

Other assessment facilities

Whilst domiciliary assessment is invaluable, further investigations are often indicated and some patients require admission for this. An assessment outpatient clinic run jointly with the geriatric physician has obvious advantages and offers a rewarding arena for mutual education and for teaching (Jolley *et al* 1980). Such clinics belong in a general hospital and should have access to the whole normal range of investigations, including X-rays and electrocardiography. Those who are more severely ill or who present complicated problems which cannot be disentangled in this setting are admitted to hospital.

There may be advantages in inpatient Psychogeriatric Assessment Units as advocated by DHSS (1970) where psychiatrists and geriatric physicians work together, or in variations ranging from a small four-bedded unit (Arie & Dunn 1973) to units of some 30 beds (Pitt & Silver 1980). Joint facilities will be further discussed in the section on the unity of services. It may be of interest that, in South Manchester, a 16 bedded ward in the General Hospital accepts some 200 admissions each year. These consist of patients with organic psychosyndromes as well as patients where there is doubt about the relative place of organic and functional components, together with patients who have functional disorders complicated by serious physical problems. Similar criteria were used for admission to the small joint unit in Ilford (Arie & Dunn 1973).

It is important that such wards should offer treatment as well as assessment. A psychiatric 'admission ward' is a more appropriate concept than an assessment unit. Practice varies as to whether such an admission ward should accept the whole range of mental disorders in old age or whether patients with functional mental disorders of old age should be nursed with younger psychiatrically ill patients. Experimentation and evaluation might be useful here.

Elderly patients with dementia

Inpatient facilities

Beds for severely demented, physically able old people have been rationed in England at 2.5–3.0 beds per 1000 of population aged 65 years and over (DHSS 1972). The basis for this allocation has been discussed and its limitations are manifest (Jolley 1977). It is probable that wards dedicated to the care of severely demented people should be no larger than 30 beds. Flexibility to accomodate men and women has many advantages and the siting of the ward should be as near to its occupants' home territory as is possible. Thus persistence with established mental hospitals may be necessary in the short-term, but most districts should aim to re-site these beds in local hospitals to assist visiting, encourage the involvement of the local community, and obviate the relegation of these wards to a backwater of the service. There is every advantage in having day hospital places for patients suffering from dementia alongside the beds for the same catchment area.

Day hospital care

The day hospital (rationed arbitrarily at 2–3 places per 1000 aged 65 and over) provides a natural link between institutional care and domiciliary care: if inpatients are encouraged to use the day hospital they are stimulated by its vigorous comings and goings, whilst day attenders get to know and trust the hospital and are less likely to be upset if they are required to stay in for a few days because of deterioration of their own function or a need for a break by those supporting them at home. The staff of the hospital, for their part, get to know the patient and their relatives as people with recognisable personalities, who demonstrate abilities as well as weaknesses. This makes for a more productive relationship than that induced when the hospital sees itself (and is seen) as taking over all responsibility for 'bodies' without backgrounds. Day hospital support for dements is usually dependent on the presence of a relative at home and is part of a spectrum of continuing care for that relative (Arie 1975). Discharge from such day care is most often by death or admission to another form of care (Bergmann *et al* 1978, Greene & Timbury 1979).

In the South Manchester service for about 28 000 elderly persons, 62 beds are available for continuing care for the severely demented. Forty-two are at a neighbouring mental hospital and without the back-up of a day hospital on site. These beds have 42 admissions and 12 deaths each year, the excess of admissions being accounted for by use of the ward for short-term relief admissions. The other 20 long stay beds are on the general hospital site and share day space with up to 20 day patients each day. Less than 10 deaths a year occur in this ward, yet more than 50 admissions are accepted mainly from the day hospital for short-term relief or rehabilitation. Thus the continuing care beds linked with day care are used more intensively than those which are not linked to day care.

Elderly patients with functional mental illness (DHSS 1971)

Inpatient facilities

Beds for mentally ill, non-demented old people are provided from the general psychiatry ration of 0.5 beds per 1000 population. Some psychogeriatric services 'pool' these beds with those for the demented and use a 'mixed' (functional and organic) admission ward for old people. An alternative is to provide beds for functionally ill old people alongside younger patients in a general psychiatric unit. This is the pattern chosen in South Manchester where 10–20 beds are being use for old people with depressions, paranoid states, etc. at any one time.

Day hospital care

This too is provided from the ration available for general psychiatry (0.65 places per 1000 population). As is the case when providing for the demented, there are advantages in siting the day hospital with the inpatient facilities, for day hospital treatment is often prolonged or recurrent and supports people quite severely disabled by chronic or relapsing symptoms. Many centres provide this day hospital care separate from that for the demented and this is the practice in South Manchester where 10 places are available daily in the general psychiatry day hospital.

Continuing care in the community

From a nucleus of beds, day hospital places, and outpatient clinics, quite a large clientele can be supported— with many more people maintaining their place at home than are admitted to hospital. Thus in South Manchester at any time the 80–90 beds and 30 day hospital places together with two active outpatient clinics are sustaining about 400 people at home. Half these 'extramural' patients are demented and their maintenance in reasonable equilibrium is dependent on teamwork involving members of the psychogeriatric service, as well as other help available from their families and other agencies.

Staffing

Each health district of 200 000–250 000 people should have among its consultant psychiatrists at least one who devotes his main interest to the elderly. The Royal College of Psychiatrists has recommended a *minimum* of the equivalent of full-time of one consultant psychiatrist (i.e. '11 sessions') for a health district, and this is often best divided between two psychiatrists who work as colleagues. Within the guidelines for future staffing agreed between the Royal College of Psychiatrists and DHSS there is a target of 18 sessions, and in teaching districts at least twice the minimum level of staffing is recommended (Royal College of Psychiatrists 1977b, 1978b). The consultant (Royal College of Psychiatrists 1977a) may devote all his time or part of it to the elderly, but either way there should be a formal commitment and a clear definition of responsibility.

The role of the 'psychogeriatrician' may be summarised as follows. *Organisation* — to take responsibility for planning, organising and deploying — in concert with other related services— his facilities and staff for the benefit of the elderly people in his district. This function includes acting as a focus for the service to which other interested people and services can relate, of acting as an 'advocate' for the service's claim for resources and for the needs of old people with mental disorders, and representing this sector of care in the committees and other forums in which planning and decision making takes place.

Clinical practice — to set standards of practice in his service and to stimulate such standards in the care of mentally ill old people in associated facilities, and to offer skilled and specialised service for 'difficult' psychogeriatric problems.
Education — to stimulate educational programmes and to participate in them for students and practitioners in all the health professions, and to contribute to general education of the public about the needs of mentally disordered old people.
Research — to conduct research, which includes studying the workings of the service itself.

Psychiatrists both in general and higher training should have the opportunity to work in services for the elderly: indeed, the Royal College of Psychiatrists has recently emphasised the need for all general psychiatrists to obtain training in the psychiatry of old age. In addition, trainee general practitioners should be given opportunities to rotate through psychogeriatric units in the course of their vocational training. Medical staffing requires at least two full-time general trainees for a district service, and further higher training posts at senior registrar level are much needed.

Nurses

Medical staff are important, and so far style of a service has generally depended upon the leadership provided by the consultant in charge; however, doctors spend relatively little time with their patients — they are 'hit and run' people, by contrast with nurses who spend hours on end with patients (Kushlick *et al* 1977). Nursing in England has undergone major changes in its thrust towards professional standing, and the implementation of new administrative arrangements following the Salmon Report (Ministry of Health 1966); it now faces the prospect of still further changes in response to EEC requirements. Arrangements under 'Salmon' have shifted status and rewards away from nurses who work with patients at ward level toward management posts. This has tended to denude wards of experienced and able nurses. Maintenance of morale has never been easy on psychiatric wards especially those for long stay and elderly patients, and disastrous developments in such areas have figured sadly and frequently in public 'scandals' (e.g. Committee of Inquiry into Whittingham Hospital 1972, Committee of Inquiry, Fairfield and Rossendale Hospitals 1975). Out of this unpromising situation psychogeriatric services have to seek to stimulate high standards of care and of job satisfaction for staff (Arie 1977). Much of the nursing must necessarily be undertaken by untrained nursing assistants, and it is important that they receive guidance and leadership from trained staff of the right calibre. Many such untrained men and women who enter nursing as assistants bring with them personal qualities and experience from previous employment or work in the home which is very relevant to the needs of dependent, frail old people. The balance between trained and untrained staff is important. One nurse to 1.5 patients on long stay wards and one to 1.5 on acute wards is recommended for geriatric wards, and the same norms should apply to psychogeriatric wards. The Royal College of Psychiatrists has also provided guidance that 'acute treatment wards' and 'heavy dependency wards' for the elderly mentally ill should be staffed by one nurse to 1.20 patients, with medium dependency wards using one nurse to 1.5 patients. In acute areas, trained staff should at least equal untrained staff and experience and qualifications in geriatric nursing are desirable. Under no circumstances should the ratio of trained and untrained staff fall below one nurse to 3 patients even in the long stay 'medium dependency' areas (Royal College of Psychiatrists 1978a).

A nursing officer should be appointed to oversee the psychogeriatric service and to work closely with the consultant psychogeriatrician.

Community psychiatric nursing

Community psychiatric nurses (CPNs) have been among the most successful innovations of recent years. They have done more perhaps than any other group to bring the hospital into the community and the community into the hospital. Their role has developed to include some of the work formerly performed by the now defunct mental welfare officers, and it also touches upon that undertaken by district nurses. The 'Nodder Report' (DHSS 1980) reviews the functions and different styles of working of CPNs (Royal College of Psychiatrists 1980, Carr *et al* 1980). In some services CPNs are based outside the hospital, relating equally to primary care and to the local psychogeriatric service; in other settings the CPN is a member of the psychogeriatric service, working outwards from a hospital base and in relation to patients who have already been referred to the service.

Social workers

Social workers are employed in Britain by local authorities and are not direct employees of the National Health Service. Social Services departments, however, have a duty to provide social work support for the Health Service and a variety of different styles of providing that support have evolved. In South Manchester one full-time social worker is attached from each of three local authority areas of 60 000–70 000 people. These relate their work to that of other field workers based in the area offices, and a senior social worker co-ordinates their activities in the psychogeriatric service, and also devotes as much time to teaching students attached by various training courses.

Occupational therapy and physiotherapy

Whilst occupational therapy has long been an accepted part of the psychogeriatric team, physiotherapists have only lately become actively

involved in the assessment of patients, in the planning of remedial programmes, and in offering advice on the use of aids and adaptations. The programme
of daily ward activity which is essential to well-being on long stay wards is
usually best accomplished by occupational therapists working together with
nursing staff. The shortage of trained personnel means that a balance has to be
struck between qualified occupational therapists and unqualified aides who,
like nursing assistants, frequently bring invaluable resources of personality
and experience. It is our experience that a much richer social environment is
created by the interaction of occupational therapy and nursing than by
increasing nursing staff alone.

Physiotherapists are only now beginning to define their role, but that there
is such a role is obvious from the high levels of infirmity and intercurrent
illness in aged people. Many patients are able to accept physical exercise when
emotional or cognitive problems make other activities difficult for them.
Success in physical therapy may ease their path to involvement in more
emotionally and intellectually challenging activity. There can be no excuse for
leaving hundreds of disabled old people without physical therapy merely
because they happen to be in the back wards of 'mental' rather than 'physical'
hospitals; and newly referred patients can often be rescued from deterioration by appropriate treatment applied early. Therein, physiotherapists in
their interaction with nursing care and indeed with occupational therapy, can
greatly enrich the quality of life and of rehabilitative resources in the wards.

Psychologists

The potential contribution of psychologists has already been discussed
(Chapter 2). Despite the enthusiasm of a few individuals, psychology has not
yet established itself as a regular contributor to psychogeriatric services. In
regard to the place of a psychologist in psychogeriatrics, it is fair to say that it is
more a case of potential than of clearly defined roles. This should add to the
challenge: there is certainly scope for new ideas throughout the whole field of
treatment, from ward regimes and their evaluation to behavioural treatments
and token economies—let alone those activities which are more clearly in the
field of research. Our impression is that psychologists are currently most
attracted by those fields of psychiatry in which potential psychotherapeutic
contributions are prominent; whilst there is plenty of scope for cultivating the
field of psychotherapy in relation to the elderly (Verwoerdt 1981), this is not
usually one of the priorities of psychogeriatric services.

Team meetings

Liaison between the members of the team is best achieved by a regular
meeting which allows time to discuss not only the management of individual
patients, but also problems or new ideas. It is particularly important to include

a 'round' of those patients who are being managed at home and whose main contact is with CPNs and social workers. In South Manchester, these patients are included in the weekly day hospital round where many difficulties can be dealt with by involving other members of the day hospital staff — either by arranging visits, or by bringing the patient up to the day hospital for review. Not least, news of patients who are doing well is a good source of morale boosting gossip! But units which are forever 'conferencing' get little work done.

Relatives' groups and other support groups

Groups for the support of relatives have been found useful (Fuller *et al* 1979). They are commonly open to relatives of patients in contact with the service, as inpatients or outpatients, and they may be led by one or more members of the staff. Shulman (1981) holds an 'open' follow-up outpatient clinic at Sunny-brook Hospital, Toronto, to which patients, and presumably relatives, can come freely without appointment. These are conducted in a group atmos-phere with supportive contact with the whole team, rather than merely as more conventional individual interviews.

Unity of services

No part of the spectrum of care of the elderly can function, or be planned, in isolation from the others. Successful psychogeriatric services must work closely with their sister geriatric services and with the social services. The planning of services must never be for a single compartment — for develop-ment in any one area of care has implications for the other parts of the spectrum.

The Standing Joint Committee of the British Geriatrics Society and the Royal College of Psychiatrists has issued 'Guidelines for Collaboration between Geriatric Physicians and Psychiatrists in the Care of the Elderly'; these are reprinted by kind permission of both bodies at the end of this chapter (Royal College of Psychiatrists 1979).

Mention has already been made of joint facilities between psychiatrists and geriatricians and of patterns of collaboration such as joint outpatient clinics. To give a personal example, in Nottingham there is a joint University Department of Health Care of the Elderly, where psychiatrists and physicians are fellow members of a joint department. This provides a medical and a psychiatric service, each separately organised but with the main facilities adjacent to each other and with an easy interchange of staff. This makes easily possible experience by trainees (and, indeed, specialists) in one or the other specialty of the work. The Nottingham department is only some three years old, but the style of work is popular with the staff and students, and is a step towards unifying services for the elderly without losing differentiated skills (Arie 1981).

Social services and residential homes

Collaboration with the Social Services department is at least as fruitful as collaboration with geriatric medicine. Personal relationships here, as in all other fields, are crucial. Of special importance is liaison in respect of the residential homes which are administered by the Special Services departments. These have always had many mentally impaired old people as residents and present trends make it clear that the proportion of confused and disabled among them will continue to increase (Wilkin *et al* 1978). This has great implications for staffing of the homes and for their support from psychogeriatric and geriatric services. Some homes specialise in the management of mentally impaired residents and there can be advantages in this provided attitudes and tolerance (as well as staffing) are right. The disadvantages are that such specialised homes in time become isolated and under-resourced hospital wards with insufficient nursing and medical support; even worse, they may become 'dumping grounds' for old people who are unwanted or unpopular on any grounds. There is evidence too that less able residents benefit from being alongside those who are more able. It is important that the most 'difficult' residents are often not mentally impaired at all but simply old people in whom difficult personality traits have become even more troublesome in old age.

Whatever the local arrangements, it is important that regular visits are paid to residential homes so that there is a regular and dependable network of contacts between the hospital services and the local authority residential homes. In some localities it has been possible to establish a joint assessment procedure involving the medical services for old people being considered for residential care (Brocklehurst *et al* 1978).

STYLE

So far we have been concerned chiefly with the different types of facilities and personnel which are now generally held to form a necessary part of the resources of psychogeriatric services. In the rest of this chapter we wish to turn to a trickier aspect, which may best be labelled 'style'. By this we mean those aspects of the service, over and above categories and levels of resources, which determine whether it actually works and, one might add, whether it is satisfying to work in. Time and again many services which have about the right resources nevertheless appear not to be effective; whilst other services which operate more or less on a shoestring (though there is no doubt whatever that a basic minimum of adequate resources is essential) are generally regarded as helpful and effective (Arie 1979, 1980).

What is it that causes this variation? Our argument is that it is due to 'style' — the way the service works and the types of people who work in it. Most important of all, perhaps, is the leadership which the personality with whom the service is most identified can bring to it; this in turn depends as much on the 'untrained' aspects of his personality, as on his formal experience and qualifications. We will not labour the point that 'good' people are likely to make good services, for it is obvious.

The staff factor

A key characteristic of successful services is that they concern themselves with the needs not only of the users of the service but of those who work in them: the 'staff factor'. For centuries perhaps until after the Second World War, most planning of statutory services was essentially a matter of philanthropy, related to the size of the available purse (Fig. 8.1). The considerations were relatively simple: need was virtually open ended and one did what one thought one was able to afford. At all events this was the scheme of private charitable initiative.

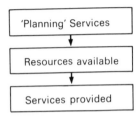

Fig. 8.1 Simple model for planning of services.

In recent decades, most particularly since the cost of services has escalated and has become largely a charge on the state, a more sophisticated planning model became established, and this involved an assessment of the likely users of the service and of their needs from it (Fig. 8.2a). This might be called the 'epidemiological model', and was clearly a considerable advance on the foregoing. But from this there was missing an element which has only been clearly identified in more recent years — the needs of those who will work in the service (Fig. 8.2b).

The needs of the staff are now seen to be as crucial as those of the users; recent experience of industrial relations in many countries makes it clear that this applies very generally indeed, but it has a quite special force in work which is generally regarded not only as unrewarding (quite wrongly we believe) but is also held in low esteem because of opinions about its content (partly realistic and partly false) and because of the low status of elderly people in modern societies (an attitude which itself tends to spread by contagion to those who work with them). It is essential, therefore, to look also at the needs of the staff, at the sources of their work satisfaction, at the components of the work which give job satisfaction to different types of staff (i.e. 'putting round pegs into round holes'). In theory, staff satisfaction and effectiveness of the service are independent variables, yet time and again experience shows that good services without contented staff rarely, if ever, exist.

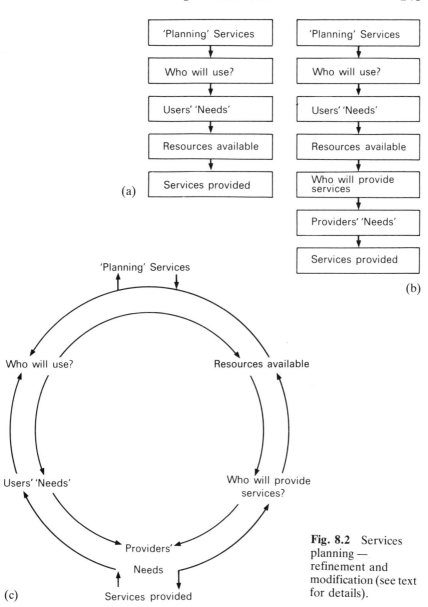

Fig. 8.2 Services planning — refinement and modification (see text for details).

Of course the path from planning to provision is not a simple linear process but is a dynamic system (Fig. 8.2c). The different components of the system constantly change and in changing, modify each other; this may produce a different end product which in turn may call for modification of the parts of the system.

'Constituencies'

Industrial psychology has much to teach us about organisation of services for the elderly. Perhaps most important is the need to create among those who depend on us — clients and staff of services — an atmosphere of availability, and of willingness to listen. We also have to remember that those who give services have at least three 'constituencies' to satisfy. First are the *users* of the service — patients, their families, the public. Second are the *staff* who man those services. Finally — and often the most difficult constituency to satisfy — are *colleagues* within our own and associated professions, for whom an effective service for the elderly can make a telling contribution to their capacity to function well within their own field. The demands of each constituency may not, indeed often do not, point in similar directions, but a successful service, which will need the political and material support of its community and its colleagues, depends on striking a happy balance to satisfy all three.

Principles

One can begin to make a tentative list of the types of consideration that govern styles of service. They have the common aim of building *confidence* in the service.

1 Flexibility

A service must constantly be trying new ways of doing things. No one has all the answers in our field, and to many questions there probably are no answers: therefore it is all the more important always to keep an open mind and to be willing to consider unusual approaches, unusual services, and unusual use of existing services. Often the best suggestions come from the clients of the services rather than from those who plan them.

2 Responsiveness and availability

A service which is not responsive and readily available generates increased demand. If the users of the service cannot get a response by moderate demands, they pitch them higher: 'cold' problems become crises, issues that can wait become immediate. Only by unfussy and prompt responsiveness will the service gain the confidence of members of the public and associated professions who use the service that, when they are in real trouble, it will quickly help them. It is the common experience of a service which makes itself readily available that crisis demands (and out-of-hours demands) become less frequent. Many, though certainly not all, 'crises' are merely testings of the service.

Inherent in this is *willingness to accept the degree of urgency on the subjective estimate of those who call for help*. If a family feels it needs help immediately, one should try to respond immediately — even if, on objective appraisal, the matter seems not so urgent. The important thing is to satisfy those who call for help that one takes them seriously. The confidence that such an approach gives to a community, and the ultimate release of pressure on the service, exceeds by far the extra work from those who abuse such ready availability.

3   Unhierarchical use of staff

Strategies such as the deliberate use of seniority also indicate 'style'—sending the top person not only because his or her skill and power of decision-making are needed objectively but because his or her appearance on the scene is likely to give maximum confidence. The obverse also applies — using relatively junior staff when it seems that they may get 'closer' to the clients of the services, and thereby again give more confidence; such staff should always be backed by the necessary skills from others where their own are insufficient.

4   Domiciliary assessment

We have discussed in some detail our reasons for identifying domiciliary assessment as a cardinal principle, in *psycho*geriatric practice. The first contact should, whenever possible, be at home unless there is a manifest 'medical' emergency.

5   Willingness to collaborate with other services and agencies

A service for the elderly depends on collaboration and its clients deserve to have easy access to the skills and resources of related services. Monopolism has no place in the care of the elderly, nor does compartmentalism. No patient should be denied access to skills and facilities that she needs simply because she has fallen into the wrong compartment of local services. Underlying this collaboration is the principle that a patient's assessed need should determine the services that she receives, rather than these being dictated merely by what is available in that compartment of care into which she happens to have fallen. Often this will mean the establishment or joint facilities or joint services.

Supportiveness, personality and education

Even the most routine act of service should be judged against two practical criteria: 1 Has the intervention been supportive, whether or not it has given those who called for help what they expected? 2 Has it left people feeling that the service understands their problem? Does it leave the clients feeling understood and helped by the service, even though it has not agreed fully their own formulation or has not got the resources to do what it would wish to do?

To achieve these two aims the personality as well as the skill of the staff has to be brought into action. Selection of the right people to man a service is crucial: if the personality is not right, experience and skill may be the only very limited assets.

Finally, every routine act should contribute to education. This is not meant in a pompous way, since the education is generally in both directions; it is simply a recognition that, ultimately, better care for the elderly depends on massive public education: education of individuals to prepare themselves for their own old age, a process which begins in the primary school by including old age in the awareness or 'life map' of individuals; education of the public about the needs of the elderly, as a necessary preliminary to persuading societies to make adequate resources available for the improvement of the life and care of old people; and finally, at a very pragmatic level, education of the users of services towards an understanding of the complexities of the care system, the issues of rationing and conflicting priorities, which, if understood, usually contribute to more rational and more moderate use of services; but which, when left unexplained, merely increase frustration and inflated demands.

DEMANDS

We have attempted to review developments in the provision of special psychiatric services for the elderly, and to look at both the material and the less tangible factors which determine the end product. We would emphasise that it is in early days in the history of these services (though there is now quite a lot of experience in work with the sick elderly in general). Thus, if we should write on this topic in ten years' time, we hope there would be many new developments. A recent survey, previously referred to, of British psychogeriatricians (Wattis *et al* 1981) shows that at the end of 1980 there were at least 120 consultant psychiatrists working chiefly in this field (some 10% of all consultants working in adult mental illness in Britain) and that there were some 87 major district services in being. Yet more than half of these doctors had started to work in psychogeriatrics only in the previous five years. Developments are recent and, though they have moved fast, we would return to our initial emphasis on the need for new directions and new ideas. For this remains an 'open field' and a challenging one; its attraction stems from many different sources and we hope we have indicated some of them. We would conclude by pointing to two in particular: first, in psychogeriatrics there is an opportunity to work in a setting that brings together closely general medicine and psychiatry, two sister disciplines which have tended to move apart in our time. We have often noted the pleasure with which young doctors coming to train in our departments have expressed satisfaction at being able not only to work so closely with physicians, but also to draw significantly both on the medical skills which form their basic training and those of psychiatry which form their chosen career.

Our final point we take from a previous review of ours (1978) '. . .the management of persistently or progressively mentally disabled old people was the psychiatry of Kraepelin, Bleuler and Pinel, yet present day psychiatry is not always at its best in this area of practice, having perhaps become mesmerised by its own power to suppress some morbid processes. Psychogeriatrics provides an opportunity to examine the issues and redefine the principles afresh.'

GUIDELINES FOR COLLABORATION BETWEEN GERIATRIC PHYSICIANS AND PSYCHIATRISTS IN THE CARE OF THE ELDERLY

A paper agreed by the Standing Joint Committee of the British Geriatrics Society and the Royal College of Psychiatrists

1 Services for the elderly should be a unity for consumers (i.e. patients, families, referrers). Patients should not be bounced back from one part of the service merely because they seem more appropriate for another part; such redistribution of referrals should be the *internal* responsibility of the service.
2 'Unity' does not mean blurring of the specificity of particular professions and facilities within the service, and the patient's right of access to them.
3 Criteria for division of responsibility must be clear, and must be known and accepted both inside and outside the service.
4 Effective collaboration depends on mutual confidence, and often frankly on personal friendships. Trust is indispensable, and people should be able at times to accept each other's judgements about their own responsibilities.
5 Mutual confidence requires basic education in each other's disciplines. Implementation of the sort of reciprocal training schemes which have been proposed at the Standing Joint Committee of the BGS/RCPsych is urgent.
6 The Statutory Instrument for the appointment of consultants allows employing Authorities to invite representation of other relevant specialties on Advisory Appointments Committee. It is always desirable that the local geriatric physician or geriatric psychiatrist should be on the Appointments Committee for his opposite number.
7 *Responsibility should be determined by the assessed needs of the patient*, and not by quirks of referral. For example, if a patient with a gross motor stroke is referred to a psychiatrist, he is no less the responsibility of the medical services through having first made contact with the psychiatrist; and vice versa with a patient with severe depression.
8 Lack of resources does not alter the definition of responsibility. Once a patient's needs are recognised as falling within the province of one service,

that service should support the patient within the limits of the feasible — even if this is less than ideal; *a 'psychiatric' patient does not become 'geriatric' simply because there are not psychiatric beds, or vice versa.*

9   Despite the foregoing, there are patients who fall in a 'grey' area where they might appropriately be dealt with by either service. This then becomes a matter of negotiation between the two services, but the service which first made contact retains responsibility until ultimate placement is agreed. *Patients must never be allowed to 'fall between stools'.*

10   The principle that responsibility is determined by the patient's needs applies equally to patients admitted under *compulsory orders.* A patient admitted under the Mental Health Act may occasionally need direct admission to a medical (or surgical) bed, and a patient admitted under the National Assistance Act to a psychiatric bed. The belief that an elderly patient who is admitted under compulsion will necessarily be disruptive or insist on leaving is understandable, but mistaken. There is rarely difficulty with such patients in general wards.

11   Criteria for division of responsibility in 'Services for Mental Illness Related to Old Age' (HM(72)71) are broadly satisfactory though the references there to the presence or absence of significant physical disease or illness may cause difficulties if common sense is not applied.

12   Experience suggests that the best criterion for the placement of demented patients needing longer term care is whether they are *ambulant* or not, always provided there is the flexibility necessary for the odd case that does not fit.

13   'Severe dementia' is used as a criterion in HM(72)71, but this can be misleading if interpreted merely in a cognitive sense. The issue turns on the presence and nature of *behaviour disturbances* associated with dementia and these may be severe in a 'mildly' demented patient, and absent in a 'severely' demented patient.

14   Practice in regard to the establishment of Joint Units, or Psycho-Geriatric Assessment Units as recommended in HM(70)11 varies from district to district. Where geriatric psychiatry and geriatrics are side by side in a District General Hospital it may not be necessary to establish a separate Joint Unit. Joint care does not depend on fixed assignment of joint beds, still less on separate joint units, though these are often desirable, especially when geriatric physician and geriatric psychiatrist have their headquarters in different hospitals. The basic principles of joint care are that patients assessed by one service as needing joint care of both should receive it; that each service should have direct access to joint care; and that 'exit responsibility' should, as in all other situations, depend on the assessed needs of the patient rather than merely on who arranged the original admission.

15   Patients with a psychiatric history who develop physical illness or gross physical deterioration at home, should be reassessed de novo. No-one should be labelled as 'a psychiatric patient' by virtue merely of some previous psychiatric episode; and vice versa for patients with previous physical illnesses who develop psychiatric disorders.

Summary of basic principles

1 Responsibility is always determined by the needs of the patient, rather than by quirks of referral.

2 Even when resources are short, as they almost always are, the service in whose responsibility the patient falls must do its best for her; a psychiatric patient does not become 'geriatric' through lack of psychiatric beds.

3 In addition to goodwill and good sense, education in each other's disciplines is essential.

4 The service must always be a unity for the consumer, though this does not mean blurring of the specific contribution of particular professions and resources within the services, and the patient's right of access to them.

REFERENCES

ARIE T. (1970) The first year of the Goodmayes psychiatric service for old people. *Lancet* ii, 1179–82.

ARIE T. (1975) Day care in geriatric psychiatry. *Gerontologia Clinica* **17**, 31–9.

ARIE T. (1977) Issues in the psychiatric care of old people. In *Care of the Elderly*, eds. A.N. Exton-Smith and J. Grimley Evans. Academic Press, New York.

ARIE T. (1979) Psychogeriatrics: How & Why? The Fotheringham Lectures in the University of Toronto. Mimeographed.

ARIE T. (1980) *Making Services Work*. Working Paper for WHO Working Group on Services & Systems of Care for the Elderly. WHO, Geneva.

ARIE T. (1981) Health Care of the Very Elderly. In *Health Care of the Elderly: Essays in Old Age Medicine, Psychiatry and Services*, ed T. Arie. Croom Helm, London.

ARIE T. & DUNN T. (1973) A do-it-yourself psychiatric–geriatric joint patient unit. *Lancet* ii, 313–16.

ARIE T. & ISAACS A.D. (1977) The development of psychiatric services for the elderly in Britain. In *Studies in Geriatric Psychiatry*, eds F. Post and A.D. Isaacs. John Wiley, New York.

BAKER A.A. & BYRNE R.J.F. (1977) Another style of psychogeriatric service. *British Journal of Psychiatry* **130**, 123–6.

BARTON R. (1965) Developing a service for elderly demented patients. In *Psychiatric Hospital Care*, ed H. Freeman. Ballière Tindall, London.

BERGMANN K. (1971) The neuroses of old age. In *Recent Advances in Psychogeriatrics*, ed D.W.K. Kay and A. Walk. British Journal of Psychiatry, special publication, no. 6.

BERGMANN K. & EASTHAM E.J. (1974) Psychogeriatric ascertainment and assessment for treatment in an acute medical ward setting. *Age and Ageing* **3**, 174–88.

BERGMANN K., FOSTER E.M., JUSTICE A.W. *et al* (1978) Management of the demented elderly patient in the community. *British Journal of Psychiatry* **132**, 441–47.

BLESSED G. (1975) Development of a psychogeriatric service. St. Nicholas Hospital, Newcastle-upon-Tyne. In *Some Models of District Psychiatric Geriatric Services*, ed R.A. Robinson. Nuffield Provincial Hospitals Trust Seminar.

BREMER J. (1951) A social psychiatric investigation of a small community in Northern Norway. *Acta Psychiatrica Scandinavica* (Suppl. 62).

BROCKLEHURST J.C. (1977) *Geriatric Care in Advanced Societies*. MTP, Lancaster.

BROCKLEHURST J.C., CARTY M.H., LEEMING J.T. *et al* (1978) Medical screening of old people accepted for residential care. *Lancet* ii, 141–2.

CARR P.J., BUTTERWORTH C.A. & HODGES B.E. (1980) *Community Psychiatric Nursing*. Churchill Livingstone, Edinburgh.

Committee of Inquiry into Whittingham Hospital (1972) Command 4861. HMSO, London.

Committee of Inquiry into the Transfer of Patients from Fairfield Hospital to Rossendale Hospital (1975) Report to the North West Regional Health Authority.

CLARKE M., HUGHES A.O., DODD K.J. *et al* (1979) The Elderly in Residential Care: Patterns of Disability. *Health Trends* **11**, 17–20.

CROSSMAN R.H.S. (1977) Diaries of a Cabinet Minister: Vol II. Hamish Hamilton, London

DHSS (1970) *Psycho-Geriatric Assessment Units*, Circular HM(70)11.

DHSS (1971) *Hospital Services for the Mentally Ill*, Circular HM(71)97.

DHSS (1972) *Services for Mental Illness Related to Old Age*, Circular HM(72)71.

DHSS (1976a) *Priorities for Health and Personal Social Services in England: A consultative document*. HMSO.

DHSS (1976b) *Health and Social Services Statistics for England 1975*. HMSO.

DHSS (1978) *A Happier Old Age: A discussion document on the elderly in our society*. HMSO.

DHSS (1979) *Patients First*. Consultative paper on the structure and management of the National Health Service in England and Wales. HMSO.

DHSS (1980) *Organisational and Management Problems of Mental Illness Hospitals*. Report of a Working Group. HMSO.

DHSS (1981) *Growing Older*. HMSO, London.

DONOVAN J.F., WILLIAMS I.E.I. & WILSON T.S. (1971) A fully integrated psychogeriatric service. In *Recent Developments in Psychogeriatrics*, eds. D.W.K. Kay and A. Walk. British Journal of Psychiatry, special publication.

EVANS G., HUGHES B. & WILKIN D., with JOLLEY D. (1981) *The management of mental and physical impairment in non-specialist residential homes for the elderly*. University Hospital of South Manchester, Psychogeriatric Unit Research Section, Research Report no. 4.

FOSTER E.M., KAY D.W.K., & BERGMANN K. (1976) The characteristics of old people receiving and needing domiciliary services. *Age and Ageing* **5**, 345–55.

FULLER J., WARD E., EVANS A. *et al* (1979) Dementia Supportive Groups for Relatives. *British Medical Journal* i, 1684–5.

GLASSCOTE R.M., GUDEMAN J.E. & MILES D.E. (1977) *Community-based Mental Health Services for the Elderly*. Joint Information Service. American Pschiatric Association, Washington.

GODBER C. (1975) Psychogeriatric services based on Moorgreen Hospital, Southampton. In *Some Models of District Psychiatric Geriatric Services*, ed. R.A. Robinson. Nuffield Provincial Hospitals Trust Seminar.

GODLOVE C., DUNN G., & WRIGHT W. (1980) Caring for Old People in New York and London: the 'nurses' aide' interviews. *Journal of the Royal Society of Medicine* **73**, 713–23.

GRAD J. & SAINSBURY P. (1968) The effects that patients have on their families in a community care and control psychiatric service. *British Journal of Psychiatry* **114**, 265–78.

GREENE J.G. & TIMBURY G.C. (1979) A geriatric psychiatry day hospital service. *Age and Ageing* **8,** 49–53.

GRUENBERG E.M. (1961) *A mental health survey of older people.* State Hospitals Press. New York.

HAS (1970–77) National Health Service Health Advisory Service. Annual Reports, 1969–75. HMSO, London.

HUGHES B. & WILKIN D. (1980) *Residential care of the elderly.* University Hospital of South Manchester Psychogeriatric Unit Research Section, Research Report no. 2.

HUNT A. (1978) *The Elderly at Home.* HMSO, London.

JOLLEY D. (1977) Hospital inpatient provision for patients with dementia. *British Medical Journal* i, 1335–6.

JOLLEY D. et al (1982) Developing a psychogeriatric service. In *Establishing a Geriatric Service*, ed. D. Coakley. Croom Helm, London.

JOLLEY D. & ARIE T. (1976) Psychiatric service for the elderly: how many beds? *British Journal of Psychiatry* **129**, 418–23.

JOLLEY D. & ARIE T. (1978) Organisation of Psychogeriatric Services. *British Journal of Psychiatry* **132**, 1–11.

JOLLEY D., KONDRATOWICZ T. & BROCKLEHURST J.C. (1980) Psychogeriatric Out-patient Clinic. Paper presented to British Geriatric Society Spring Conference, Isle of Man.

JONES K. & SIDEBOTTOM R. (1962) *Mental Hospitals at Work.* Routledge and Kegan Paul, Henley-on-Thames.

KAY D.W.K., BEAMISH P. & ROTH M. (1962) *Some Social and Medical Characteristics of Elderly People Under State Care.* Sociological Review Monograph no. 5, Keele.

KAY D.W.K., BEAMISH P. & ROTH M. (1964a) Old Age mental disorders in Newcastle-upon-Tyne: Part 1: A study of prevalence. *British Journal of Psychiatry* **110**, 146–58.

KAY D.W.K., BEAMISH P. & ROTH M. (1964b) Old Age mental disorders in Newcastle-upon-Tyne: Part 2: A study of possible social and medical causes. *British Journal of Psychiatry* **110**, 668–82.

KAY D.W.K., BERGMANN K., FOSTER E.M. et al (1970) Mental illness and hospital usage in the elderly. *Comprehensive Psychiatry* **1**, 26–35.

KUSHLICK A., PALMER J., FELCE D. et al (1977) *Summary of Current Research in Mental Handicap Work.* Health Care Evaluation Research Team, Wessex Regional Health Authority, Research Report no. 126.

LANGLEY G., WRIGHT W.B., SOWDER R.R. et al (1975) The Exe Vale Joint Psychogeriatric Assessment Clinic. *Age and Ageing* **3**, 125–8.

LEVITT R. (1976) *The Re-organised National Health Service.* Croom Helm, London.

MACMILLAN D. (1960) Preventive geriatrics. *Lancet* ii, 1439–40.

MEACHER M. (1972) *Taken for a Ride.* Longman, London.

MILLAR H.R. (1981) Psychiatric morbidity in elderly surgical patients. *British Journal of Psychiatry* **138**, 17–20.

Ministry of Health (1966) Report of the Committee on Senior Nursing Staff Structure. HMSO, London.

NIELSEN J. (1962) Geronto-psychiatric period prevalence investigation in a geographically delimited population. *Acta Psychiatrica Scandinavica* **38**, 307–30.

Office of Population Censuses and Surveys (1975) *The General Household Survey 1972.* HMSO, London.

PARSONS P.L. (1965) Mental health of Swansea's old folk. *British Journal of Social and Preventive Medicine* **19**, 43–7.

PASKER P., THOMAS J.P.R. & ASHLEY J.S.A. (1976) The elderly mentally ill — whose responsibility? *British Medical Journal* ii, 164–6.

PITT B. (1974) *Psychogeriatrics*. Churchill Livingstone, Edinburgh.

PITT B. & SILVER C.P. (1980) The combined approach to Geriatrics and Psychiatry. *Age and Ageing* **9**, 33–7.

PORTSMOUTH O.H.D. (1973) The organisation of psychogeriatric care. *Modern Geriatrics* **3**, 553–6.

ROBINSON R.A. (1962) The practice of a psychiatric geriatric unit. *Gerontologia Clinica* **1**, 1–19.

Royal College of Psychiatrists
  (1973a) *News and Notes*, January, p.9. Formation of a Group for the Psychiatry of Old Age.
  (1973b) *News and Notes*, August, p.2. Joint Report of the British Geriatrics Society and the Royal College of Psychiatrists on matters relating to the care of Psycho-Geriatric Patients.
  (1976) *New and Notes*, September, p.10. Memorandum on Residential Homes for the Elderly Mentally Infirm.
  (1977a) *The Bulletin*, September, p.4. The responsibilities of Consultants in Psychiatry within the National Health Service.
  (1977b) *The Bulletin*, December, p.5. Providing a District Service for General Psychiatry, its Special Interests and Related Specialties — Modern Manpower Priorities.
  (1978a) *The Bulletin*, January, p.4. Memorandum on Nursing Needs for the Elderly Mentally Ill.
  (1978b) *The Bulletin,* December, p.201. Medical Manpower Requirements of Teaching Hospitals.
  (1979a) *The Bulletin*, May, p.85. A Happier Old Age: the College's Comments.
  (1979b) *The Bulletin*, November, p.168. Guidelines for Collaboration between Geriatric Physicians and Psychiatrists in the Care of the Elderly.
  (1980) *The Bulletin*, August, p.114. Community Psychiatric Nursing.

SHEPHERD M., COOPER B., BROWN A.C. *et al* (1966) *Psychiatric Illness in General Practice*. Oxford University Press.

SHULMAN K. (1981) Service Innovations in Geriatric Psychiatry. In *Health Care of the Elderly: Essays in Old Age Medicine, Psychiatry and Services*, ed. T. Arie. Croom Helm, London.

SHULMAN K. & ARIE T. (1978) Fall in admission rate of old people to psyciatric units. *British Medical Journal* i, 156–8.

SLATTERY M. & BOURNE A. (1979) Norms and recent trends in Geriatrics. *Journal of Clinical and Experimental Gerontology* **1**, (1), 79–99.

TOWNSEND P. (1962) *The Last Refuge*. Routledge and Kegan Paul, Henley-on-Thames.

VERWOERDT A. (1981) Psychotherapy for the Elderly. In *Health Care of the Elderly: Essays in Old Age Medicine, Psychiatry and Services*, ed. T. Arie. Croom Helm, London.

WATTIS J., WATTIS L. & ARIE T. (1981) Psychogeriatrics: A National Survey of a New Branch of Psychiatry. *British Medical Journal* **282**, 1529–33.

WHITEHEAD J.A. (1972) Services for old people with mental symptoms. *Community Health*, 83–6.

WILLIAMSON J., STOKOE I.H., GRAY S. *et al* (1964) Old people at home: their unreported needs. *Lancet* i, 1117–20.

WILKIN D., MASHIAH T. & JOLLEY D. (1978) Changes in behavioural characteristics of elderly populations of local authority homes and long-stay hospital wards, 1976–77. *British Medical Journal* ii, 1274–6.

CHAPTER 9

Psychogeriatric Care in the Community

Loïc Hemsi

CARE AND CONTEXT

In any country, the practice of medicine is greatly influenced by the cultural and social conditions prevailing. This is particularly true for those diseases and handicaps which are not readily self-limiting or quickly remedied by such physical means as drugs or operations. That is the case for mental disorders and disabilities, especially in the elderly and those with chronic brain disorders.

The author is intimately familiar with the health and social services only as they operate in Great Britain—in fact only in England—and this chapter has been written from that standpoint. The views and opinions expressed will certainly in part not be valid in other contexts, at any rate so far as the *route* to objectives is concerned, the objectives themselves probably having a wider application and acceptability. Even within a single country the patterns of local services are very diverse, and may be dictated by imperatives, for example, of geography. Uniformity is neither possible nor desirable, especially as the evaluation of services is a complex task and one which is as yet hardly begun. There is a need to set out and to clarify principles in the hope that there will be little difficulty in agreeing them. Translation into practice can then follow, in accordance with the requirements of the local population and with the resources which are available to it.

This then is the framework of the chapter: a consideration of general principles and a detailed exposition of one approach to individual patients. It is concerned primarily with clinical care and not with the organisation of a service, which the author has described elsewhere (Hemsi 1980).

THE SPECIALIST TEAM IN THE COMMUNITY

Necessity is without doubt a strong incentive to development and innovation in the health and social services! The impetus provided by wars to advances in many branches of medicine is well known. Under the conditions of civilian life, social factors vie with technical advances in determining the course and the application of clinical practice. This is happening in the psychiatry of late life, with technology lagging far behind the demands of the population.

Two factors are pre-eminent in the planning of services for this population. The first is demography, with the huge increase in the number of the very old now taking place and expected to continue (Office of Population Censuses and Surveys 1980); tied in with this is an increase in the number of very disabled (Hunt 1978). The second factor is epidemiology, or the distribution and pattern of disabilities and diseases in the total population. The vast majority of old people, many of them seriously handicapped, live outside institutions. It is therefore most important that the specialist teams operate substantially outside the hospital.

There are many reasons for a community emphasis in psychogeriatrics. The nature of the mental disorders is such that often no hospital investigations are necessary and little or nothing is to be gained by the elderly patient, as opposed to other people, by admitting him to hospital; indeed much may be lost! Then there is the crucial fact, not infrequently overlooked in hospital practice, that old people are integral members of social networks; it is therefore essential to have a good working knowledge of that network for each patient. It is in the community that these people are to be found so that it is best to see them there. Whether or not the patient has a remediable condition, he is likely to need support and in turn those supporting him will require help in many cases. To provide that help it is necessary, among other things to understand and to handle the psychological processes in operation within and around the patient, to understand that his situation is in part the result of lifelong interaction between his personality and that of others. Moreover, there are enormous problems in caring for old people in institutions, quite apart from the scarcity and the high cost of places there. It is therefore not realistic to expect that there will be a large shift towards institutional care in the foreseeable future.

For all these reasons, and for others too, if the specialist service is to be worthwhile and comprehensive, it must be centered in the community. It must assess the old people in their own homes and in their own social setting, and the other people in their group also. It must take part in the management of a total situation, of which the old person is only one variable and his disease (if any) only one component. It must act on the basis that assessment outside the old person's environment is at best incomplete and may be grossly misleading. It must be readily available, particularly in times of crisis.

The implications of having a multidisciplinary hospital-based specialist team working regularly outside the well-charted and clearly-demarcated waters of the hospital are many and profound. They involve questions of skills, roles and professional boundaries; of responsibility, authority and control; of availability and of communication. They are of importance in the working relationships between general practitioners and consultants and between medical teams and social work teams. Such considerations exist, of course, outside the psychiatry of old age but, given the nature of the task, they are particularly sensitive in this field. It is necessary, therefore, to describe that task and to look at the consequences which follow from it.

The tasks in psychogeriatrics

These can be summarised as *assessment* (of the designated patient and of those around him), *treatment* (of disease, where present and treatable), *management* (of a situation, including the psychodynamics), and effective, efficient, and economic *use of resources* (including the allocation of priorities). It is the aim of this chapter to deal with that task in detail, but it is as well in this introduction to highlight the themes relating to each of its constituent parts.

Assessment

Assessment is the most important step as it forms the basis for all decisions in a case; it should therefore be comprehensive. Often it is not; indeed there may not even be an explicit and clear understanding of what is required!

Assessment involves a detailed statement of the presenting problem, as perceived by those concerned, set against the background of the (designated) patient's biographical history and followed by an examination of his mental, physical, and social state. It involves the making of a diagnosis, including sometimes that the 'patient' is normal, but must go beyond the diagnosis of disease into a description of disability and an understanding of manifest behaviour, of its determinants and consequences. Nor is it sufficient to look at the patient only: those in his social orbit must be assessed as well. Initially this may require tact and caution if they are not to be irretrievably antagonised.

To state these essential requirements is to say that what is needed is a working knowledge of people and of the range of normality in the elderly; of normal and abnormal individual and group psychology; of physical and mental diseases; and of the interplay of these forces in creating situations around disabled old people. No single professional group encompasses all the necessary skills in depth. However, the psychiatrist, with his training in medicine, in psychology, and in the social sciences, has a potential breadth of approach which is unmatched by any other group. Therefore, provided his vision is not obscured by a distaste for old people and for organic psychosyndromes, the trained psychiatrist should be able to make the requisite comprehensive assessment with a greater expertise than others. This indeed is his foremost role and assessment of cases is the aspect which most heavily engages the specialist in this field.

When it is applicable, no model is simpler and more useful for understanding and assisting people in distress than that of disease. All too often, physical diseases lead to decompensation of brain function and to abnormal behaviour in the elderly, who may present first to the psychiatrist. Similarly, the concept of disease is helpful in the management of depressed and paraphrenic old people. In such cases, the relief of symptoms and the restoration of behaviour to normal may require no more than the conceptually simple treatment of a disease process: an antibiotic, an antidepressant, a tranquilliser. Hence the importance of accurate diagnosis in the course of the assessment and the irreplaceable advantage of a medical training.

However, there are dangers in this model. For example, it may lead to the assumption that where disease is present it is of necessity responsible for the problem, rather than possibly coincidental or even a red herring and a hook upon which to hang other difficulties. Too much store may be placed upon physical therapies, particularly drugs, when in fact social and psychological approaches are more important, as in dementia. When the disease is not treatable, e.g. senile dementia, the case may be dismissed as 'social' only, not the concern of doctors, let alone specialists. This is to deny the essence of psychiatry, which is to deal in emotions, in abnormal behaviour, and in interpersonal relationships. There is no difference in principle between psychiatry in the old and in others, merely a difference in the mix and in the emphasis — not in the approach.

Treatment

Treatment does not need elaboration in this introduction. In the decision on the allocation of roles, so important and so complex, as will be shown later, treatment is clearly situated in the sphere of the health professions.

Management

Next to assessment, management is the most complex part of the task. Its difficulty comes in part from the problem of coping for long periods with very abnormal people and with normal people under great stress. In part also, it derives from the fact that there are multiple helpers and helping agencies in the field, with differences in perception of, and approaches to, cases. It is essential to co-ordinate efforts and this is not easy.

Management entails consultation in order to set out realistic objectives for the patient and others and the working out of how they are to be attained; the handling of risk; the discovery of who is involved in a helping capacity and the decision of who does what (allocation of roles); the limitation of those involved to a reasonable number and the establishment of good communication between them; the setting out of a policy on dealing with crises which are bound to arise; and, finally, a mechanism for reviewing and altering policy.

Resources and priorities

The last part of the task is to look at the needs and the demands in an individual case against the background of those of others in the population served. As need and demand usually exceed the supply of services available, priorities must be decided consciously, deliberately, and explicitly. Resources must be carefully husbanded and their use thought out, in the knowledge that waste in one case will mean unnecessary deprivation for others. Difficult medical and ethical decisions must be faced. It has to be acknowledged that equitable rationing is an integral part of the task: this means doing less than the best for some, in order to avoid doing nothing for others. There must be an overall view of what is required by the population and what is available by way of services: the worm's eyeview and the bird's eyeview are both essential, the former for the individual and the latter for the population! In the final analysis, only the head of a psychogeriatric unit can discharge that function for the services which it provides: delegation is possible only within fairly narrow limits and then only to other members of the specialist team.

The granting to outsiders of decision-making on the use of the resources of the service is not desirable where scarcity exists, as it always will. For example, if the right of deciding on admissions to a tiny pool of beds were to be extended to general practitioners, the perceived needs of the individual could not be weighed by that practitioner against those of patients unknown to him. There would be no consideration of priorities and possibly no thought of alternatives to admission.

With the refusal to share the authority for the use of resources there must be a readiness to share the burden of presenting need and demand. The specialist team must not use the security of the hospital and the inadequacy of facilities to deny its part of responsibility. When the hospital-based staff really believe in and practice the responsibility that they have for people outside the hospital and work in concert with those whose base is in the community, many of the frictions and differences between colleagues which otherwise can sap a comprehensive service can be avoided or dissipated.

THE ELDERLY IN THE COMMUNITY: THEIR PSYCHIATRIC DISABILITIES AND THEIR SOURCES OF SUPPORT

So strong is the effect of tradition and of labelling that there is a tendency to think of old people as if they form a homogeneous group comprising all those aged 65 and over. For example, statistics published annually in the Department of Health and Social Security document *Health and Personal Social Services Statistics* (DHSS 1980) give figures of the population '65 and over' without further breakdown and show tables of residents in accommodation provided by and on behalf of local authorities by the age groups 'under 65' and 'over 65'. Similarly, planning guidelines for the elderly mentally ill (DHSS 1972) are for the group aged 65 and over without any subgroup within the elderly. The White Paper *Growing Older* (DHSS 1981) applies the term 'elderly people' generally to those aged 65 and over.

This may be appropriate so far as employment and old age pensions are concerned, but it is not when it comes to population numbers and to the planning of health and social services for those with disabilities related to old age. Demographically, the elderly include subgroups which will alter in their distribution in different ways in the next 30 years. Psychiatrically, the nature and the rates of psychiatric disabilities change with advancing age and different types of service are required for the younger elderly and the very old.

Demography

The last census of the United Kingdom population for which figures are available was conducted in 1971; until the data of the 1981 census are published, we have to depend upon estimates for more up-to-date information. In 1978 the estimated total population of the United Kingdom was just under 56 000 000. It is projected that it will rise to 57 000 000 in 1991 and to 58 000 000 in 2001 (increases of 1.8% and 3.6% respectively).

Among the elderly, the changes are not even. The group aged 60–74 is expected to fall from 8 000 000 to 7 700 000 ($-$ 3.8%) and to 7 142 000 ($-$ 10.7%) in 1991 and 2001 respectively. In contrast, the population over the age of 74 years is due to rise by 21% and 24% respectively by 1991 and 2001 (from 2 988 000 in 1978 to 3 621 000 and 3 694 000) (Office of Population Censuses and Surveys 1980). The rise in the over-85 population is expected to be even greater, well above 40%.

Thus, demographically, the elderly constitute populations with differing trends: the very old increasing in number and in proportion but the younger old falling significantly in the next twenty years. These trends are of particular importance in as much as there are substantial differences in the prevalence and in the nature of disabilities respectively in the first decade of old age and later.

Prevalence and nature of disabilities

Isaacs & Neville (1975) measured need in old people in three communities in the west of Scotland in 1971. The need studied was for basic care, i.e. the provision of food, warmth, cleanliness and security. The authors found that, whereas only 16% of the subjects aged 65–74 were unable, as a result of physical or mental disease or disability, to perform for themselves all or some of the basic activities of daily living, the proportion for the group aged 75–84

Loïc Hemsi

was 41%, and for those aged 85 and over it was 64%. The association between age and potential need was highly significant for all types of need.

The published data on the prevalence of psychiatric disorders in the elderly are unfortunately reported mostly with respect to the population over 60 or over 65 as a whole. However, there is some information from a Danish study and from Newcastle-upon-Tyne on prevalence within age subgroups in old people.

Nielsen (1962) studied the prevalence of mental disorders over a period of six months in the 994 persons aged 65 and over who were living on the Danish island of Samso in 1961. His findings are summarised in Tables 9.1, 9.2 and 9.3, and show how important it is not to regard the elderly as a homogeneous group.

Table 9.1 Six-month prevalence rates (cases per 1000) for mental disorders in 1961 in Samso (Denmark). Men and women ($n = 370$). (Adapted from Nielsen 1962.)

Diagnosis	65 and over	65–74	75–84	85 and over
Organic mental disorders				
Severe dementia	30.7	6.3	54.9	178.6
Mild dementia	154.3	73.0	277.9	428.8
Cerebrovascular disease	28.6	22.2	41.2	35.7
Functional mental disorders				
Manic-depressive psychosis	12.3	14.3	6.9	17.9
Psychogenic psychoses	18.4	19.0	20.6	0
Paranoid psychoses	6.1	7.9	3.4	0
Neuroses	38.9	49.2	24.0	0
Character disorders	27.6	30.1	27.4	0
Alcoholism	5.1	7.9	0	0
Mental deficiency	14.3	19.0	3.4	17.9
Not specified	38.9	47.9	27.4	0
All diagnoses	378.3	298.2	490.6	696.4

Table 9.2 Six-month prevalence rates (cases per 1000) for organic and functional mental disorders by age group in 1961 in Samso. Men and women ($n = 370$). (Adapted from Nielsen 1962.)

Diagnostic group	65 and over	65–74	75–84	85 and over
Organic mental disorders	213.6	101.5	374	643.1
Functional mental disorders	103.3	128.4	82.3	17.9

Table 9.3 Organic mental disorders as a percentage of total diagnosed mental disorders in the population of Samso aged 65 and over in 1961. (Adapted from Nielsen 1962.)

	65 and over	65–74	75–84	85 and over
All cases	370	188	143	39
Cases with organic mental disorders	209	64	109	36
Percentage with organic mental disorders	56.5	34	76	92

The following observations can be made from his figures.

1 The overall prevalence rate for all diagnoses for all the elderly subjects subsumes great differences between the age subgroups. Thus, the total rate is 378.3 per thousand for all aged 65 and over, 298.2 for the group aged 65–74, 490.6 for the group aged 75–84, and 696.4 at age 85 and over. The total morbidity *rate* rises sharply with age (Table 9.1 and 9.2).

2 Because the number in the population groups fall with advancing age — about two-thirds of the population over 64 is in the age-group 65–74 — the numbers of *cases* of mental disorders are *highest* in the decade 65–74 even though the *rates* are *lowest* in that group. Similarly, the numbers are lowest and the rates highest in the over-85 population.

3 The proportion of cases of organic mental disorders in the psychiatrically abnormal population rises markedly with age: 34% in the years 65–74, 76% between 75 and 84, and 92% after the age of 85. Whereas psychiatry in old people under 75 is concerned predominantly with the functional disorders and the possibility of treatment and cure, after that age increasingly its subject matter is organic illness, with the need for management and care (Table 9.3).

4 Within the group of organic psychosyndromes, it is the diagnosis of mild dementia which provides the greatest number of cases and which accounts for the highest rates at all ages. The terms 'mild' and 'severe' apply to the degree of intellectual impairment. They should not be read as 'easy' and 'difficult' management: old people with 'mild' dementia can behave very abnormally as a result of the dementia and thus present many management problems.

5 As the demographic changes described earlier take effect, with a relative and absolute increase of the very old, the total morbidity and the emphasis on dementia will rise also. Planning must therefore be for an elderly population with changing needs and increasing disabilities.

Bergmann (1977) also provides evidence from surveys in Newcastle-upon-Tyne in the early 1960s (Table 9.4) of the increasing prevalence of the chronic brain syndrome with advancing age, again demonstrating the importance of dividing the elderly into smaller age subgroups in quantifying morbidity and planning for it.

Table 9.4 Prevalence of chronic brain syndrome by age. Newcastle-upon-Tyne 1960 and 1964 (Bergmann 1977).

Age	Number in sample	Chonic brain syndrome	%
65–69	253	6	2.3
70–74	243	7	2.8
75–79	144	8	5.5
80+	118	26	22.0
Total	758	47	6.2

Table 9.5 Population aged 65 and over in England (1977) and place of residence.

	Number	%
Persons aged 65 and over	6 733 000	100.00
Persons aged 65 and over in accommodation provided by or on behalf of local authorities	116 564	1.73
Persons aged 65 and over in registered voluntary homes	23 788	0.35
Persons aged 65 and over in registered private homes	21,320	0.32
Average occupied geriatric beds daily	51 800	0.77
Residents aged 65 and over in mental illness hospitals and units	40 446	0.60
Total number of persons aged 65 and over in institutional care	253 918	3.77
Total number of persons aged 65 and over living outside institutions	6 479 082	96.23

Sources
1   Department of Health and Social Security: Health and Personal Social Services Statistics for England 1978. (HMSO 1980)
2   Department of Health and Social Security: Inpatient Statistics from the Mental Health Enquiry for England 1977.

Living circumstances

In 1977, the population of England aged 65 and over was 6 733 000, of whom 254 000 (less than 4%) were resident in institutions (Table 9.5). Thus, the vast majority of old people live in private households. Hunt (1978), in her survey of the elderly at home in 1976, provides a wealth of information on their circumstances.

Whereas 25% of the men and women aged 65–74 live alone, that proportion rises to 37.4% for the group aged 75–84, and to 44% for those aged 85 and over. Fewer men, and smaller proportions, live alone than is the case with women, 47% and 50% of whom in the age groups 75–84 and over 85 respectively live alone.

The geographical stability of old people is shown by the fact that 80% of the elderly in the survey had been in their current neighbourhood for more than ten years and fewer than 4% for less than two years.

The social networks and contacts were studied. Nearly 95% of the old people had living close relatives (apart from those in the same household, if they lived with relatives). Almost 90% were visited by relatives, 32.9% several times a week and 21.5% at least once a week. Where relatives did not visit or visited rarely, this was because they lived abroad or too far away in Britain in two-thirds of the cases. Visiting relatives gave help to over half of the elderly over the age of 75 years. Contacts with neighbours were the next highest source of social interaction and occurred in half the cases.

Against this background of contact with kin and neighbours, statutory and other formal services can be seen to be a much smaller source of visiting for the generality of the elderly (Table 9.6). Doctors formed the highest single group visiting, especially for the very old (49.2% of the over 85 group visited) and for the housebound (71.3%). District nurses visited 19.6% of those 85 and over and 36.8% of the bedfast and housebound. Involvement of the Social Services consisted primarily of the provision of home helps (for 27.3% of the over 85 and 31% of the bedfast and housebound) and meals-on-wheels (for 11.5% of the over 85 and 12.1% of the bedfast and housebound).

Table 9.6 Visits received during past six months. Persons aged 65 and over living at home (Hunt 1978).

Visits received from	Lives alone %	Lives with others %
Doctor	28.4	35.5
Health visitor	5.6	3.8
District nurse	7.6	7.9
Home help	18.9	4.0
Council welfare officer	5.9	3.0
Social security/supplementary benefits visiting officer	9.0	4.7
Meals on wheels	6.4	1.0
Mobile library	2.8	2.9
Other official person	3.8	3.4
Voluntary organisation	2.8	2.6
Minister of religion	17.6	15.6
Insurance man	36.5	53.8
None of these	28.5	23.5
Insurance man is the only visitor	17.0	26.2

Hunt's survey was not concerned specifically with disabled old people. Obviously, where there is no disability and no need, there is no reason for statutory and other formal helping agencies to become concerned with the elderly. Nevertheless, what her figures do show is that even when there is disability and dependence, much of the support is provided by informal networks—family and neighbours. Her evidence is not presented by cause of disability and cannot therefore tell us how the mentally abnormal elderly who are dependent in their homes are supported. There is in fact no detailed published information on this question, although, if for no better reason than the weight of numbers, it is an important one.

In their survey of the prevalence of old age mental disorders in Newcastle-upon-Tyne, Kay and his co-workers found that those with identifiable mental disorders were, to an overwhelming extent, living at home and not in institutions (Kay *et al* 1964). Thus, for every old person with a severe organic brain syndrome in an institution there were six at home; for every one with a functional psychosis there were twelve at home; and for every one with a mild brain syndrome, a neurotic, or a character disorder in an institution there were 23 in private households. That survey was carried out more than 20 years ago and no similar study has been repeated more recently. It is nonetheless commonplace clinical experience that its conclusions as to the distribution of mentally disordered old people are still true. A knowledge of the social network of the elderly in the community is therefore necessary.

Social networks in old age

Mitchell (1969) has defined a social network as ' . . . a specific set of linkages among a defined set of persons, with the property that the characteristics of these linkages as a whole may be used to interpret the social behaviour of the persons involved'.

The assessment of a disabled, and therefore dependent, old person must include the analysis of her social network, as this provides the means of support, given a handicap. Social support systems have both formal and informal components (Cantor 1979). The older person can be viewed as at the core of, and interacting with, a series of subsystems (network sets) which usually operate independently but at times intersect.

First, there is the set of basic entitlements available to the elderly who qualify, e.g. retirement pensions, supplementary pension, attendance allowance, invalidity allowance, etc. (DHSS 1981). Then, there are the statutory and other agencies which carry out the economic and social policies of the government by actually providing the services, e.g. the Department of Social Services in a local authority. Third are the non-service, formal or quasi-formal organisations (or their representatives), e.g. church groups. These three sources of support constitute the formal network. The informal network or primary group consists of kin (nuclear family and extended family), friends, and neighbours.

There are differences in the tasks performed respectively by the formal and the informal systems. The informal primary group is small in size, with non-instrumental and diffuse roles, continuous face-to-face contact, affective bonds, and long-term commitment. It is best able to handle 'non-uniform tasks': unanticipated events, i.e. those which are subject to many contingencies and those which do not require anything more than everyday socialisation to master. This informal group is more likely than formal organisations to be available for unpredictable events; more familiar with the contingencies of the situation; and more motivated to act under conditions of uncertainty where objective evaluation and instrumental rewards are not possible. In contrast, the formal agencies can draw potentially on a larger pool of people and possess technical expertise, skill, and resources (Dono *et al* 1979).

There are three major requirements of a social network acting as a successful support system: socialisation, the carrying out of tasks of daily living, and assistance in illness or crisis. To a considerable extent, these requirements are fulfilled by the informal network.

Cantor (1975) conducted a survey of the elderly living in the inner part of New York City using a sample of 1552 persons aged 60 and over. She found that two-thirds had living children and had not been abandoned by them and that familial bonds were strong. At least two-thirds of the old people received help from their children in the case of illness and in the chores of daily living. Friends and neighbours were also important in the social support system, particularly in emergency situations or in crisis intervention and when there were no children available. She concludes from her extensive data that ' . . . kin are clearly considered the primary source of help, regardless of the task. Only to the extent that family, particularly children, are not available and with respect to certain well-defined tasks do friends, neighbours and formal organisations become important in the provision of informal social supports. Thus, for example, in the arena of socialisation and the provision of day-to-day companionship, friends and neighbours play a highly significant role. Likewise, friends and neighbours are helpful for short-term emergency service, such as . . . help when one is ill. But their most important function appears to be as compensatory support elements when kin and children are non-existent or unavailable.'

Because the survey was of old people living in the community and did not consider the institutionalised elderly, it could not provide information on the social factors influencing admission to institutions. Obviously, these include the absence and the failure of informal support systems and the inability of the formal networks to compensate. No doubt the level and the nature of disabilities are also important in leading to institutional care. Nevertheless, as the very old and the very disabled increase in number and in proportion, it is essential that the statutory agencies learn from the coping strategies and procedures adopted by the families, neighbours, and friends, which form the preponderant support for the elderly; in particular, they need to devise methods for improving their availability in crisis situations and their long-term commitment. They need to incorporate flexibility in the performance of the tasks required by and for the elderly and to avoid the rigidity of staff roles which exists in formal agencies and in the professions. Such inflexibility militates against the best care of individuals and the most efficient use of the limited resources which exist to serve a total community. While the convenience of professionals and the preservation of status are understandable motives, they may well stand in the way of the primacy of excellence in the provision of care. There is a danger of undue subordination of the needs of consumers in this field to the needs of the providers! The pendulum should perhaps move some way in the direction of availability and flexibility of individual workers if we are to cope best with the needs of old people whose informal networks of support are inadequate.

THE PRACTICE OF PSYCHOGERIATRICS IN THE COMMUNITY

To be effective, safe, and efficient, the care outside institutions of old people with mental disorders must be comprehensive and painstaking in its attention to detail, both in the assessment and in the treatment and management of cases.

Infact that requirement is often overlooked or else tacitly recognised but ignored. The deficiency finds its origins primarily in the low regard with which the elderly are held by many practitioners in the health and the social services and in the limitations of their training; in addition, there is a certain lack of curiosity beyond the making of a diagnosis of the disease, which seldom presents a problem in psychogeriatrics. The results of this deficiency may be unnecessary distress to patients and to those supporting them, waste of resources, occurrence of avoidable crises, and inappropriate or premature admission of old people to institutions.

For these reasons, this section — intended as a severely practical guide to day-to-day clinical work — will deal with the relevant issues in some detail. It will consider the method of assessment and the formulation following this initial step. It will then refer briefly to treatment and at length to the management, in its complexity and variety of approaches, in the light of conflicts of interest and of priorities.

Assessment

Location — home or hospital

Assessment, initially should be in *the patient's home*, particularly in the case of the old old and where the information on referral suggests the presence of an organic mental syndrome. There are good reasons for this opinion, some of them applicable also to psychiatric practice with younger people.

In the first place, a much fuller view of patients as people, as well as of people as patients, is gained by seeing them in their home than can be obtained from a description, however good and however full this may be. The understanding of personality and of the person's past and present way of life, is central in psychiatry and much of it is expressed by the manner in which he keeps his home and by his behaviour within it.

The physical environment can be studied in a few minutes and give an important picture of failing performance, of adequate adjustment despite impaired mental function, or of a successful compensatory supportive mechanism for someone no longer able to cope independently. One can quickly examine such factors as risk (uneven floors, steep and winding stairs, faulty electrical and gas appliances); warmth of house and method of heating; cleanliness or its opposite; the supply and storage of food; the tell-tale wet and soiled patches of the incontinent; the standard of the sanitation, of bathing and of water-heating facilities; the accumulation of unpaid bills, etc.

The identity of other key people can be established conveniently during the visit: family, neighbours visiting friends, home helps, home nurses, etc. Thus the membership of the social network can be ascertained, together with the knowledge which the members have of the situation, their views and their attitudes. Such people can much less easily be assembled in the hospital and the planning of care, especially for the confused, is very uncertain without first gauging the contribution which can be expected from them.

The hospital consulting room, and the hospital itself, is foreign territory to the patient. It can be intimidating. It can induce anxiety together with other abnormal feelings and behaviour. Brain-damaged individuals have a very fragile equilibrium with their surroundings and find it difficult to cope with change in it; their behaviour in the hospital thus gives only slight insight into their behaviour elsewhere, which may be the relevant issue. Such influences obtain also for the consultation process itself, wherever conducted, but they are usually less pronounced on the familiar ground of the patient's own home. Allowance of course is made for such distorting influences, but even so the artificiality of the situation adds an avoidable complication to the process of assessment.

The hospital, as a place of assessment as opposed to treatment and management, functions best where the disease model is the most useful one, where special investigations are required in order to reach a diagnosis and where the patient's condition is expected to be remedied or palliated by instituting treatment based on the diagnosis. The hospital is therefore of the greatest importance for old people whose illness is primarily physical, for those with mental disorders which may result from physical disease, and for those who also have, or are suspected of also having, physical disease which is significant and treatable.

For many, however, especially the very old and those with clear-cut dementia, few tests may be required and even those can be performed from the patient's home, e.g. blood and urine tests. Where the initial assessment points to the need for more extensive, particularly radiological, investigations, these can be arranged later by planned outpatient attendance or admission to hospital.

For the great majority of the patients, treatment for functional disorders, or care for those with organic disorders, will be in their own home for most or all of the illness. It is therefore essential to have as full a direct knowledge of that environment as possible. It is much more convenient for the elderly patients, and for their often equally elderly relatives/friends/neighbours, to be seen at home. They then avoid the tiring journeys and long waits for ambulances which are so characteristic of visits to outpatient departments. Similarly, the Health Service avoids ambulance costs and has a lesser need for outpatient premises and staff. The specialist gains from the convenience of not being tied to rigid clinic times and by the limited availability of clinic space.

What has been said about outpatient clinics holds all the more strongly for admission to hospital. This, for the elderly mentally ill, is a major management decision, whose consequences can be far reaching. It therefore requires a *prior* assessment of commensurate thoroughness: the adage that diagnosis should normally precede treatment applies, *mutatis mutandi*, to assessment before management.

However, such a policy is not without its problems and, in the first place, it requires a readjustment of medical attitudes and availability. The specialist must be prepared to set up a system within his service which is able to deal with referrals speedily, including emergency referrals at all times. If he decides to assess at home rather than by bringing the patient to an emergency clinic or to a routine outpatient clinic (let alone by admitting for assessment), he must be readily available — directly or through other members of his team who are familiar with the assessment procedure and who are themselves prepared to deputise for him outside the hospital. Registrars in the community is still a novel concept! For his part, the general practitioner must learn, and be willing to make contact with or to be re-channelled to the specialist team rather than expecting whoever happens to be on duty for the hospital to deal with his request. He must also be willing to have his own assessment and resulting management decision—which frequently is a request for immediate admission—subjected to independent scrutiny and not necessarily endorsed. Tact is needed to impart the message that admission to hospital as a decision lies in the consultant's prerogative and not in the general practitioner's. It is of course right and proper for the general practitioner to demand, and to expect to receive, assistance as soon as he requests it. In an ideal service assessment must be not only expert but also quick (Chapter 8). Such a service throws a heavy burden upon the specialist team, in a field already full of crises and lacking in resources of all types.

Finally, such a system of domiciliary assessment is greatly hampered by the long distances of rural practice and the traffic congestion of urban life. This may well prevent the consultant from being able to make the bulk of the assessments personally. Under such conditions, there may have to be more sharing of the assessment function within the specialist team or more training in it of outside workers, e.g. general practitioners, home nurses, social workers, etc.

Procedure

Assessment means gathering information about the person referred and about those concerned with him, in order to determine what the problem is, how it came about, and what is to be done about it. It is made by obtaining the history, examining and understanding the patient and the other relevant persons and, sometimes, requesting further investigations — medical, social, or psychological. The process of assessment is a continuing one, to be deepened and revised in the light of increasing familiarity and of evolving situations. It begins with receiving the referral.

Receiving the referral

The quality of the initial assessment and of the decisions flowing from it can be enhanced by judicious preparation. The team's secretary is usually the first person contacted; she must have clear instructions as to what to ask, preferably completing a form with appropriate headings. In addition to the identifying details, this information should include an explicit description of the problem for which help is being sought (behaviour being more important than diagnosis); the names, addresses and telephone numbers of those already involved (family, neighbours, friends, voluntary and statutory workers); what has been done already and by whom (e.g. medication, hospital contacts in detail, Social Services intervention); what is required specifically from the psychiatric team (as opposed to, say, from the Department of Social Services); and the speed which the referral has to be dealt with.

The patient

A standard _full psychiatric history_ is the starting point, supplemented by details of relevance to the elderly as a group and by information connected with the possible presence of brain pathology. The designated patient should be approached first but, if it becomes clear that the reliability of his history is doubtful or that communication is going to be difficult and excessively time consuming, the factual framework should be obtained from the other informants, whose presence will have been arranged prior to the visit. Time must be husbanded and it is pointless to be groping after facts from those who are memory-impaired, severely depressed, deluded, paranoic, very deaf, etc., though tact and discretion must be used in turning to others. When the patient is interviewed to take his mental state, his version of the history will, of course, also be obtained.

The more specific points are those concerned with the patient's behaviour, risk factors, his physical health, and his financial arrangements. The aim is to determine whether the necessities of daily life are being provided and if so how.

Behaviour should be described over a typical 24-hour period, beginning with the time the patient wakes one day to the same time on the following day. This quickly gives invaluable insights into the patient's disabilities, their effects upon others, who these others are and how they react. It may be very important to go into great detail in analysing how abnormal behaviour arises. For example, aggression is often cited as a major problem; it can almost as often be traced to restraints placed upon the patients, especially those with dementia. Some of these may be unavoidable but others may be unnecessary and reflect undue anxiety or overprotectiveness on the part of others. Such knowledge is then helpful when it comes to deciding on management, which may achieve more normal behaviour of the patient indirectly by altering the way he is handled by others.

The *factors of risk* must be enquired into specifically, the principal ones being: heating arrangements and hypothermia; wandering out of the house; handling of gas and electrical appliances; fire; and risk to property by allowing strangers into the home. Here again an accurate description is essential, not only of what *might* happen but of what *has* infact happened. Many people are at risk from many hazards, all of which cannot be removed. Some, however, can be lessened once known and it is obviously unwise to incur a serious risk again once a mishap has passed from a potential to an actual event.

Information on *physical health* will have been obtained from the general practitioner on referral, but it can be brought up to date, with particular reference to how the activities of daily living are affected and how the administration of any drugs prescribed is handled.

Finally, with tact and sensitivity but again in the greatest detail that the patient will allow, an enquiry should be made into his *financial circumstances*. This is in order to ensure that he is receiving his entitlements; that he is discharging his commitments and paying his service bills; that, if his mental state impairs his ability to manage his affairs, proper arrangements have been made for another person to do so on his behalf; and in order to determine what assets and income he has, to improve his amenities and support at home if necessary and to seek alternative accommodation if advisable.

By the end of the process of history taking, an outline of the patient as a person should be available: of his family, life, health, personality, and relationships and of his current mode of existence and world. It should be clear how the basic necessities of food, warmth, cleanliness, and security are being provided or are lacking. In nine cases out of ten the diagnosis of the psychiatric disorder present, if any, will have been made. These bones of the case can usually be put together in half an hour or so; much else needs to be added over time and cannot be known after a single meeting, however long. This matters little at that stage, provided the essentials above have been collected.

This history is followed by an examination of the patient's *mental state*, by a *physical examination* if time allows (and in all cases where the history points to its being particularly important), and by the collection of a *sample of blood* for a full count, measurement of the erythrocyte sedimentation rate, and of the blood urea. These further steps normally take another half hour or so and the initial diagnostic assessment of the patient is thus completed in approximately one hour.

The social network

In the course of questioning the person referring the designated patient and of obtaining the history, much information will have been collected about the social network of which the patient is a member. That information should be organised in such a way as ' . . . to mobilise the family, members of the larger kinship system, friends and others of significance to the individual or family in order to promote supportive and curative actions from network members and to bring about changes in ... the debilitating or destructive aspects of particular relationships' (Snow & Gordon 1980).

It is useful to set out that social network diagrammatically as a circle, with the patient at the centre and the members of the social network on the circumference. The network can then be analysed (Snow & Gordon 1980) with respect to the following.

Structural features: number of people in the network; their geographical location; their frequency of contact; whether family, neighbours, friends, representatives of formal agencies etc.; and the tasks which they perform.
Dynamic features: emotional bonds between the patient and the individual network members; interactions between the patient and the individual network members; interactions between the network members and the patient; effect of the patient upon the lives of others and vice versa; and attitudes, wishes and expectations of others with regard to the patient.
The patient's subjective view of the network.
The influence of *significant life events.*
The individual's behaviour including coping, defensive and problem-solving styles.

Such analysis is particularly important in the case of old people with dementia because, as will be shown later, much of the management has to be planned for the members of the social network rather than for the designated patient, whose demands may be none, whose needs may be small and met relatively easily, but about whom there may be intense feeling in the social network.

Formulation

As was stated above, the assessment aims to determine what the problem is, how it came about, and what is to be done about it. The formulation is a statement intended to answer those three questions; like the assessment itself it is open to revision at any time. In general, it should:

1   Summarise the relevant points in the *history* and in the *examination* with respect to the patient and to others in the social network.

2   Set out the nature of the *problem* as perceived by the patient, by others in the social network, and by the assessor.

3   Consider the *factors leading to the problem*. Is there a disease/illness? If there is, what could it be (differential diagnosis)? Is further information necessary? Would this be helpful in deciding which is the most likely diagnosis? Should it be sought in the interest of the patient and/or those in her social network rather than to satisfy the assessor's curiosity? If there is no disease/illness or if this does not entirely account for the problem perceived on referral, what does?

4   Consider what *treatment* should be given—physical, psychological, social — to the patient and/or others, in order to remedy the problem, so that it is no longer experienced as a problem. If it cannot be removed, can it be eased by palliative measures? What can realistically be expected of the treatment approach?

5   Consider the *care* for, and the *management* of, the patient and those about her if the problem leading to referral cannot be resolved.

6   Determine the *priority* to be given to the individual case for the allocation of resources, in the light of the demands of the population and the availability of staff and other facilities.

In essence, the formulation can be construed in terms of four concentric circles, one inside the other: the disease/illness, the person, the social network and, finally, the total community. It must always deal with each in turn if it is to do justice to the case.

Treatment

Treatment has been dealt with elsewhere in this book and little more has to be said here. What does need to be stressed is the importance of realising how important are the details of treatment with drugs in the home setting: who is to obtain the prescription and have it dispensed; can the patient be relied upon to take the medication; if not, who is to administer it; are the risks of unwanted effects worth the benefit of possible control of symptoms and return to normality? Each case must obviously be judged on its merits, in the light of the facts at the time. It may well be appropriate to arrange day hospital attendance, or even inpatient admission, in order to initiate the drug therapy and to assess response through the observations of qualified staff, despite the comparative mildness of a particular illness.

It is rare in psychogeriatric patients for the intervention of the professional to be limited to the treatment of disease. This is often either irremediable, as in dementia, or only partially and temporarily responsive, as in depression and paraphrenia. Similarly, neurotic patterns of reaction and maladjustments of personality are usually of longstanding and not substantially reversible. The approach to be adopted is therefore one which concerns itself with the person-in-his-world — the designated patient and with all those about him also. This is the process of management and of care. It entails planning, on the one hand, for the designated patient and, on the other hand, for the other people around the patient.

MANAGEMENT AND CARE

The professional relationship

The traditional relationship between doctor and patient is frequently modified in psychogeriatric practice and this fact has enormous impact upon the handling of the care and management.

Normally the adult patient more or less of his own accord consults the doctor. He has symptoms which distress him and for which he seeks assistance. He is (usually) clear about what he wants, asks for it, and is able to give an informed decision on whether he accepts or rejects what is offered. He can then judge whether what has been done satisfies him. In other words, he is a full party to the processes of consultation, treatment, management and evaluation. The helper is the second party and the contract, tacit or explicit, is between the two of them: other people obviously may be involved and affected and they are then brought into the situation if the patient agrees. However, they have no *right* of involvement and none of deciding *for* the patient. Where there are conflicts of interest, those of the consulting patient take precedence, with the uncommon exceptions of cases where other persons need to be protected (primarily against violence) and cases where the Mental Health Act is invoked for the benefit of other persons. and not the patient.

That pattern of relationship does, of course, apply to many elderly people, particularly the young old who suffer predominantly from functional psychiatric disorders and who as a group are fitter than the old old. However, in many other cases it is not the old person who requests the assistance but others, acting for and in the interest, as they perceive it, of the designated patient. The reasons for this intercession are obvious enough. They amount to the perception by others of a disability in the patient, which calls for assistance and which is not sought by the patient himself, either because he does not understand the need for it or because he is prevented from so doing by the very nature of the handicap.

It follows that all the factors which shape the views of the person seeking the help have also to be taken into account. The definition of the problem and the assistance requested being *on behalf* of the patient and not *by* him, it follows that the doctor (or other helper) must consider not only whether the service requested for the patient is *feasible* but also whether it is *desirable*. In other words he must begin by determining what the objectives should be, first and foremost for the patient and then for the other people in the case.

The typical patient is the one with moderate, or even severe, dementia. It is on such a patient that the remainder of this discussion of management will focus, though it will also often apply to patients in other diagnostic groups where a persistent disability exists which cannot be corrected by treatment or other measures.

Objectives — the patient

The objectives for the patient can be stated simply: to relieve distress, to ensure that the necessities of life are provided to a reasonable standard, and to avoid making matters worse.

Distress in the functional psychiatric disorders means symptoms, and they are treated in the standard way (see Chapter 7). In chronic brain failure signs are abundant but symptoms are uncommon, except in the early stages when insight into failing faculties is still present. Such gross abnormalities as self-neglect, incontinence, nocturnal restlessness, incoherence, etc., are rarely distressing to the patient. Occasionally visual hallucinations, illusions, or paranoid ideas stemming from the cognitive impairment may upset the patient but they are almost always transient and usually call for nothing more than patience, tolerance, and reassurance until they recede.

The *basic necessities* are shelter, food, warmth, cleanliness, drugs for certain physical diseases, and money. It is essential in the supervision of these dependent old people to check these points. It is equally important to be realistic, not to expect perfection and to accept some risk while reducing hazards as far as possible.

Whereas there is little that can be done to improve the mental state and, where impaired, the well-being of old people with dementia, it is extremely easy to make the patient worse and to affect his behaviour adversely. The commonest way of so doing is by harbouring or expressing high emotion about him (as will be described in the next section) and by taking injudicious steps as a result, for example, moving the patient from a familiar environment, restraining him unnecessarily or excessively, giving him medication inappropriately, etc. All elderly people, but the brain-damaged especially, have a reduced ability to cope with change and with stress. The manner in which they are handled by others is therefore of crucial importance; a major part of the management consists in protecting them from such harmful, albeit well intentioned, feelings and actions.

Thus, the primary objective is to construct an effective support system for the patient or to make more effective what exists already. The informal network members may need assistance from formal agencies; in the latter, the less expert require the support of the more expert, the less secure the help of the more secure and self-confident.

Objectives — other persons

In the words of Caplan (1974) ' . . . the essential elements in a marital or family group from the point of view of its acting as a support system are attitudes of sensitivity and respect for the needs of all its members and an effective communication system.' These words apply very well to the whole group of people who may be concerned with a particular old person. What are the needs of those people? Primarily, they are emotional but in part they are for factual information and in part also for practical assistance, readily accessible when required.

Understanding the psychodynamics

There is a wide range of possible feelings, attitudes, and views which can be held by those involved with mentally disabled old people — kin, neighbours, friends, voluntary and professional workers. These psychodynamic factors must now be considered; it is the major management task of the specialist in psychogeriatrics to work with them so as to benefit the supporters of the old person and thus, indirectly, the old person himself.

Anxiety is the commonest emotion. This is helpful for the patient in as much as it signals danger but potentially also unhelpful if it is excessive or unjustified. The anxiety is experienced as concern for the patient; although sometimes it is perceived by the other person as being also about himself. More often the latter source of anxiety is not recognised; instead it is repressed, denied and rationalised — the patient being viewed as the only focus and origin of the worry. In such a situation, what is really for the benefit of others is seen and put over as being for the patient's good; the wrong conclusions are then drawn as to what is to be done. It is one of the objectives of management to utilise helpful anxiety and as far as is possible to detect and lower excessive concern; where the line is drawn is of course a matter of opinion in an individual case but that such a line does indeed exist must be appreciated.

There are five channels to excessive and damaging anxiety; they are all amenable to change by information-giving, by practical measures, and by counselling. The first is *ignorance:* of the nature and aetiology of the disability; of the potential and limitations of the treatment approach; of the options available in the management; and of the complexities of the social, health, social security and legal systems. To elicit that ignorance and then to reduce it by the unhurried exposition of facts and explanation is a part both of the assessment and the management.

The second is the feeling of an *unending and unshared burden.* All too often, unfortunately, there is plenty of justification for that feeling. The prospect of partial relief— provided promises made are kept— may transform a situation which has not festered without help for too long. Similarly, the reduction of certain symptoms, notably insomnia, by appropriate treatment, may increase substantially the tolerance of supporters who are basically willing or even eager to look after the patient (Sanford 1975).

The third is distress felt at the *falling standards* in which the patient lives: less clean, less active, less fit, less well turned-out, developing unpleasant habits or idiosyncrasies, etc. The other person mourns the passage of one personality into another, deteriorated but not itself distressed. So far as possible and provided outside help is accepted by the patient and does not itself cause distress, standards can be hoisted by others. It is, however, part of the counselling process to help those around the patient to adjust to the reduced standards and to enable them not only to work through their grief but also to accept that alternatives may well be very upsetting to the patient.

The fourth is the *risk of harm to the patient* (and others) arising out of his disability. That risk should be reduced as far as possible but it cannot be totally removed, any more than it can for normal and for younger people. It may lessen anxiety to explain authoritatively that mishaps from fire, explosion, road accidents, and wandering are in fact exceedingly uncommon in such old people living on their own; that institutionalisation (the 'solution' frequently requested) does not remove the risk (fires and deaths in institutions are by no means rare, and old people can and do wander out of such places); that the loss of independence and control over one's life that institutionalisation entails can be very distressing to an old person; and the rights and risks have to be balanced after exhaustive assessment by people of suitable training and competence (Norman 1980). Again, patient discussion can be very helpful in placing the risk factor in the right perspective and in getting the members of the social network to accept that a reasonable risk is a fact of life in these cases. Thus overprotectiveness can be lessened.

Finally, there is the *anxiety felt by the other people about their own position* in the face of current or future criticism: are they being unkind or negligent in not 'doing something', i.e. removing the patient; may their promotion and career be blighted by 'something going wrong', by a calculated risk which in the event does lead to an undesirable happening? Such motivation is a potent and not uncommon (albeit unadmitted or unvoiced) factor in precipitate or inappropriate admissions to homes or to hospital. Again, it must be recognised during the assessment procedure, brought out into the open and dealt with. One way of doing so is by thorough discussion; another is by having an experienced professional assuming responsibility for the decision not to institutionalise and being prepared to 'face the music'. This is one of the functions of the Consultant Psychiatrist, not only because of his expertise but also because he remains a practitioner despite his seniority, whereas in the nursing and social work professions senior staff are purely managerial or administrative and do not have personal knowledge or take personal responsibility in these difficult cases.

There are a number of other important psychodynamic factors to be taken into account.

Depression is common (Sanford 1975) but it too can be alleviated by reducing the burden through partial relief from total care, by psychological support, and sometimes by medication.

Guilt may be a major problem, particularly where the total demand from different sources upon one person is beyond their capacity, e.g. a married daughter pulled in different directions by an aged mother, by her own husband and her children. Whatever the distribution and extent of that daughter's effort, someone remains unsatisfied and the guilt smoulders chronically, albeit unjustified.

Aspects of the patient's behaviour may cause intense *irritation*, e.g. constant repetitions of the same question or following others around. This may lead to outright *rejection*. Sometimes there is unalloyed *hostility* to the patient but this rarely develops anew and is usually born of many years of friction — the deteriorating behaviour merely making the feeling acceptable and respectable. The disability now affords a pretext for getting rid of the patient, ostensibly in his own interest! Such a wish may well be understandable and evoke sympathy, given the difficult personality of some old people, but in such cases that it must be made clear that the professional worker is ethically bound to put the interests of the patient first.

In practice is it much more usual to witness *ambivalence* towards the patient in the members of the network — the negative features possibly masked by intense reaction formation. Superficially, there is an outward appearance of overwhelming devotion and commitment, whose true nature becomes evident only through a sudden explosion of resentment.

Dissension and *division* may occur within a family, regarding the share of the burden borne by its different members. On the other hand, friction may antecede the patient's disabilities and demands which become a screen and the patient a scapegoat. In such cases, much can be achieved by bringing the family together with the therapist: exploration and ventilation of family interactions and feelings may have a cathartic effect. Where the process is effective, there may a dramatic clearing of the air, a newly-found joint approach to the problems, and a sharing or reallocation of family work. The feeling 'we are all in it together' may emerge, to the advantage of the patient, especially when the professional can be seen by the family as a partner in this task.

Just occasionally, pure *venality* is the operative psychodynamic, actuating families to try — prematurely — to take what is the old person's. Fortunately, this is a very uncommon motive, save where admission to an institution has been agreed by all to be essential but the family exerts pressure towards the inferior facilities of a long-stay hospital ward, which are free, rather than in the direction of a Home, which is fee-paying and dents the future inheritance.

Many of these reactions and mechanisms can affect not only family members and other informal contacts but also professionals themselves so that, where conflicts of interest arise between the patient and others, those of the former may go unprotected. This is liable to occur as a result of *identification with the healthy people in the social network* — a process which is insidious, unconscious, and yet all-pervasive. It may lead to an assessment and decisions which in fact are those of the informant, although they appear to be those of the professional worker. If a problem is viewed entirely through one pair of eyes, the solution is also likely to be the one advocated by that beholder! Ethical issues are never far from the surface in psychogeriatrics and it is necessary not to cause patients avoidable distress and harm, when they cannot actually be helped, in order primarily to assist others. Fortunately, such conflicts of interest are by no means universal and intervention can often be to the benefit of all concerned.

PRACTICAL DETAILS

It will be readily understood that old people can thus be at the centre of a maelstrom of emotions and that these can be very damaging. After an assessment it is not always possible to be certain what it is best to do and, not infrequently, the answer may be: very little. Paradoxically, this can be very difficult; much skill and perseverance may be required to achieve that objective, while at the same time developing a relationship with the supporters which continues to harness their goodwill and their beneficent involvement.

It now remains to go through the nature of the decisions to be made in an individual case, to indicate who should make them, and to sketch the background problem of how to apportion insufficient resources.

When the assessment has been made, treatment has been found impossible or only partially effective, and an old person is left with a persistent abnormality which impairs his ability to cope independently, what follows is the construction of two support systems — one for the patient and the other for those concerned with him. These systems must see to it that a number of essential needs are met. In most instances they are supplied largely by family and neighbours, as has been shown above; however, it is as supplements to these (or in their place when they are not available) and in the performance of specialised tasks that the statutory social and health services operate. Hand in hand with the degree of disability, support is initially given entirely within the home setting, then partially in the home and partially elsewhere (day-care and/or intermittent admissions to an old people's home or hospital), and finally, in a minority of cases, by permanent admission.

Providing the essential needs

Most of these are delivered under the umbrella of the Department of Social Services through home helps: shopping; drawing the pension where appropriate; cleaning; visiting, supervision and companionship. Meals on wheels are also provided by that department. Similarly, the Department has powers, for example to make adaptations to the home and to provide a vast range of aids following assessment by an occupational therapist, or to help financially with the installation and rental of a telephone in defined cases (Family Welfare Association 1981).

Other services come within the province of nurses: dressing; dressings; drug administration and other physical treatments; bathing, etc. These nurses are mostly trained in general nursing but community psychiatric nurses are playing an increasing role in the care of mentally abnormal old people at home (Ainsworth & Jolley 1978).

These services are never delivered in a mechanical manner: there is always some kind of relationship. Therefore, refusal by a patient of something offered by one person does not necessarily mean that it cannot be provided by another person. For example, a bath may not be accepted if the helper is a competent but overinvolved or hostile daughter and this may then be a major problem in the total care which is readily overcome by the introduction of a bath attendant. The importance of this point cannot be overemphasised; skill may be needed to ensure that apparently trivial, but infact vital, tasks are performed. As will be mentioned when roles are considered, a good relationship may be so useful and so specific that professionals may have to be prepared to undertake apparently non-professional tasks, or some belonging more properly to professions other than their own, in the interests of the patients and their supporters. Otherwise a need will unnecessarily go unmet or will be met in a less desirable way.

Finance

The questions to be answered in this area are as follows:
1 Can the patient cope unaided with his finances; if not, is he obtaining appropriate help?

2 Is he receiving the benefits and other moneys to which he is entitled?
3 Is he discharging his financial obligations?

In response to the first question, if the patient is lucid, he can seek or be offered information and advice but the decisions are entirely his. If he is unable physically to deal with his affairs or chooses not to do so, he may make arrangements for someone else to take over that function, either informally or more formally by giving that person *power of attorney*. That power enables the other person to deal on behalf of the patient and is best established with the advice of a solicitor. The giver must fully understand what he is doing; he can revoke the authority at any time and it lapses in law if the patient ceases to be lucid. The power of attorney is not endorsed or supervised by a court: it is a private arrangement between the parties concerned. It is *not* appropriate or valid where the patient is not lucid. In that event, the case should be referred to the Court of Protection.

The Court of Protection (25 Store Street, London WC1E 7BP) is an office of the Supreme Court of Judicature. It derives its statutory authority from Part VIII of the Mental Health Act, 1959. Judges of the Supreme Court are nominated to it by the Lord Chancellor. Its function is to protect and control the administration of the property of persons who become mentally incapable of doing so themselves.

The Court can be notified (through its Chief Clerk) by anyone that the patient is incapable of managing his affairs because of mental disorder but this is usually done by relatives through a solicitor. The Court then makes enquiries into the circumstances of the patient and seeks medical evidence, namely a certificate on a standard form that the patient ' . . . is incapable, by reason of mental disorder, of managing and administering his property and affairs' (Mental Health Act, 1959, Section 101). That certificate can be given by any doctor who knows the patient. The Court usually makes an order appointing a Receiver to receive the income and administer the property under the direction of the Court during the patient's inability to do so. In certain cases, the appointment of a Receiver may not be necessary — the matter being dealt with by a single order authorising the application of the patient's property for his benefit. Where urgent need exists, an interim order may be made by the Court. In the exercise of its powers, the Court has regard first of all to the requirements of the patient. A receivership order can be discharged by the judge on his being satisfied that the patient has become capable of managing and administering his property and affairs.

It is most important to advise patients and their families on the need to approach the Court where the patient has significant assets and income and is either clearly incapable of looking after his affairs or fluctuates in his capacity so to do. The making of a Receivership Order may take several months and the procedure should therefore be initiated without delay where it appears that an Order may be necessary. The person appointed as Receiver is normally a member of the patient's family but it may be any fit person.

Occasionally the patient has no family, friends, or other suitable person known to him; the Court then may appoint the Official Solicitor or an officer of the Local Authority.

The ability to deal with financial matters including the making of a will, i.e. testamentary capacity, is assessed by seeking answers to two questions: 1 Does the person grasp and understand the nature of the transaction? If he does not, then he is incapable; 2 If he does grasp and understand, is he exercising substantially adequate judgement? In other words, is he making decisions which are reasonable for him, given his circumstances, and which he can be expected to have made were he not suffering from a disease or illness? If the answer is negative, then he is incapable.

The validity of this second question may appear more controversial than that of the first but it becomes clear if we consider patients with, for example, mania or severe depression who understand intellectually but misjudge facts and events.

The evidence upon which the opinion is formed must be set down not only in general terms relating to the diagnosis of any abnormal mental state but also as answers to specific questions asked of the patient to test his understanding and his judgement.

In response to the second question concerning finance, the next step is to ensure that the patient and his family know of their entitlements to social security benefits, are assisted, if they wish, in applying for them, and that the benefits granted to them are infact being collected.

The Department of Health and Social Security issues free leaflets on social security matters; they explain what benefits and grants are available and how to apply for them. These leaflets are listed in a catalogue (NI 146) and they are available at local security offices or by post (DHSS Leaflets, PO Box 21, Stanmore, Middlesex, HA7 1AY). Another very useful source of information is the booklet *Your Rights* published by Age Concern (Bernard Sunley House, 60 Pitcairn Road, Mitcham, Surrey) and revised at frequent intervals.

The main state benefits for which elderly people may be eligible are: retirement pension; supplementary pension; attendance allowance; mobility allowance; invalidity allowance; and invalid care allowance. These benefits are too complex to be considered in detail in a book such as this. However, because of the nature of the disabilities of patients who form the subject matter of this book, it is appropriate to give some information on the attendance allowance (DHSS Leaflet NI 205). It is payable to those who are so severely disabled that for six months they have needed, by day, frequent attention in connection with bodily functions (e.g. eating, drinking, walking, keeping clean and warm) or continual supervision in order to avoid substantial danger to themselves or others; by night the patient must require prolonged or repeated attention in connection with bodily function, or continual supervision in order to avoid substantial danger to themselves or others. The rate of the allowance for day or night (June 1982) is £15.75

per week and for day and night £23.65. Old people with dementia often qualify. The allowance is payable for as long as the disability remains and the person is not living in a place which is provided or helped by public money.

Finally, on the question of finance, someone in the support system must check that ordinary bills are being paid, when the patient himself cannot be relied upon to do so. This should be obvious and yet it is surprising how often disabled old people can be visited at home and receive active care from statutory agencies without this simple point being dealt with.

The management of risk

This involves five main points. 1 The systematic enquiry into possible sources of risk (uneven floors; falls; fire; gas; cold and hypothermia; wandering; exposure and road accidents; side-effects of drugs; infection and infestation in unhygenic conditions). 2 The reduction and avoidance of risk so far as possible (levelling floors; checking and correcting unsafe appliances; appropriate heating; careful assessment of the need for drugs and control of their administration; improvement of hygiene so far as possible). 3 Measures to enable the early discovery of accidents and incidents once they have occurred, especially in the case of those living alone (frequent visiting; telephone checks; use of alarm systems—though these have their problems; labelling of clothing to identify wanderers abroad). 4 The deliberate weighing up of whether it is best to accept risk which cannot be lessened or to take alternative steps, e.g. moving into sheltered or communal accommodation, with the potential disadvantages which this carries. 5 The psychological support of those who are themselves at risk or have to live with risk to those close to them, so as to help them to adjust to the situation.

Planning for emergencies

Psychogeriatric practice in the community means not only long-term care within it but also a lot of crisis management. It is therefore necessary to have an agreed, clear, and known policy on who should be summoned in an emergency and on what the availability and role of the specialist team should be at such times. This point will be further considered when role allocation comes to be discussed.

Handling the psychodynamics around the patient

The nature of some of the reactions evoked by mentally disabled and dependent old people, particularly those with dementia, has been described already (p. 273), together with aspects of their management. In this section, additional points will be made on how the interests of such patients can be directly promoted, by assisting their supporters.

First, the worker must be clear in his own mind what the objectives should be for the patient: the relief of distress as far as possible, the provision of basic needs, the planning for emergencies, and the continuing review of the situation — these constitute reasonable and realistic care, not perfection. They are not infact unduly difficult to achieve! The worker must thus examine his own feelings in the face of limited aims, which he may find difficult to accept. He must avoid aiming too high, both because this may be counter-productive and because it is not the function of the medical and social services to achieve the ideal for the individual but only the reasonable, having regard to what is possible and also to the needs of other people. One of the major points in the management is to get the workers involved to do neither too little nor too much: only in this way can they help the members of the informal network to the same posture. They need self-confidence to undertake what is subsumed in the word 'support'.

What this means is the formation of a trusting relationship between workers and supporters, with empathy, availability, accessibility, and reliability being required from the former. Within that secure relationship problems, feelings, attitudes, responses, and expectations can be expressed and ventilated. There may then develop a greater awareness of how and why problems arise (especially abnormal behaviour) with resulting changes in the handling of the patient by non-patients. Practical and more general information is supplied, explanations are provided, feelings are worked with, and negotiation is undertaken on what infact is to be done at any one time. This process of counselling is open-ended; it may involve not only an individual but a whole family group. Psychological and practical support may also be obtained from self-help and relatives' groups.

Day-care and intermittent admissions

So far, the whole management has been described as if the patient were in his own home for the whole time. This is true for many but not all: some patients and/or their supporters benefit from day-care, provided its purpose is under-stood and provided the distances in rural practice do not make this form of support impracticable.

Day-care may serve one or more of several functions: assessment, treat-ment and support, or maintenance. It has been stated already that assessment is very largely a domiciliary procedure. Occasionally, however, the diagnosis is not certain and further observation or physical, psychological, or social investigations may be necessary. Day-care allows for these needs, without endangering the patient's hold on his home and without drawing on scarce beds. Similarly, treatment for functional mental disorders or for concomitant physical disease may be given under observation. This function predomin-antly concerns the younger old. However, for the majority of patients, attendance is for the purpose of providing for the basic needs of old people with dementia and to enable their supporters to have partial relief from their presence (Arie 1975, Greene & Timbury 1979, MIND 1980).

For the patient, such an arrangement has the advantage of making survival in his own home environment possible, despite severe disability, and this may well be preferable in terms of quality of life and of his own choice. For the family, ordinary activities can be continued without the constant worry of an unattended old person or the irritation of disturbing behaviour. For the service, provided the day-places and the transport which is essential are available, a lesser and probably more economical care than admission is adequate. Nevertheless, for some patients and situations day-care is used simply as a holding measure, when admission to a long-term bed is necessary but no such bed is available.

The problems in psychogeriatric day-care hospitals are largely for the nursing staff. They have to adjust to caring for a succession of old people who are not going to improve and who require heavy physical, and sometimes distressing psychiatric, nursing. While many nurses infact find the care of such very dependent old people rewarding, some become demoralised by an apparent lack of objective. It is thus undoubtedly helpful to them to be able to see the therapeutic effect of such day-care for the supporters and it is highly desirable that such day-hospital nurses (and inpatient nurses also) should be able to see the patients and their families not only in the hospital setting but also in their homes, so as the better to appreciate the immense good that their work does.

In a local service which aims to be efficient as well as comprehensive, psychogeriatric day-hospitals must be closely integrated with day-centres for the elderly run by local authorities and by voluntary organisations (Edwards *et al* 1980) but they tend not to be (MIND 1980). There is overlap between the therapeutic and social functions of day-care (Martin & Millard 1978). Day facilities provided in hospitals for the functionally, the organically, and the physically ill elderly; and in day centres for the less disabled, all have a mixed population in practice. Movement between them should be smooth, as the needs of the old people change and as the mix in a given setting may become inappropriate for its primary purpose.

Another way of affording relief is by temporary admission to hospital or home, either ad hoc or on a recurrent and regular basis.

Leaving home

Whenever an old person has a disability which is persistent and which impairs his independence, alternatives to his remaining at home may have to be considered, especially when he lives alone. Where the patient can make an informed decision and has the means to make arrangements privately, there is no need for the professional worker to become involved, save when his advice is sought. Unfortunately, the patients with whom we are concerned here are seldom in that position. How then are we to proceed, and what are the alternatives?

First it must be established by a suitably trained and experienced doctor that the disability cannot be reversed. Unfortunately this elementary point is often ignored (British Medical Journal 1981) and old people continue to be admitted to homes for long-term care when what they need is treatment for disease.

Next, before arranging for an elderly person to leave his home permanently, it must be ascertained that everything possible has been done to support him there, using *all* the available services and not merely those of the services which happen to be on the scene!

Then, it must be understood that there can be no certainty as to how the change of environment is going to affect the old person, particularly if he is confused or if he has an awkward personality. Every admission to a sheltered home or to an old people's home is a trial, an experiment, and one must therefore plan what to do in the event of failure before the step is taken. This means not only considering a return to the previous position but also the possible need for hospitalisation if this will be feasible.

Sometimes the old people are moved to live with other members of the family; this too carries a major risk of failure, with disruption of the family. Like other moves, this must be as a trial at first and the patient's house should remain available to them.

All in all, the risks of failure and of added unhappiness are so great that the greatest caution is necessary in making the recommendation that the patient should leave home. If he does, and does not make private or family arrangements, he can go into sheltered, warden-supervised accommodation (normally administered by the local housing authority); into a local authority home (Part III accommodation); or into a voluntary home (registered with, and sometimes financed in part by, the local authority) — depending upon the degree and nature of the disability and upon local policies. Homes are fee-paying and there is a means test in the determination of what proportion of the full cost the old person has to pay. Entry into such homes is by free and voluntary application by the patient/client. He should therefore appreciate what he is doing, although in fact a smaller or greater element of confusion often impairs his judgement in this respect. In rare instances (see below) the admission to a home or a general hospital is involuntary, under the provisions of Section 47 of the National Assistance Act, 1948. Finally, where the disability, or the behaviour, is such as to require skills which are properly those of nursing staff, a long-stay psychiatric hospital bed is the last alternative.

Long-stay institutional care is full of problems for staff and residents alike: in policy (Godlove & Mann 1979) and in practice. This applies both in homes for the elderly (Wilkin *et al* 1978, DHSS 1979b) and in hospitals. It is uncommon for the quality of life, admittedly a subjective but nevertheless a most important factor, to be as good in institutions as in the old person's own home — unsatisfactory though that may be. Therefore, except where the person can make a fully informed judgement, has an opportunity of first sampling institutional life, and decides to opt for it permanently, every effort should be made to sustain him in his own home or in sheltered accommodation, which enables him to retain much of his freedom and independence.

Where the patient does not, or cannot, himself make the decision to seek admission to a home or a hospital, a difficult judgement must then be made on his behalf, taking into account whether he will be able to tell the difference between one environment and another; assessing the balance of the risks and the availability of support and of alternative accommodation; and, not least, the ethical aspects raised by conflicts of interest between the old person and others (Norman 1980).

Compulsory admission

Requests for compulsory admission may be made by the family or by other people who are worried about or exasperated by an old person. There are two statutes which enable this to be effected: the Mental Health Act and the National Assistance Act, 1948 (amended in 1951).

With the exceptions of patients with an insight-impairing functional psychosis (who may well respond to physical treatment but who refuse it and then can be detained ' . . . in the interests of (their) own health and safety'), the Mental Health Act compulsory provisions are rarely justified in these patients, either in their own interest or for the protection of other persons (from substantial danger as opposed to nuisance or anxiety). In patients with dementia the only thing that can be offered of significance in the institution is basic care; observation is not required and treatment is not possible. In such cases, either the patient is too impaired to give a valid refusal (or acceptance) and compulsion is not necessary for admission or he can give a valid refusal, in which case it is highly unlikely that the requirements for an Order will be satisfied.

Section 47 of the National Assistance Act, 1948 applies to persons who are firstly suffering from grave chronic disease or, being aged, infirm, or physically incapacitated, are living in insanitory conditions, and who secondly are unable to devote to themselves, and are not receiving from other persons, proper care and attention. The Act enables the Medical Officer of Health, now a Community Physician, to certify to the Health Authority that he is satisfied after thorough enquiry that, in the interests of any such person or for preventing injury to the health of, or serious nuisance to, other persons, it is necessary to remove that person from the premises in which he is residing. An application is then made to a court of summary jurisdiction which may order the removal of the person to a suitable hospital or other place for a period of not more than three months, renewable by the court for a further period not exceeding three months. Seven days' notice of the application is required.

That period of notice was done away with by the National Assistance (Amendment) Act, 1951, which requires two medical certificates instead of one; enables the order to be made by a single justice as well as by the court; and restricts the duration of the order to three weeks.

It will be noted that, in contrast to the Mental Health Act, these provisions are applicable to people without or with mental disorder and that orders are made by a court or a justice. Doctors merely certify the presence of the stated conditions; they are not signatories to the Order.

On the basis of a questionnaire sent by Muir Gray (1980) to all the community physicians in England responsible for Section 47, it appears that about 200 people are removed from their homes each year by that procedure, to hospitals or old people's homes. In the Northern Regional Health Authority area, the ratio of requests to compliance was 6.7:1 in the years 1975–78 (Forster & Tiplady 1980).

These statutory powers are a double-edged sword: they can lead both to abuse of patients' rights and to their protection against the pressures for informal, but not necessarily voluntary, admission to institutions (Muir Gray 1980, Norman 1980). Individuals will sometimes differ on whether compulsion is justified and it is useful for a psychiatrist unwilling to compel under the Mental Health Act to be able to point to the alternative of the National Assistance Act and to recommend another opinion to act as a check on his own.

Roles in management

Who does which of the above-mentioned tasks in caring for these patients? This question of roles can be difficult and it causes many of the conflicts which unhappily are common in practice. It has been well reviewed by Sladden (1974) in her study of psychiatric nursing in the community.

Some roles and responsibilities are clearly defined: the provision of social workers, home helps, meals-on-wheels, house adaptations, admission to day centres and to Part III accommodation are the prerogative and the responsibility of the Department of Social Services. Similarly, decisions about hospital care, compulsory admission, fitness to manage finances, are exclusively or largely those of doctors.

Much less clear-cut are the responsibilities for counselling. This is an activity in practice undertaken to a greater or lesser extent by general practitioners, psychiatrists, geriatricians, district nurses, community psychiatric nurses, health visitors, social workers, psychotherapists, home helps and many others. Other 'grey areas' include the roles of day centres as against day hospitals and of old people's homes as against hospital wards; the degree to which one worker should stray into the province of another when he is the only person already involved or when his good relationship with the patient/relatives makes it likely that he will do better than the 'proper' person;

and the advisability of a policy leaving emergencies which arise out of hours and in known patients to a stranger who happens to be on duty for emergencies rather than attempting to reach the regular worker.

In the opinion of the author, the only reasonable approach is one of negotiations with colleagues, with the patient, and with their relatives to define what is to be done and then, by agreement, to decide who should do it. In difficult situations, where many people are involved, it may be best to call a case conference to plan management. One possibility is to appoint a key worker to undertake the overall management of the case, doing himself as much as he is competent and empowered to do, and arranging the remainder through the appropriate others.

It goes without saying that a plan of management must be subject to *constant review* and the way in which this is to be done must also be part of the plan.

Determining priorities

The final step in working with a patient and those supporting him is to view them as one group among many in the locality who have needs and to make an explicit, if subjective and to some extent arbitrary, judgement as to how much of what is available they should receive, and how soon. Obviously, everything depends on the case, the place, and the time and nothing more can be said here, except to stress how vital is a statement of the priority of each case in the running of a total service.

REFERENCES

AINSWORTH D. & JOLLEY D. (1978) The community nurse in a developing psychogeriatric service. *Nursing Times* **74**, 873–4.

ARIE T. (1975) Day care in geriatric psychiatry. *Gerontologia Clinica* **17**, 31–9.

BERGMANN K. (1977) Chronic brain failure — epidemiological aspects. *Age and Ageing* **6** (suppl.) 4–8.

British Medical Journal (1981) leading article. *British Medical Journal* **282**, 1817–18.

CANTOR M.H. (1975) Life space and the social support system of the inner city elderly of New York. *Gerontologist* **15**, 23–7.

CANTOR M.H. (1979) Neighbours and friends — an overlooked resource in the informal support system. *Research on Aging* **1**, 434–63.

CAPLAN G. (1974) *Support systems and community mental health.* Behavioural Publications, New York.

DHSS (1972) *Services for Mental Illness Related to Old Age.* HM (72) 71. HMSO, London.

DHSS (1979) *In-patient statistics from the mental health enquiry for England, 1977.* HMSO, London.

DHSS (1979b) *Residential Care for the Elderly in London: a study by DHSS*, Social Work Service London Region. HMSO, London.

DHSS (1980) *Health and Personal Social Services Statistics for England (with summary tables for Great Britain), 1978.* HMSO, London.

DHSS (1981) *Growing Older*. HMSO, London.

DONO J.E., FALBE C.M., KAIL B.L. *et al* (1979) Primary groups in old age — structure and function. *Research on Aging* 1, 403–33.

EDWARDS C., SINCLAIR I. & GORBACH P. (1980) Day centres for the elderly: variations in type, provision and user response. *British Journal of Social Work* 10, 419–30.

Family Welfare Association (1981) *Guide to the Social Services*. London.

FORSTER C.P. & TIPLADY (1980) Doctors and compulsory procedures. Section 47 of the National Assistance Act 1948. *British Medical Journal* i, 739–40.

GODLOVE C. & MANN A. (1979) Residential care of the elderly in Britain today. *Psychological Medicine* 9, 417–9.

GREENE J.B. & TIMBURY G.C. (1979) A geriatric psychiatry day hospital service: a five year review. *Age and Ageing* 8, 49–53.

HEMSI L.K. (1980) Psychogeriatric care in the community. *Health Trends* 12, 25–9.

HUNT A. (1978) *The elderly at home: a study of people aged 65 and over living in the community in England in 1976*. HMSO, London.

ISAACS B. & NEVILLE Y. (1975) *The measurement of need in old people*. Scottish Health Service Studies no. 34, Scottish Home and Health Department. HMSO, London.

KAY D.W.K., BEAMISH P. & ROTH M. (1974) Old age mental disorders in Newcastle-upon-Tyne. I: a study of prevalence. *British Journal of Psychiatry* 110, 146–58.

MARTIN A. & MILLARD P.H. (1978) *Day hospitals for the elderly — therapeutic or social?* Geriatric Teaching and Research Unit, St. George's Hospital, London.

MIND (1980) *Caring from day to day:* a report on the development of the day hospital within the service for elderly people who are mentally infirm. London.

MITCHELL J.C. (1969) The concept and use of social networks. In *Social networks in urban situations: analyses of personal relationships in central African towns*, ed. J.C. Mitchell. Manchester University Press, Manchester.

NIELSEN J. (1962) Geronto-Psychiatric Period — prevalence investigation in a geographically delimited population. *Acta Psychiatrica Scandinavica* 38, 307–30.

MUIR GRAY J.A. (1980) Section 47. *Age and Ageing* 9, 205–9.

NORMAN A.J. (1980) *Rights and risk: a discussion document on civil liberty in old age*. National Corporation of the Care of Old People. London.

Office of Population Censuses and Surveys (1980) *Population Projection 1978—2018*. HMSO, London.

SANDFORD R.A. (1975) Tolerance of debility in elderly dependents by supporters at home: its significance for hospital practice. *British Medical Journal* iii, 471–3.

SLADDEN S. (1979) *Psychiatric Nursing in the Community*. Churchill Livingstone, Edinburgh.

SNOW D.L. & GORDON J.B. (1980) Social network analysis and intervention with the elderly. *Gerontologist* 20, 463–7.

Index

passim means 'here and there throughout'